Recent Advances in Angiogenesis and Antiangiogenesis

Domenico Ribatti
Department of Human Anatomy
University of Bari Medical School
Italy

FOREWORD

It has been known for a very long time that blood vessels are essential to deliver oxygen, nutrients and key regulatory signals to the tissues. Early pioneers like Glenn Algire and Isaac Michaelson observed several decades ago that tumor growth and certain eye disorders resulting in impaired vision, including proliferative diabetic retinopathy, are accompanied by increased vascular proliferation and proposed that the new vessels play a pathogenic role in these disorders. In 1971 Judah Folkman was the first to appreciate the therapeutic potential of the field, proposing that anti-angiogenesis might represent a therapy for solid tumors. This vision has been, at least in part, fulfilled by the recent approval of several anti-angiogenic drugs for the treatment of advanced tumors and age-related macular degeneration. Also, as of February 2009, almost 40,000 Medline citations are found under the keyword "angiogenesis", reflecting the interest among basic scientists and clinicians in this field.

The progress in basic biology and in the clinical applications notwithstanding, much more needs to be done. Indeed, the clinical results with anti-angiogenic agents posed a series of questions that will need to be addresses before the field can advance in a meaningful way. To mention a few, it will be of great importance to identify the molecular pathways mediating tumor resistance to angiogenesis inhibitors, establish the most effective combinatorial therapies and identify the patients that are more likely to benefit from such treatments.

The book edited by Prof. Domenico Ribatti provides a broad overview of the molecular and clinical aspects of angiogenesis and addresses the aforementioned questions. Chapters written by experts in their respective fields will make the reader acquainted with a variety of topics ranging from the role of axon guidance molecules in angiogenesis, the role of circulating endothelial cells in tumorigenesis, to the characterization of novel cellular and pharmacological approaches to inhibit angiogenesis. As such, the volume should be particularly useful to basic investigators, oncologists, opthalmologists and clinicians interested in the latest advances in this exciting field.

Napoleone Ferrara, *M.D.*
Genentech Inc
San Francisco, CA
USA

PREFACE

Angiogenesis, the process by which new blood vessels are formed, is an important event in both physiological and pathological conditions. Angiogenic and antiangiogenic molecules released by accessory cells control neovascularization, notably the migration and proliferation of endothelial cells, their morphogenetic differentiation in capillaries and the concurrent remodeling of the extracellular matrix. Under physiological conditions, these steps are tightly controlled, and loss of such control is an important feature of several diseases.

Increased production of angiogenic stimuli and/or reduced production of angiogenic inhibitors leads to abnormal neovascularization, such as occurs in cancer, chronic inflammatory diseases, diabetic retinopathy, macular degeneration and cardiovascular disorders.

Starting with the hypothesis of Judah Folkman that tumor growth is angiogenesis dependent, this area of research now has a solid scientific foundation. Several clinical studies have shown a positive correlation between the number of vessels in the tumor, metastasis formation and disease prognosis.

Many solid and hematologic tumors in advanced stages are not curable with the currently available anticancer treatments, which primarily target the tumor cells. The genetic instability of tumor cells permits the occurrence of multiple genetic alterations that facilitate tumor progression and metastasis, and cell clones with diverse biological aggressiveness may coexist within the same tumor. These two properties allow tumors to acquire resistance to cytotoxic agents, which is still the main cause of treatment failure in cancer patients.

Whereas conventional chemotherapy, radiotherapy, and immunotherapy are directed against tumor cells, antiangiogenic therapy is aimed at the vasculature of a tumor and will either cause total tumor regression or keep tumors in a state of dormancy.

A number of approaches have been proved to inhibit tumor angiogenesis. Since tumor-associated angiogenesis develops as a physiological mechanism, its inhibition should not lead to emergence of resistance; and since each neovessel supplies hundreds of tumor cells, inhibition of angiogenesis should potentiate the oncostatic effect. By contrast, vascular targeting focused on specific molecular determinants of the neovasculature to be used for local delivering of a toxic effect that leads to a vascular damage and tumor necrosis.

Numerous compounds inhibit angiogenesis, but few of them proved effective *in vivo* and only a couple of agents were able to induce tumor regression. Antiangiogenic tumor therapy has gained much interest in preclinical and clinical assessment.

It has been estimated that over 10000 cancer patients worlwide have received experimental form of antiangiogenic therapy. However, the results from these clinical trials have not shown the dramatic antitumor effects which were expected following preclinical studies. This may be because of inadequate trial design in earlier studies. From the results obtained so far in clinical trials it can be concluded that the future clinical success of angiogenesis inhibitors could be related to their use in combination with chemotherapy or radiotherapy.

The main problem in the development of antiangiogenic agents is that multiple angiogenic molecules may be produced by tumors, and tumors at different stages of development may depend on different angiogenic factors for their blood supply. Therefore, blocking a single angiogenic molecule was expected to have little or not impact on tumor growth. Currently, most of the FDA-approved drugs as well as those in phase III clinical trials target a single proangiogenic protein. However, in apparent contrast with this view, experiments with neutralizing antibodies and other inhibitors demonstrated that blockade of vascular endothelial growth factor (VEGF) alone can substantially suppress tumor growth and angiogenesis in several models. Therefore, eventually other angiogenic proteins may be expressed by a tumor in which only VEGF is inhibited and give the clinical appearance of acquired "drug resistance".

A clinical challenge in antiangiogenesis is the finding of biological markers that help to identify subsets of patients more likely to respond to a given antiangiogenic therapy, as well as to determine optimal dosing of therapy, to detect early clinical benefit or emerging resistances and to decide whether to change therapy in second-line treatments.

An ideal angiogenesis inhibitor should be orally bioavailable with acceptable short-term and long-term toxicity and have a clinically useful antitumor effect. Moreover, carefully constructed clinical trials with valid endpoints need to be executed. Finally, cancer genomics and proteomics are likely to identify novel tumor-specific endothelial targets and accelerate drug discovery. With the advent of specific and potent new agents, oncologists have a variety of direct and indirect antiangiogenic agents to choose from when designing therapy protocols.

This book was undertaken to discuss the biological process and molecular mechanisms involved in angiogenesis and to discuss some agents that have shown to inhibit angiogenesis. I express my gratitude to all my colleagues who have contributed to this book.

Domenico Ribatti
University of Bari

CONTRIBUTORS

Francesco Bertolini	Unit Director,European Institute of Oncology, Milan, Italy
Katiuscia Bonezzi	Assistant, Tumor Angiogenesis Unit Department of Oncology, Mario Negri Institute for Pharmacological Research, Bergamo, Italy
Paola Braidotti	Assistant Professor, Department of Medicine, Surgery and Dentistry, University of Milan Medical School and "San Paolo" Hospital, Milan, Italy
Federico Bussolino	Full Professor, Institute for Cancer Research and Treatment, Department of Oncological Sciences, University of Torino Medical School, Candiolo, Italy
Anca Maria Cimpean	Assistant Professor, Department of Histology and Molecular Pathology, "Victor Babes" University of Medicine and Pharmacy, Timisoara, Romania
Enrico Crivellato	Assistant Professor, Section of Anatomy, Department of Medical and Morphological Researches, University of Udine Medical School, Udine, Italy
Maria Fico	Postdoctoral Researcher, Department of Biomedical Sciences and Human Oncology, University of Bari Medical School, Bari, Italy
Eberhard Gunsilius	Assistant Professor of Medicine, Tumor Biology & Angiogenesis Laboratory, Department of Internal Medicine V, University of Innsbruck Medical School, Innsbruck, Austria
Irene M. Ghobrial	Assistant Professor in Medicine, Department of Medical Oncology, Dana-Farber Cancer Institute and Harvard Medical School, Boston, USA
Chyso Kanthou	Tumour Microcirculation Group, Section of Oncology, School of Medicine & Biomedical Sciences, University of Sheffield, Sheffield, UK
Robert S. Kerbel	Full Professor, Sunnybrook Health Science Centre, Molecular and Cellular Biology, Department of Medical Biophysics, University of Toronto, Toronto, Canada
Daria Leali	Postdoctoral Researcher, Unit of General Pathology and Immunology, Department of Biomedical Sciences and Biotechnology, University of Brescia Medical School, Brescia, Italy
Sandra Liekens	Postdoctoral Researcher, Department of Microbiology and Immunology, Rega Institute for Medical Research, Leuven, Belgium
Giuseppe Mangialardi	Postdoctoral Researcher, Department of Biomedical Sciences and Human Oncology, University of Bari Medical School, Bari, Italy
Patrizia Mancuso	Unit Vice Director, European Institute of Oncology, Milan, Italy
Michele Moschetta	Postdoctoral Researcher, Department of Biomedical Sciences and Human Oncology, University of Bari Medical School, Bari, Italy
Antonella Naldini	Associate Professor, Unit of Neuroimmunophysiology, Department of Physiology, University of Siena, Siena, Italy
Fabio Pastorino	Fellow, Fondazione Italiana per la Lotta al Neuroblastoma, "G. Gaslini" Children's Hospital Genoa, Italy

Vito Pistoia	Head, Laboratory of Oncology, G. Gaslini Children's Hospital, Genoa, Italy
Mirco Ponzoni	Head, Experimental Therapies Unit, Laboratory of Oncology,"G. Gaslini" Children's Hospital, Genoa, Italy
Marco Presta	Full professor, Unit of General Pathology and Immunology, Department of Biomedical Sciences and Biotechnology, University of Brescia Medical School, Brescia, Italy
Lizzia Raffaghello	Fellow, Fondazione Italiana per la Lotta al Neuroblastoma, "G. Gaslini" Children's Hospital Genoa, Italy
Marius Raica	Full Professor, Department of Histology and Molecular Pathology, "Victor Babes" University of Medicine and Pharmacy, Timisoara, Romania
Roberto Ria	Assistant Research, Department of Biomedical Sciences and Human Oncology, University of Bari Medical School, Bari, Italy
Domenico Ribatti	Full Professor, Department of Human Anatomy and Histology, University of Bari Medical School, Bari, Italy
Aldo M. Roccaro	Instructor in Medicine, Department of Medical Oncology, Dana-Farber Cancer Institute and Harvard Medical School, Boston, USA
Guido Serini	Assistant Researcher, Insitute for Cancer Research and Treatment, Department of Oncological Sciences, University of Torino Medical School, Candiolo, Italy
Yuval Shaked	Assistant Professor, Technion Israel Institute of Technology,and Department of Molecular Pharmacology, Rappaport Faculty of Medicine, Haifa, Israel
Giulia Taraboletti	Head, Tumor Angiogenesis Unit, Department of Oncology, Mario Negri Institute for Pharmacological Research, Bergamo, Italy
Gillian M. Tozer	Full Professor, Tumour Microcirculation Group, Section of Oncology, School of Medicine & Biomedical Sciences, University of Sheffield, Sheffield, UK
Gerold Untergasser	Assistant Professor, Tumor Biology & Angiogenesis Laboratory, Department of Internal Medicine V, Universty of Innsbruck Medical School, Innsbruck, Austria
Angelo Vacca	Full Professor, Department of Biomedical Sciences and Human Oncology, University of Bari Medical School, Bari, Italy
Donatella Valdembri	.Fellow, Insitute for Cancer Research and Treatment, Department of Oncological Sciences, University of Torino Medical School, Candiolo, Italy

CHAPTER 1

Plexins and Neuropilins Regulate Integrin Conformation and Trafficking in Endothelial Cells

Guido Serini, Donatella Valdembri and Federico Bussolino

Institute for Cancer Research and Treatment, Department of Oncological Sciences, University of Torino, I-10060 Candiolo, Italy

Address correspondence to: Dr. Federico Bussolino, Institute for Cancer Research and Treatment- Strada provinciale di Piobesi 142, Km 3.95 10060 Candiolo, Italy; Tel: 0039 011 9933347; Fax: 0039 011 9933524; E-mail: federico.bussolino@ircc.it

Abstract: Integrin the are major extracellular matrix receptors and their functional state with respect to the affinity for extracellular matrix proteins is pivotal for their biological activities in physiologic and pathological settings. Integrins' machinery depends on the dynamic regulation of their adhesive function in space and time. In cells, integrins exist in different conformations which determine their affinity for extracellular matrix proteins and are continuously endocytosed, trafficked through endosomal compartments, and recycled back to the plasma membrane. Therefore real-time modulation of cell - extracellular matrix adhesion can result from two interconnected phenomena: the regulation of integrin conformation and traffic in response to extracellular stimuli. This review summarizes recent data highlighting the different mechanisms by which semaphorins and their receptors plexins and neuropilins regulate integrin functions in vascular system.

1. INTRODUCTION

Cell adhesion to the extracellular matrix (ECM) is mainly mediated by integrins, a protein family that signs the evolution from protozans to metazoans. A functional integrin is composed of non-homologous transmembrane α and β subunits that control cell adhesion through complex molecular mechanisms. Outside-in signaling informs the cell about the ECM environment, while inside-out signaling promotes modifications in integrin functional activity [1, 2]. In the last 10 years, an increasing body of evidences has demonstrated that integrins are not mere adhesion receptors, but interact and influence the biological activity of several other molecular systems within the cell [3].

Vascular system represents an outstanding example to understand how the dynamic interactiona between cells and ECM influence tissue behaviors both in physiologic and pathological conditions. Vascular cells (*i.e.* endothelium, pericytes and smooth muscle cells) express a wide range of integrins including $\alpha1\beta1$, $\alpha2\beta1$, $\alpha4\beta1$, $\alpha5\beta1$, $\alpha v\beta1$, $\alpha v\beta3$, $\alpha v\beta5$, $\alpha v\beta8$, $\alpha6\beta1$ and $\alpha6\beta4$ [4]. During angiogenic remodeling of pre-existing vessels, endothelial cells (ECs) move and change their reciprocal positions and interactions in response to the several guidance cues that control their motility. As a result of a balanced response to fluid shear stress, chemoattractant and chemorepulsive agents, ECs dynamically regulate their adhesiveness both in terms of cell-to-cell and cell-to- ECM contacts. Integrin-mediated cell-to-ECM adhesion play a deterministic role in vascular development by contributing to cell movement, to protect cells from *anoikis* and to endow the vasculature with the ability to sense and respond to changes in physical forces [4, 5]. The mechanisms regulating the interactions between cells and ECM are mainly based on the specific ECM composition that characterizes organs and tissues [6], on diverse integrin conformational states endowed with different binding affinity for ECM proteins [1, 2] and on integrin membrane trafficking [7].

Many elegant experiments have explained the molecular mechanisms supporting integrin activation by growth factors, chemokines and shear stress [1, 2]. On the contrary the molecular events switching-off activated integrins are under extensive investigation. Recent evidences strongly indicate that semaphorins (Sema) and their receptors plexins (Plx) and neuropilins (Nrp) play a determinant role in counterbalancing the growth factor activity on integrin functional state.

2. SEMAPHORINS, PLEXINS AND NEUROPILINS

Firstly identified as chemorepulsive axon guidance cues, Sema constitute one of the largest phylogenetically conserved family of pleiotropic molecules acting in a wide range of biological processes, including central and peripheral nervous system development and regeneration, cardiovascular development, and immune system function [8, 9].

Sema are charatecerized by the presence of five specific types of domain: a ~500- amino-acid conserved Sema domain that constitutes the family hallmark, PSI (plexins, semaphorins and integrins) domains, Ig-like domains, thrombospondin domains and a basic C-terminal domain. Eight different classes have been described: classes 1,2 and 5 in invertebrates; classes 3, 4,6 and 7 in vertebrates; class V classifies virally encoded proteins. Some classes (1,4,5,6 and 7) are characterized by membrane-bound molecules (transmembrane or glycosyl - phosphatidylinositol linked), while classes 2, 3 contain secreted Sema. Some membrane-associated semaphorins are proteolytically cleaved to generate soluble proteins, generating further diversity [reviewed in ([8, 9]] (Fig. 1).

By far the most prominent Sema receptors are the Plx proteins. Plx are large conserved transmembrane

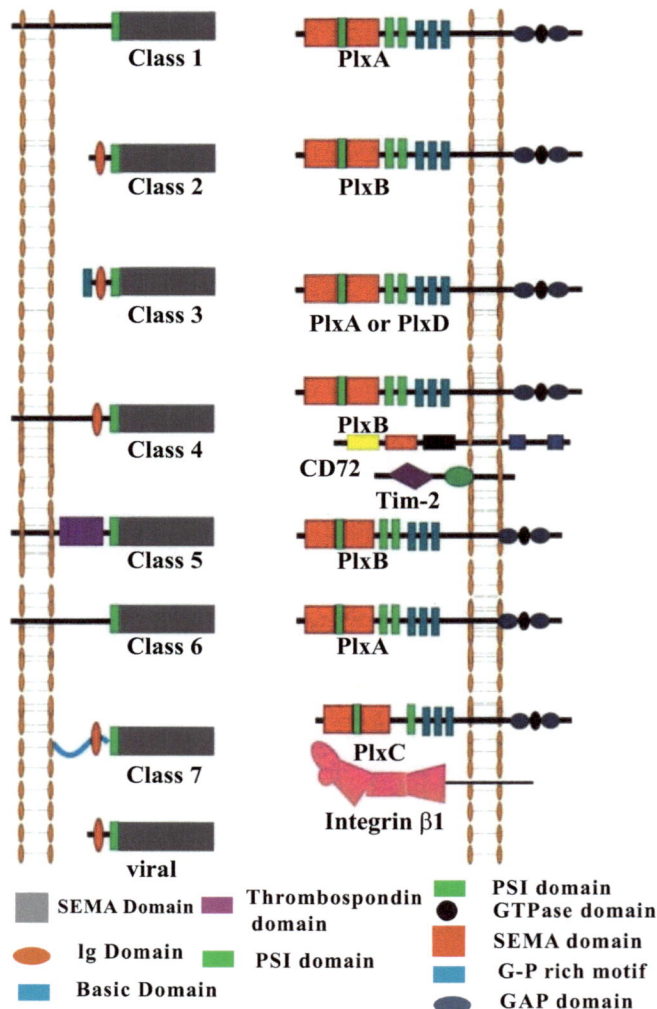

Fig. (1). Semaphorins and their receptors. Sema include transmembrane, secreted, and glycosyl phosphatidyl-inositol -linked proteins, most of which bind to Plx receptors. Class 1 and 2 and Sema5c Sema are invertebrate, and class 1 and 2 Sema utilize PlexA and PlexB receptors. The coreceptor D-OTK functions with PlexA. Sema in classes 3–7 are found in vertebrates. Class 3 and 6 Sema utilize PlexA receptors; however, most Sema3s require an obligate Nrp coreceptor. Sema6s interact directly with PlexAs. Other coreceptors that can function with PlexAs are L1CAM (L1 cell adhesion molecule), VEGFR2, and Offtrack. Class 4 and 5 Sema associate with PlexB1–3, and the receptor tyrosine kinases Met and ErbB2 can function as a coreceptor with PlexBs for certain class 4 Sema functions. Class 4 Sema directly bind to CD72 or Tim-2 in the immune system. Sema7A and a viral sema function together with PlexC1, and Sema7A also utilizes β1 integrin.

belonging to four classes (A–D), contain a divergent extracellular Sema domain and a conserved cytoplasmic domain unique to Plx with sequence similarity to a group of Ras-family-specific GTPase-activating protein (GAP) activity. In addition to Plx, Sema holoreceptor complexes contain numerous coreceptors. Some of them are modulatory subunits (for example, Ig superfamily cell adhesion molecules), or provide further diversity to semaphorin function, such as such as CD72, T cell immunoglobulin and mucin-domain-containing 2 (Tim-2), vascular-endothelial growth factor (VEGF) receptor R-2, c-Met and Erb-2 receptors, tyrosine kinase- like transmembrane protein offtrack or integrins [10-15]. However, most secreted Sema, including Sema3A and Sema3F do not bind directly to Plx receptors, but they use Nrp-1 or Nrp-2 as coreceptor ligand-binding subunits [16]. Interestingly, Nrp-1 and -2 are coreceptors of VEGFR-1,-2 and -3 engaged by different VEGF forms [17-19]. The extracellular region of Nrp1 contains two repeated complement-binding domains (CUB domains; a1–a2 domains), two coagulation factor-like domains (b1–b2 domains), and a juxtamembrane 5 meprin/A5/μ-phosphatase (MAM) homology domain. The Nrp1 intracellular region is only 50 amino acids long, and its function is poorly characterized [8, 9]. Domains b1-b2 have been implicated in the binding with VEGF-A165 [20], a1-a2 and b1-b2 domains with Sema3A. The MAM/c domain instead mediates the Sema3A elicited Nrp1 oligomerization [8, 9] that is required for Sema3A

biological activity. The cytoplasmic tail includes about 42–44 amino acids and does not display catalytic activity of its own, but presents a binding site for the PDZ domain of Nrp-1-interacting protein [21] (Fig. **2**).

3. ROLE OF SEMAPHORINS IN VASCULAR SYSTEM

The first evidences for a role of Sema/Nrp/Plx system in vascular biology were provided by the groups Klagsbrun and Fujisawa, which respectively demonstrated that in ECs Nrp-1 acts a VEGFR-2 co-receptor [19] and found that Nrp-1 is required for mouse cardiovascular development [22]. Afterwards, several reports confirmed and extended these observations. In zebrafish, knockdown of *sema3aa* affects the migration of Nrp-1[+] angioblasts, finally impairing dorsal aorta formation and normal circulation [23]. Additionally, single morpholino knockdown of either *sema3aa* or *sema3ab* in TG(fli1:EGFP)[y1] embryos results in a less dramatic phenotype with patterning defects of intersomitic vessels [24]. Knockdown of Sema3a gene in outbred CD-1 mouse strain and over-expression of dominant negative Sema3 receptor mutants [25] or delivery of anti-Sema3A antibodies [26] in chick embryos were found to cause angiogenic remodeling defects. By studying the positive effect exerted by a specific Sema3A inhibitor in axonal regeneration into the injured spinal cord it has been observed an enhancement of angiogenesis in the injured tissue, reinforcing the concept of the negative modulatory role of Sema3A in angiogenesis [27]. In ECs PlxD1[28] and, albeit to lesser extent, PlxA2 [29] are the most abundant Plxs. Both Sema3A and Sema3C bind with a significantly higher affinity to a receptor complex formed by the association of Nrp-1 and/or -2 with PlxD1 than to a complex in which Nrps associates with PlxA1 [28].

Therefore, the Nrp/PlxD1 complex could represent the most efficient transducer of the chemorepulsive effect of Sema3A [30, 31]. Different from other Sema3, Sema3E can directly bind to PlxD1 [32]. Mainly based on defects in the intersomitic vessel patterning of Sema3E and PlxD1, Sema3E/PlxD1 has been proposed to be the major signaling pathway regulating vascular development [32, 33]. However, while *Sema3e* null mice are viable and do not show any gross abnormality [32], all *PlxD1*[-/-] pups become cyanotic shortly after birth and succumb within 24 hrs because of severe cardiovascular defects [28]. Therefore, it is likely that in ECs PlxD1 transduces signals not only from Sema3E, but also from other Sema3 likely employing Nrp as co-receptors, as originally proposed by Epstein and colleagues [28]. Based on the fact that ECs express high levels of both Nrp1 and PlxD1 and on observations that Sema3E promotes tumor angiogenesis [34, 35], at present these

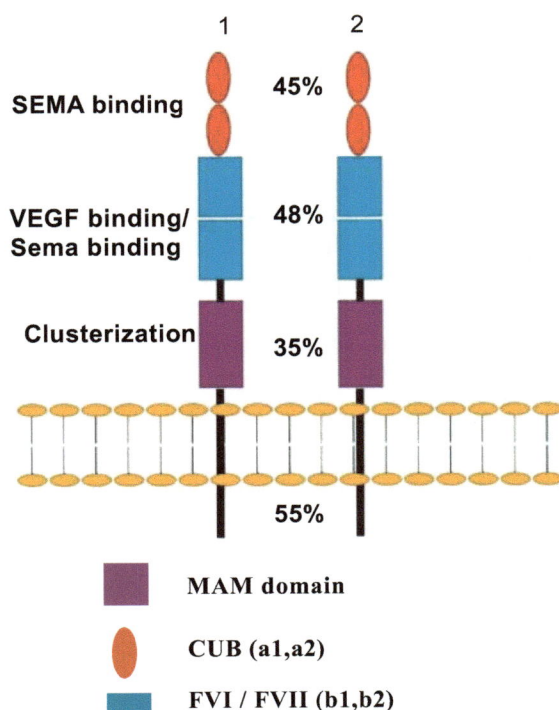

SEMA binding   45%

VEGF binding/ Sema binding   48%

Clusterization   35%

55%

■ **MAM domain**

● **CUB (a1,a2)**

■ **FVI / FVII (b1,b2)**

Fig. (2). Neuropilins structure. For details see text. Numbers indicate the homology percentage between Nrp-1 and Nrp-2.

findings cannot be easily reconciled with the proposed chemorepulsive effect played by Sema3E *via* PlxD1 on ECs of developing mouse embryos [32].

The controlling role of class 3 Sema on vascular functions has been further confirmed by *in vitro* studies. Independently from a competitive activity with VEGF-A, Sema3A and Sema3F inhibit EC migration and adhesion and promote apoptosis [25, 31, 36-38]. Interestingly, Sema3F has been reported to be an oncosuppressor gene under the control of p53. Loss of functional p53 in tumour cells results in downregulation of Sema3F and induction of tumour angiogenesis[39]. The complexity of Sema class 3 system in vasculature is further supported by the recent data showing that Sema3A is a powerful vasopermeabilizing molecule through a mechanism that involves VE-cadherin phosphorylation [40].

Besides Sema class 3, molecules belonging to class 4 regulate angiogenesis. Sema4D is a potent pro-angiogenic molecule [41, 42]. Sema4D, originally discovered in the immune system where it controls T-cell activation[43], can be found either as soluble or membrane-bound molecule [44]. Sema4D acts by binding to PlxB1 or to PlxB2, or to a low affinity receptor, CD72, expressed mainly by cells of the hematopoietic lineage[45]. It has been previously shown that activation of Plx-B1 through Sema4D binding transactivates c-Met and promotes angiogenesis both *in vitro* and *in vivo*[41]. More recently, these observations have been extended to tumor angiogenesis by proving the pro-angiogenic and pro-tumorigenic role of Sema4D produced by macrophages of the tumor microenvironment [46]. In contrast to Sema4D, Sema4A upon binding to PlxD1 inhibits EC migration and *in vivo* angiogenesis [47].

4. REGULATION OF INTEGRIN CONFORMATION AND FUNCTION BY SEMAPHORIN / PLEXIN / NEURO-PILIN SYSTEMS.

By analyzing the biological activities of Sema3A on ECs, we firstly noticed that it inhibited cell adhesion to different ECM protein by acting on integrins [25]. By using antibodies able to specifically recognize the bend inactive or straight active form of β1 or αvβ3 we demonstrated that Sema3A and Sema3F promote a conformational change leading to the functional inhibition of these integrins [25, 48]. Accordingly, after stimulation with either Sema3A or Sema3F adherent ECs lose their focal adhesions [31]. High affinity integrins are highly concentrated at adhesion sites and at the leading edge of migrating ECs [49] where they promote new adhesions to support directed cell motility. Major determinants of vascular remodeling, such as fluid shear stress and angiogenic growth factors, activate integrin adhesive function[5].

Notably, during angiogenesis and in cultured ECs opposing autocrine loops of Sema3A [25, 50-52] and VEGF-A [53-55] have been found. These chemorepulsive signals of Sema class 3 endow the vascular system with the plasticity required for reshaping by inhibiting integrins. The final result is a continuous and subtle modulation of integrin function *versus* an all-or-none activation. Such a fine-tuning of integrin-mediated adhesion to the ECM allows a graded control of EC migration and redirectioning during physiological vascular remodeling. The observed loss of autocrine Sema3A in favor of VEGF-A in ECs during malignant tumor progression [52] could account at least in part for the structural and functional abnormalities of tumor vasculature.

The mechanism by which Sema3A inhibits integrin activity has been extensively investigated. In the low affinity state, the large extracellular domain of integrins is bent over the cell surface, whereas α and β transmembrane and cytoplasmic domains tightly interact and are probably stabilized through a juxta-membrane salt bridge [56]. Interaction of phosphotyrosine-binding (PTB) domain containing proteins, such as talin[57], with the two NPxY tandem repeats located in the cytoplasmic tail of the integrin β subunit causes its separation from the α subunit cytodomain, the extension of the extracellular domain, and the uncovering of the ECM binding site of integrins [56]. Talin PTB domain is part of a larger trefoil Protein 4.1/ezrin/radixin/moesin (FERM) domain and can be involved in an intramolecular association with the rod domain that impairs talin binding to the integrin β subunit [57]. Such an inhibition can be relieved upon binding of plasma membrane phosphatidylinositol-4,5 bisphosphate (PIP2) to the talin rod domain, thus allowing talin activation, head-to-tail dimerization and integrin binding [57]. In addition, activated talin can also bind the FERM domain of phosphatidyl - inositol- 4-phosphate 5- kinase (PIPKIγ661), increase PIP2 levels at adhesion sites, and thus trigger a positive feed-back loop supporting cell adhesion to the ECM [58].

The small GTPase R-Ras, which *in vivo* is largely expressed by vascular ECs and smooth muscle cells [59], has been found to promote integrin-mediated cell adhesion to different ECM proteins[60]. Remarkably, integrin function is activated by R-Ras and TC21/R-Ras2 and inhibited by H-Ras [60]. Intriguingly, H-Ras and R-Ras display a significantly different plasmamembrane compartmentalization [61, 62]. The fact that R-Ras localizes both in focal adhesions and lipid rafts is compatible with the recent observation that integrin signaling regulates lipid rafts distribution [63]. All together, these data indicate that both targeting to focal adhesions and interaction with specific downstream effectors, such as Nck, must be involved in defining the unique capability of R-Ras-GTP to promote integrin function. Activated R-Ras-

GTP is thought to promote cell adhesion by favoring the activation of other small GTPases such as Rap1 [64] and Rac1 [61, 64].

The cytoplasmic domain of Plx is endowed with an R-Ras GAP activity. Specifically, the juxtamembrane basic sequence of class A Plxs directly interacts with FARP2, a Rac guanosine exchange factor (GEF). Sema3A binding to the Nrp-1/PlxA1 complex induces the dissociation of FARP2 from PlxA1[65]; next, FARP2 GEF activity elicits a rapid increase of active Rac1-GTP that in turn facilitates the binding of the small GTPase Rnd1 to the linker region of PlxA1 cytodomain [66]. This event finally activates the R-Ras GAP activity of PlxA1 that that impairs the function of the small GTPase R-Ras and is required for Sema3A inhibition of integrins. In addition, FARP2 holds a FERM domain that mediates its binding to PlxA1 [65]. Upon dissociation from PlxA1, the FERM domain of FARP2 competes with talin for binding to PIPKIγ661 and hence impairs the talin/PIPKIγ661/PIP2/talin positive feedback that supports the formation of ECM adhesion sites.

5.   NEUROPILIN-1 SPECIFICALLY REGULATES THE MEMBRANTE TRAFFICKING OF α5β1 INTEGRIN

Defects of developing blood vessels caused by *Nrp1* gene knockdown in mice[22, 67] are different from vascular malformations displayed by mice lacking either Sema3A [68] or VEGF-A165 [69]. Furthermore, it has been recently reported that Nrp-1 is required for EC responses to both VEGF-A165 and VEGF-A121 isoforms, the latter being incapable of binding Nrp1 on the EC surface [70]. Therefore, it is conceivable that the vascular abnormalities of *Nrp1-/-* mice could be due at least in part to the disruption of a Sema3A / VEGF-A165-independent Nrp-1 function(s). This suggestion was further supported by the data that Nrp1 regulated EC adhesion independently from VEGFR-2[71]. Prompted by these observations we investigated the mechanisms by which Nrp-1 modulated EC adhesion to different ECM proteins [72] by Nrp-1 silencing experiments and we discovered that loss of Nrp1 greatly reduced EC adhesion to fibronectin (FN), but not to other proteins, indicating that Nrp-1 is selectively involved in adhesion to FN. By using extracellular and cytosolic mutants of Nrp-1 we dissected the domains involved in this mechanism and firstly we excluded a role for the extracellular domains and their binding activities to VEGF-A and Sema3A. The C-terminal SEA sequence of Nrp-1 interacts with the PDZ domain of the endocytic adaptor protein GIPC1[21], whose knockdown during development results in altered arterial branching [73]. By a combined strategy based on Nrp-1 silencing and rescues experiments with cDNAs encoding for cytosolic mutants we definitively demonstrated the

role the SEA sequence in regulating EC adhesion to FN.

α5β1 integrin is the main FN receptor in ECs [4]. Therefore we examined whether in ECs Nrp-1 could interact physically with this integrin. By co – immuno - precipitation experiments, microscope confocal studies and fluorescence resonance energy transfer analysis we found that both the C-terminal SEA and cytoplasmic domain of Nrp1 were fully dispensable for its interaction with α5β1 integrin. Besides a co-localization between Nrp-1 and α5β1 integrin at the focal adhesions, confocal fluorescence analysis surprisingly revealed the two proteins were inside Rab-5 positive vesicles. All together, these data indicate that in living cells Nrp-1 physically associates with α5β1 at or near sites of cell-ECM contact, and that this interaction is likely maintained following internalization of the complex.

The efficiency of cell adhesion and spreading on ECM is generally thought to be proportional to the amount of either active or total (*i.e.* active and inactive) integrin at the cell surface [1, 2]. By analyzing the different subcelluar compartimentalizations of total and active forms of α5β1 integrin, we found that the down-modulation of Nrp-1 does not affect endocytosis of the cell-surface pool of total α5β1 integrin but markedly reduced the quantity of active heterodimers internalized by ECs.

Taken together, these data indicate that on the cell surface Nrp-1 interacts with active α5β1 heterodimers at adhesion sites and acts to promote their internalization and localization to intracellular vesicles.

To visualize the post-endocytic trafficking of the α5β1/Nrp1 complex, we deployed a photoactivatable α5-GFP probe connected with the use total internal reflection fluorescence. However, the multitude of fluorescent vesicles travelling to restrict the plane of activating fluorescence. By this technique we showed that photoactivated α5β1 was then rapidly (<6 sec.) internalized and co-transported with Nrp-1 in small endocytic vesicles that moved away from the adhesion sites and then (~80 sec) it comes back to the adhesion sites. These data indicate that α5β1 integrin and Nrp-1 are co - internalized into intracellular vesicles, which are then rapidly returned or recycled to the plasma membrane. Interestingly, both the internalization and recycling of Nrp-1-associated α5β1 integrin occurs at site of adhesion to the ECM (Fig. **3**).

6. CONCLUSIONS

During angiogenesis ECs undergo activation of autocrine circuits by chemoattractant and chemorepulsive molecules, *e.g.* angiogenic growth factors and Sema. The final result is a fine-tuning of endothelial integrin function, which contributes in the

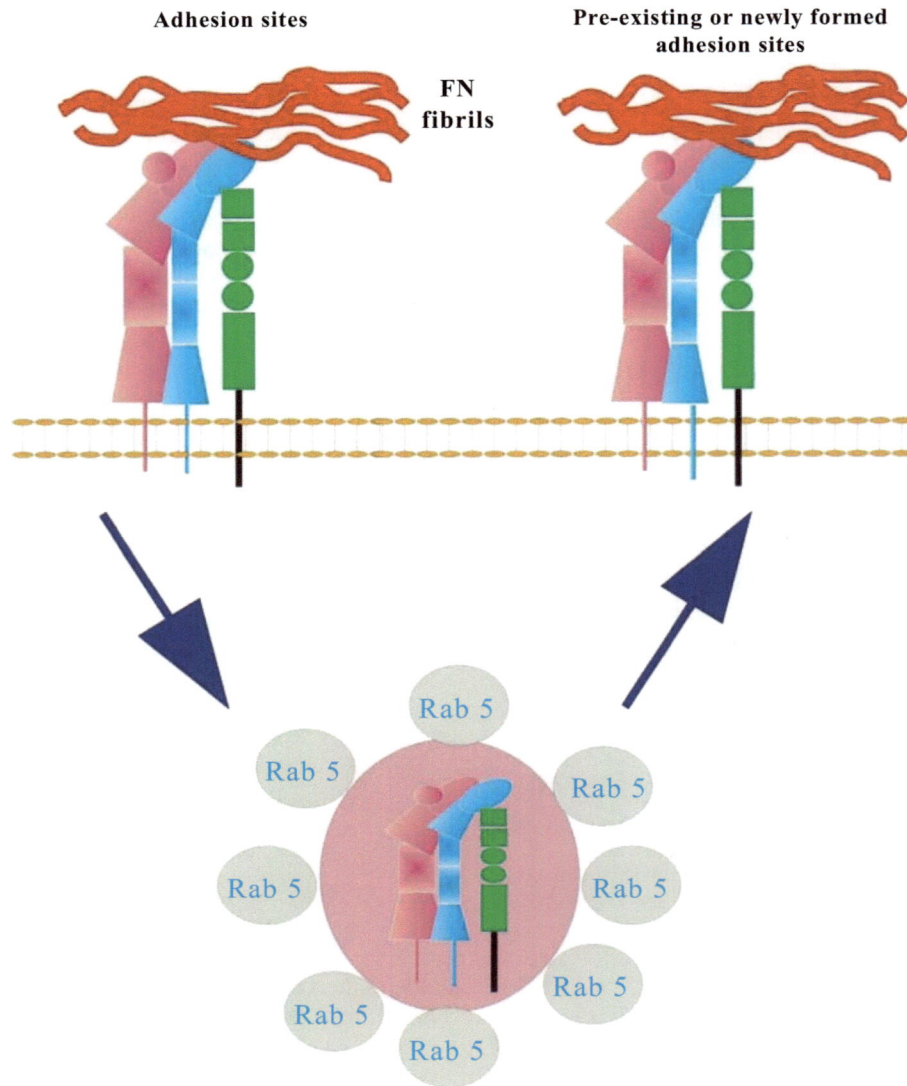

Fig. (3). At adhesive sites of ECs spreading on FN, Nrp1, *via* its cytoplasmic association with oligomers of the endocytic adaptor GIPC1, promotes the Rab5/Rab21 dependent internalization of active α5β1 1 integrin. Once endocytosed, active α5β1 is then recycled back from Nrp1 positive vesicles to the cell surface, thus favoring the dynamic re-handling of newly forming adhesion sites.

proper assembly of vascular tree. Such a fine-tuning of endothelial integrin function is likely to be disrupted in pathological angiogenesis, including solid tumors. Indeed, opposite autocrine loops of VEGF-A and Sema3A are present in angiogenic ECs and an imbalance in the ratio of autocrine VEGF-A/Sema3A in ECs could support cancer progression and contribute to the defects of tumor blood vessels. Notably, resistance to VEGF-A-targeted therapies, due to loss of responsivity to VEGF-A inhibitors, has been reported [74]. Recently, Vacca and colleagues uncovered that tumor ECs can lose autocrine loops of Sema3A in favor of endogenous VEGF-A [52]. Thus, restoring Sema3A in tumors could synergize with VEGF-A blockers and help to improve the efficacy of current anti-angiogenic therapies.

7. ACKNOWLEDGMENTS

Research in the authors'labs is supported by Telethon Italy (GGP04127 to GS), Fondazione Guido Berlucchi (to GS); Associazione Augusto per la Vita (to G.S.); Associazione Italiana per la Ricerca sul Cancro (to G.S. and F.B.); Ministero della Salute - Programma Ricerca Oncologica 2006 and Ricerca Finalizzata 2006 (to G.S. and F.B.) and 2007 (to F.B.); Regione Piemonte - Ricerca Sanitaria Finalizzata 2006 and 2008, Ricerca industriale e sviluppo precompetitivo 2006: grants PRESTO and SPLASERBA (to G.S. and F.B.) grant Ricerca Tecnologie convergenti 2007: grant PHOENICS (to F.B.); Sixth Framework Programme of European Union Contract LSHM-CT-2003-503254 (to F.B.); Fondazione Cassa di

Risparmio di Torino (to F.B) and MiUR (PRIN 2007) (to F.B.).

8. REFERENCES

1. Luo B H, Carman C VSpringer T A. Structural basis of integrin regulation and signaling. Annu Rev Immunol 2007; 25: 619-647.

2. Banno AGinsberg M H. Integrin activation. Biochem Soc Trans 2008; 36 (Pt 2): 229-234.

3. Serini G, Napione L, Arese MBussolino F. Besides adhesion: new perspectives of integrin functions in angiogenesis. Cardiovasc Res 2008; 78 (2): 213-222.

4. Hynes R O. Cell-matrix adhesion in vascular development. J Thromb Haemost. 2007; 5 Suppl 1: 32-40.

5. Serini G, Valdembri DBussolino F. Integrins and angiogenesis: A sticky business. Exp Cell Res 2006; 312: 651-658.

6. Kalluri R. Basement membranes: structures, assembly and role in tumor angiogenesis. Nature Rev. Cancer 2003; 3: 422-433.

7. Pellinen TIvaska J. Integrin traffic. J Cell Sci 2006; 119 (Pt 18): 3723-3731.

8. Tran T S, Kolodkin A LBharadwaj R. Semaphorin regulation of cellular morphology. Annu Rev Cell Dev Biol. 2007; 23: 263-292.

9. Zhou Y, Gunput R APasterkamp R J. Semaphorin signaling: progress made and promises ahead. Trends Biochem Sci 2008; 33 (4): 161-170.

10. Falk J, Bechara A, Fiore R, Nawabi H, Zhou H, Hoyo-Becerra C, Bozon M, Rougon G, Grumet M, Puschel A W, Sanes J RCastellani V. Dual functional activity of semaphorin 3B is required for positioning the anterior commissure. Neuron 2005; 48 (1): 63-75.

11. Kumanogoh AKikutani H. Immune semaphorins: a new area of semaphorin research. J Cell Sci 2003; 116 (Pt 17): 3463-3470.

12. Giordano S, Corso S, Conrotto P, Artigiani S, Gilestro G, Barberis D, Tamagnone LComoglio P M. The semaphorin 4D receptor controls invasive growth by coupling with Met. Nat Cell Biol 2002; 4 (9): 720-724.

13. Toyofuku T, Zhang H, Kumanogoh A, Takegahara N, Suto F, Kamei J, Aoki K, Yabuki M, Hori M, Fujisawa HKikutani H. Dual roles of Sema6D in cardiac morphogenesis through region-specific association of its receptor, Plexin-A1, with off-track and vascular endothelial growth factor receptor type 2. Genes Dev 2004; 18 (4): 435-447.

14. Pasterkamp R J, Peschon J J, Spriggs M KKolodkin A L. Semaphorin 7A promotes axon outgrowth through integrins and MAPKs. Nature 2003; 424 (6947): 398-405.

15. Winberg M L, Tamagnone L, Bai J, Comoglio P M, Montell DGoodman C S. The transmembrane protein Off-track associates with Plexins and functions downstream of Semaphorin signaling during axon guidance. Neuron 2001; 32 (1): 53-62.

16. Fujisawa H. From the discovery of neuropilin to the determination of its adhesion sites. Adv Exp Med Biol 2002; 515: 1-12.

17. Favier B, Alam A, Barron P, Bonnin J, Laboudie P, Fons P, Mandron M, Herault J P, Neufeld G, Savi P, Herbert J MBono F. Neuropilin-2 interacts with VEGFR-2 and VEGFR-3 and promotes human endothelial cell survival and migration. Blood 2006; 108 (4): 1243-1250.

18. Fuh G, Garcia K Cde Vos A M. The interaction of neuropilin-1 with vascular endothelial growth factor and its receptor flt-1. J Biol Chem 2000; 275 (35): 26690-26695.

19. Soker S, Takashima S, Miao H Q, Neufeld GKlagsbrun M. Neuropilin-1 is expressed by endothelial and tumor cells as an isoform-specific receptor for vascular endothelial growth factor. Cell 1998; 92 (6): 735-745.

20. Mamluk R, Gechtman Z, Kutcher M E, Gasiunas N, Gallagher JKlagsbrun M. Neuropilin-1 binds vascular endothelial growth factor 165, placenta growth factor-2, and heparin via its b1b2 domain. J Biol Chem 2002; 277 (27): 24818-24825.

21. Cai HReed R R. Cloning and characterization of neuropilin-1-interacting protein: a PSD-95/Dlg/ZO-1 domain-containing protein that interacts with the cytoplasmic domain of neuropilin-1. J Neurosci 1999; 19: 6519-6527.

22. Kawasaki T, Kitsukawa T, Bekku Y, Matsuda Y, Sanbo M, Yagi TFujisawa H. A requirement for neuropilin-1 in embryonic vessel formation. Development 1999; 126 (21): 4895-4902.

23. Shoji W, Isogai S, Sato-Maeda M, Obinata MKuwada J Y. Semaphorin3a1 regulates angioblast migration and vascular development in zebrafish embryos. Development 2003; 130 (14): 3227-3236.

24. Torres-Vazquez J, Gitler A D, Fraser S D, Berk J D, Van N P, Fishman M C, Childs S, Epstein J AWeinstein B M. Semaphorin-plexin signaling guides patterning of the developing vasculature. Dev Cell 2004; 7 (1): 117-123.

25. Serini G, Valdembri D, Zanivan S, Morterra G, Burkhardt C, Caccavari F, Zammataro L, Primo L, Tamagnone L, Logan M, Tessier-Lavigne M, Taniguchi M, Puschel A WBussolino F. Class 3 semaphorins control vascular morphogenesis by inhibiting integrin function. Nature 2003; 424 (6947): 391-397.

26. Bates D, Taylor G I, Minichiello J, Farlie P, Cichowitz A, Watson N, Klagsbrun M, Mamluk RNewgreen D F. Neurovascular congruence results from a shared patterning mechanism that utilizes Semaphorin3A and Neuropilin-1. Dev Biol 2003; 255 (1): 77-98.

27. Kaneko S, Iwanami A, Nakamura M, Kishino A, Kikuchi K, Shibata S, Okano H J, Ikegami T, Moriya A, Konishi O, Nakayama C, Kumagai K, Kimura T, Sato Y, Goshima Y, Taniguchi M, Ito M, He Z, Toyama YOkano H. A selective Sema3A inhibitor enhances regenerative responses and functional recovery of the injured spinal cord. Nat Med 2006; 12: 1380-1389.

28. Gitler A D, Lu M MEpstein J A. PlexinD1 and semaphorin signaling are required in endothelial cells for cardiovascular development. Dev Cell 2004; 7 (1): 107-116.

29. Herzog Y, Guttmann-Raviv NNeufeld G. Segregation of arterial and venous markers in

subpopulations of blood islands before vessel formation. Dev Dyn 2005; 232 (4): 1047-1055.

30.   Kusy S, Funkelstein L, Bourgais D, Drabkin H, Rougon G, Roche JCastellani V. Redundant functions but temporal and regional regulation of two alternatively spliced isoforms of semaphorin 3F in the nervous system. Mol Cell Neurosci 2003; 24 (2): 409-418.

31.   Guttmann-Raviv N, Shraga-Heled N, Varshavsky A, Guimaraes-Sternberg C, Kessler ONeufeld G. Semaphorin-3A and semaphorin-3F work together to repel endothelial cells and to inhibit their survival by induction of apoptosis. J Biol Chem 2007; 282 (36): 26294-26305.

32.   Gu C, Yoshida Y, Livet J, Reimert D V, Mann F, Merte J, Henderson C E, Jessell T M, Kolodkin A LGinty D D. Semaphorin 3E and plexin-D1 control vascular pattern independently of neuropilins. Science 2005; 307 (5707): 265-268.

33.   Zhang Y, Singh M K, Degenhardt K R, Lu M M, Bennett J, Yoshida YEpstein J A. Tie2Cre-mediated inactivation of plexinD1 results in congenital heart, vascular and skeletal defects. Dev Biol 2009; 325 (1): 82-93.

34.   Christensen C, Ambartsumian N, Gilestro G, Thomsen B, Comoglio P, Tamagnone L, Guldberg PLukanidin E. Proteolytic processing converts the repelling signal Sema3E into an inducer of invasive growth and lung metastasis. Cancer Res 2005; 65 (14): 6167-6177.

35.   Roodink I, Raats J, van der Zwaag B, Verrijp K, Kusters B, van Bokhoven H, Linkels M, de Waal R MLeenders W P. Plexin D1 expression is induced on tumor vasculature and tumor cells: a novel target for diagnosis and therapy? Cancer Res 2005; 65 (18): 8317-8323.

36.   Bielenberg D R, Hida Y, Shimizu A, Kaipainen A, Kreuter M, Kim C CKlagsbrun M. Semaphorin 3F, a chemorepulsant for endothelial cells, induces a poorly vascularized, encapsulated, nonmetastatic tumor phenotype. J Clin Invest 2004; 114 (9): 1260-1271.

37.   Kessler O, Shraga-Heled N, Lange T, Gutmann-Raviv N, Sabo E, Baruch L, Machluf MNeufeld G. Semaphorin-3F is an inhibitor of tumor angiogenesis. Cancer Res 2004; 64 (3): 1008-1015.

38.   Miao H Q, Soker S, Feiner L, Alonso J L, Raper J AKlagsbrun M. Neuropilin-1 mediates collapsin-1/semaphorin III inhibition of endothelial cell motility: functional competition of collapsin-1 and vascular endothelial growth factor-165. J Cell Biol 1999; 146 (1): 233-242.

39.   Futamura M, Kamino H, Miyamoto Y, Kitamura N, Nakamura Y, Ohnishi S, Masuda YArakawa H. Possible role of semaphorin 3F, a candidate tumor suppressor gene at 3p21.3, in p53-regulated tumor angiogenesis suppression. Cancer Res 2007; 67 (4): 1451-1460.

40.   Acevedo L M, Barillas S, Weis S M, Gothert J RCheresh D A. Semaphorin 3A suppresses VEGF-mediated angiogenesis yet acts as a vascular permeability factor. Blood 2008.

41.   Conrotto P, Valdembri D, Corso S, Serini G, Tamagnone L, Comoglio P M, Bussolino FGiordano S. Sema4D induces angiogenesis through Met

recruitment by Plexin B1. Blood 2005; 105: 4321-4329.

42.   Basile J R, Barac A, Zhu T, Guan K LGutkind J S. Class IV semaphorins promote angiogenesis by stimulating Rho-initiated pathways through plexin-B. Cancer Res 2004; 64 (15): 5212-5224.

43.   Hall K T, Boumsell L, Schultze J L, Boussiotis V A, Dorfman D M, Cardoso A A, Bensussan A, Nadler L MFreeman G J. Human CD100, a novel leukocyte semaphorin that promotes B-cell aggregation and differentiation. Proc Natl Acad Sci U S A 1996; 93: 11780-11785.

44.   Elhabazi A, Delaire S, Bensussan A, Boumsell LBismuth G. Biological activity of soluble CD100. I. The extracellular region of CD100 is released from the surface of T lymphocytes by regulated proteolysis. J Immunol 2001; 166: 4341-4347.

45.   Suzuki K, Kumanogoh AKikutani H. Semaphorins and their receptors in immune cell interactions. Nat Immunol 2008; 9: 17-23.

46.   Sierra J R, Corso S, Caione L, Cepero V, Conrotto P, Cignetti A, Piacibello W, Kumanogoh A, Kikutani H, Comoglio P M, Tamagnone LGiordano S. Tumor angiogenesis and progression are enhanced by Sema4D produced by tumor-associated macrophages. J Exp Med 2008; 205 (7): 1673-1685.

47.   Toyofuku T, Yabuki M, Kamei J, Kamei M, Makino N, Kumanogoh AHori M. Semaphorin-4A, an activator for T-cell-mediated immunity, suppresses angiogenesis via Plexin-D1. Embo J 2007; 26 (5): 1373-1384.

48.   Maione F, Molla F, Meda C, Latini R, Zentilin L, Giacca M, Serini G, Bussolino FGiraudo E. Semaphorin 3A is an endogenous angiogenic inhibitor that blocks tumor growth and normalizes the vasculature in a mouse model of multistage tumorigenesis. submitted to J. Clin. Invest 2009.

49.   Kiosses W B, Shattil S J, Pampori NSchwartz M A. Rac recruits high-affinity integrin alphavbeta3 to lamellipodia in endothelial cell migration. Nat Cell Biol 2001; 3 (3): 316-320.

50.   Ito T, Kagoshima M, Sasaki Y, Li C, Udaka N, Kitsukawa T, Fujisawa H, Taniguchi M, Yagi T, Kitamura HGoshima Y. Repulsive axon guidance molecule Sema3A inhibits branching morphogenesis of fetal mouse lung. Mech Dev 2000; 97 (1-2): 35-45.

51.   Damon D H. Vascular endothelial-derived semaphorin 3 inhibits sympathetic axon growth. Am J Physiol Heart Circ Physiol 2006; 290: H1220 - H1225.

52.   Vacca A, Scavelli C, Serini G, Di Pietro G, Cirulli T, Merchionne F, Ribatti D, Bussolino F, Guidolin D, Piaggio G, Bacigalupo ADammacco F. Loss of inhibitory semaphorin 3A (SEMA3A) autocrine loops in bone marrow endothelial cells of patients with multiple myeloma. Blood 2006; 108 (5): 1661-1667.

53.   Yonekura H, Sakurai S, Liu X, Migita H, Wang H, Yamagishi S, Nomura M, Abedin M J, Unoki H, Yamamoto YYamamoto H. Placenta growth factor and vascular endothelial growth factor B and C expression in microvascular endothelial cells and pericytes. Implication in autocrine and paracrine regulation of angiogenesis. J Biol Chem 1999; 274 (49): 35172-35178.

54. Lee S, Chen T T, Barber C L, Jordan M C, Murdock J, Desai S, Ferrara N, Nagy A, Roos K PIruela-Arispe M L. Autocrine VEGF signaling is required for vascular homeostasis. Cell 2007; 130 (4): 691-703.

55. Serini G, Ambrosi D, Giraudo E, Gamba A, Preziosi LBussolino F. Modeling the early stages of vascular network assembly. EMBO J 2003; 22: 1771-1779.

56. Arnaout M A, Goodman S LXiong J P. Structure and mechanics of integrin-based cell adhesion. Curr Opin Cell Biol 2007; 19 (5): 495-507.

57. Campbell I DGinsberg M H. The talin-tail interaction places integrin activation on FERM ground. Trends Biochem Sci 2004; 29 (8): 429-435.

58. Ling K, Schill N J, Wagoner M P, Sun YAnderson R A. Movin' on up: the role of PtdIns(4,5)P(2) in cell migration. Trends Cell Biol 2006; 16 (6): 276-284.

59. Komatsu MRuoslahti E. R-Ras is a global regulator of vascular regeneration that suppresses intimal hyperplasia and tumor angiogenesis. Nat Med 2005; 11 (12): 1346-1350.

60. Kinbara K, Goldfinger L E, Hansen M, Chou F LGinsberg M H. Ras GTPases: integrins' friends or foes? Nat Rev Mol Cell Biol 2003; 4 (10): 767-776.

61. Furuhjelm JPeranen J. The C-terminal end of R-Ras contains a focal adhesion targeting signal. J Cell Sci 2003; 116 (Pt 18): 3729-3738.

62. Hansen M, Prior I A, Hughes P E, Oertli B, Chou F L, Willumsen B M, Hancock J FGinsberg M H. C-terminal sequences in R-Ras are involved in integrin regulation and in plasma membrane microdomain distribution. Biochem Biophys Res Commun 2003; 311 (4): 829-838.

63. del Pozo M A, Alderson N B, Kiosses W B, Chiang H H, Anderson R GSchwartz M A. Integrins regulate Rac targeting by internalization of membrane domains. Science 2004; 303 (5659): 839-842.

64. Self A J, Caron E, Paterson H FHall A. Analysis of R-Ras signalling pathways. J Cell Sci 2001; 114 (Pt 7): 1357-1366.

65. Toyofuku T, Yoshida J, Sugimoto T, Zhang H, Kumanogoh A, Hori MKikutani H. FARP2 triggers signals for Sema3A-mediated axonal repulsion. Nat Neurosci 2005; 8: 1712-1719.

66. Garrity P A. Tinker to Evers to Chance: semaphorin signaling takes teamwork. Nat Neurosci 2005; 8 (12): 1635-1636.

67. Gu C, Rodriguez E R, Reimert D V, Shu T, Fritzsch B, Richards L J, Kolodkin A LGinty D D. Neuropilin-1 conveys semaphorin and VEGF signaling during neural and cardiovascular development. Dev Cell 2003; 5 (1): 45-57.

68. Shankar S L, O'Guin K, Cammer M, McMorris F A, Stitt T N, Basch R S, Varnum BShafit-Zagardo B. The growth arrest-specific gene product Gas6 promotes the survival of human oligodendrocytes via a phosphatidylinositol 3-kinase-dependent pathway. J Neurosci 2003; 23 (10): 4208-4218.

69. Ruhrberg C, Gerhardt H, Golding M, Watson R, Ioannidou S, Fujisawa H, Betsholtz CShima D T. Spatially restricted patterning cues provided by heparin-binding VEGF-A control blood vessel branching morphogenesis. Genes Dev 2002; 16 (20): 2684-2698.

70. Shraga-Heled N, Kessler O, Prahst C, Kroll J, Augustin HNeufeld G. Neuropilin-1 and neuropilin-2 enhance VEGF121 stimulated signal transduction by the VEGFR-2 receptor. Faseb J 2007; 21 (3): 915-926.

71. Murga M, Fernandez-Capetillo OTosato G. Neuropilin-1 regulates attachment in human endothelial cells independently of vascular endothelial growth factor receptor-2. Blood 2005; 105 (5): 1992-1999.

72. Valdembri D, Caswell P T, Anderson K I, Schwarz J P, Konig I, Astanina E, Caccavari F, Norman J C, Humphroes M J, Bussolino FSerini G. Neuropilin-1/GIPC1 signaling regulates α5β1 integrin traffic and function in endothelial cells. Plos Biol 2009; in press.

73. Chittenden T W, Claes F, Lanahan A A, Autiero M, Palac R T, Tkachenko E V, Elfenbein A, Ruiz de Almodovar C, Dedkov E, Tomanek R, Li W, Westmore M, Singh J P, Horowitz A, Mulligan-Kehoe M J, Moodie K L, Zhuang Z W, Carmeliet PSimons M. Selective regulation of arterial branching morphogenesis by synectin. Dev Cell 2006; 10 (6): 783-795.

74. Kerbel R S. Tumor angiogenesis. N Engl J Med 2008; 358 (2039-2049).

CHAPTER 2

The Role of Osteopontin in Angiogenesis

Daria Leali[1] and Antonella Naldini[2]

[1]Unit of General Pathology and Immunology, Department of Biomedical Sciences and Biotechnology, University of Brescia, Brescia, Italy; [2]Unit of Neuroimmunophysiology, Department of Physiology, University of Siena, Siena, Italy

Address correspondence: Prof. Antonella Naldini, Department of Physiology, University of Siena, Via Aldo Moro 2, 53100 SIENA, ITALY. Tel.: +39-0577-234212. Fax: +39-0577-234219. E-mail: Naldini@Unisi.it

Abstract: Osteopontin (OPN) is a phosphorylated acidic (Arg-Gly-Asp) RGD-containing glycoprotein, which exists both as an immobilized extracellular matrix component and as a soluble molecule. The biological functions of OPN are extensively regulated on the post-transcriptional and post-translational levels and many of the signaling pathways mediated by secreted OPN are activated by ligation of the integrin and CD44 families of receptors. Such a multifaceted glycoprotein, that is expressed by numerous different cells and tissues, is expected to exert pleiotropic functions. Indeed, OPN is implicated in tumor metastases, tissue remodeling, inflammation, and cell-mediated immunity. Recently, substantial evidence suggests that OPN positively regulates angiogenesis. However, the mechanisms that define the role of this molecule in angiogenesis are incompletely understood. The following review will discuss the biochemical and biological properties of OPN in the context of its role in the modulation of angiogenesis.

1. INTRODUCTION

Osteopontin (OPN) is an arginine-glycine-aspartate (RGD)-containing acidic member of the small integrin-binding ligand N-linked glycoprotein (SIBLING) family of proteins [1]. OPN was originally isolated as a protein secreted by transformed mammalian cells [2]. Due to independent isolation from different sources, and with recognition of its diverse biological roles, OPN has also been known as "bone sialoprotein I (BSP-1)", "secreted phosphoprotein 1 (Spp1)", "2ar", "uropontin" and "early T-lymphocyte activation (ETA-1) factor" [3-7]. As immobilized extracellular matrix (ECM) molecule and soluble cytokine, OPN is implicated in tumor metastases, tissue remodeling, inflammation, and cell-mediated immunity [8,9] and exerts its biological activity by interacting with integrin receptors and several CD44 variants expressed on target cells [9]. Nevertheless, an intracellular form of OPN has also been described [10]. Such a multifaceted glycoprotein, that is expressed by numerous different cells and tissues (see below), is expected to exert pleiotropic functions. Indeed, OPN acts as a pro-inflammatory cytokine that plays important roles in monocytes/macrophage functions [9]. Experiments performed on OPN null mice implicate OPN in T helper (Th)1 cell-mediated immunity during infection, autoimmune demyelinating disease, rheumatoid arthritis, wound healing, and bone resorption [11-13]. On the other hand, OPN exerts cell-adhesive and chemotactic activity for endothelial cells that are protected from apoptosis via αvβ3 integrin-induced NF-κB activation [14]. Also, OPN upregulation occurs in endothelial cells treated with interleukin (IL-1), interferon (IFN)-γ, glucocorticoids, or vascular endothelial growth factor (VEGF) [14,15] during angiogenesis in vitro, and during endothelium regeneration in balloon-injured artery [9]. The latter reports suggest that OPN may play an important role in angiogenesis.

Angiogenesis is a complex process, where several cell types and mediators interact to establish a specific microenvironment suitable for the formation of new capillaries from pre-existing vessels [16]. Such biological processes occur in several physiological conditions, such as embryo development and wound healing, as well as in pathological conditions, including tumors and diabetic retinopathy.

Inflammatory cells, such as T lymphocytes, neutrophils and monocytes, fully participate in the angiogenic process by secreting cytokines, that could control endothelial cell proliferation, their survival and apoptosis, as well as their migration and activation [17]. On the other hand, recent studies on cytokines released by T lymphocytes support the hypothesis that Th cells may control angiogenesis by switching to different phenotypes, which promote or antagonize the angiogenic process [18]. Thus, angiogenesis is the result of a net balance between the activities exerted by positive and negative regulators. Cytokines released by monocytes have been extensively studied in that context. Indeed, monocytes/macrophages produce direct and indirect inducers of angiogenesis, including

IL-1, tumor-necrosis factor (TNF)-α, IL-8 and VEGFs, as well as angiogenic inhibitors, such as angiostatin, inhibitory chemokines, and thrombospondin [17,19,20]. There is mounting evidence for the role of another cytokine, secreted by activated macrophages, in providing a link between inflammation and angiogenesis and that cytokine is OPN.

While it is widely accepted the definition of OPN as metastasis gene for tumor progression [21,22], information regarding the role of OPN in angiogenesis is still scant. Here, the biochemical and biological properties of OPN will be reviewed in the context of its role in the modulation of angiogenesis.

2. OPN GENE STRUCTURE AND EXPRESSION

Comparative analysis of cDNA isolated from different species (human, mouse, rat, bovine and chicken) revealed a high omology degree in OPN sequence [23]. The human OPN gene occurs at the long arm of chromosome 4 (4q21–4q25). Of the seven exons present, six of them (exons 2–7) contain coding sequences which are about 954 bp and the first exon is untranslated. The 5' upstream sequence of OPN gene contains a number of potential regulatory sequences. Regulatory sequences include a TATA-like sequence found at position −27 to −22 [24], CCAAAT-like sequence scattered throughout the 5' upstream region from −73 to −2190 [24,25], and the vitamin D responsive element at positions −698 to −684 and −1892 to −1878. An interferon regulatory factor-1 binding sequence, AACTGA, is also identified at positions −1270 to −1264 [26]. In addition, potential binding sites for transcription of OPN gene include AP-1, AP-2, Ets-1, E2A, E2BP, TCF, and Myb which are characterized near the 5' cap site of rat and human OPN promoter (see [27] for a recent review).

The biological functions of OPN are extensively regulated on the post-transcriptional and post-translational levels. Human OPN cDNA analysis suggests the existence of three splicing isoforms (hOPNa, hOPNb e hOPNc) [28]. OPN-b lacks exon 5 and OPN-c lacks exon 4 [29]. The shortest splice variant, OPN-c, is a selective marker of breast cancer and may support breast tumor progression[30]. Furthermore, an intracellular form of OPN (iOPN), is generated as a consequence of translation initiation from a non-AUG site residing 40-nt downstream of the canonical AUG sequence [31]. This mechanism, which does not involve alternative mRNA transcription initiation or splicing, generates a full-length secreted OPN (sOPN) and a smaller product (iOPN) that lacks the signal peptide from a single full-length mRNA species. In contrast with secreted OPN isoforms, iOPN presumably interacts with the cytoplasmic domain of CD44, thus partecipating to CD44 signaling [31] (see below).

Cell types which express OPN include osteoclasts, osteoblasts, kidney, breast and skin epithelial cells, nerve cells, vascular smooth muscle cells and endothelial cells [23,28,32-34]. In the immune system, OPN is expressed by many different cell types, including macrophages, neutrophils, B- and T lymphocytes, NK cells, Kuppfer cells, mast cells and plasmacytoid dendritic cells [10,35-40]. The induced expression of OPN has been detected in T lymphocytes, epidermal cells, bone cells, macrophages and tumor cells in remodeling processes such as inflammation, ischemia-reperfusion, bone resorption and tumor progression [27,28,33,34,41-44]. Furthermore, a variety of stimuli including phorbol 12-myristate 13-acetate (PMA), 1,25-dihydroxyvitamin D, basic fibroblast growth factor (FGF2), platelet derived growth factor (PDGF), TNF-α, IL-1, IFN-γ and lipopolysaccharide (LPS) upregulate OPN expression [9,28,33,34,45].

It has been proposed that distinct cell types differ in their post-translational modifications of OPN (see below), which may underlie cell-type specific differences in the functions of OPN [46].

3. OPN PROTEIN STRUCTURE

The complete amino acid sequences of OPN for human, rat, mouse, pig, cow and chicken [24] have been deduced from their cDNA sequences. OPN protein consists of a single chain of 264-333 amino acid, rich in sialic acid, glutamic acid and serine residues, depending on species (297 in mouse; 314 in human) [24].

Human OPN contains a hydrophobic leader sequence typical of secreted protein [9,47] (Fig. **1**). A protease-hypersensitive site separates the NH2-terminal/integrin binding from the COOH-terminal/CD44 binding domains, which carry out distinct signaling functions. The thrombin cleavage motif in this region has a conserved sequence, ^{168}RSK^{170}, present in most species [48].

The NH2-terminal region of OPN contains most of the well-conserved functional domains of the protein, such as an aspartate-rich region and several integrin binding sites. Via the RGD sequence located in the ^{158}GRGDS^{162} motif near the centre of the protein, OPN interacts with a variety of α_v integrin receptors (including $\alpha_v\beta_1$, $\alpha_v\beta_3$, $\alpha_v\beta_5$, $\alpha_v\beta_6$), $\alpha_8\beta_1$ and $\alpha_5\beta_1$ [9,28,49-51]. Furthermore, the RGD-dependent interaction of OPN with $\alpha_v\beta_3$ integrin requires phosphorylation of the protein [52]. A cryptic binding site located immediately downstream of the RGD domain (^{162}SVVYGLR^{168} in human, SLAYGLR in mouse) is exposed upon thrombin cleavage between the R^{168} and S^{169} residues and mediates an RGD-indipendent interaction of OPN with $\alpha_9\beta_1$ and $\alpha_4\beta_7$ integrins [28,51,53]. Earlier reports indicated that

OPN acts also as a substrate for matrix metalloproteases MMP-3 and MMP-7, and the cleaved fragments enhanced adhesion and migration *in vitro* through ligation of receptors including β1 integrin [54]. Indeed, there are two different binding sites for $\alpha_4\beta_1$ integrin present in a 38-amino acid domain within the N-terminal thrombin fragment, corresponding to both ^{162}SVVYGLR^{168} and ^{131}ELVTDFPTDLPAT^{143} motifs [55]. Furthermore, the sequence ^{43}WLNPDP^{48} has been recently described as a novel functional motif of OPN, involved in migration and survival of human lymphocyte, although the corresponding interacting receptor has not been identified [56].

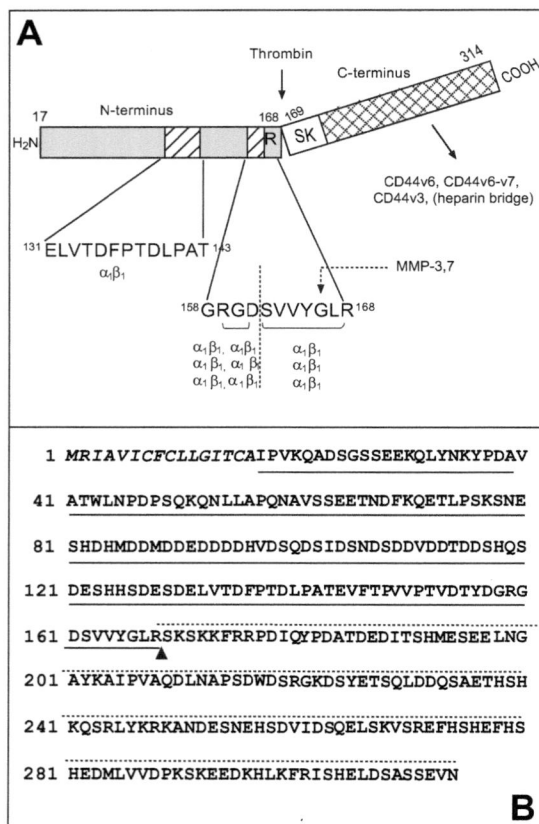

NH$_2$-terminal and the C-terminal regions of the protein, has been recently identified as "collagen binding motif", corresponding to the ^{166}GLRSKSKKFRRPDIQYPDATDEDITSHM^{193} sequence in human OPN [59].

The C-terminal fragment of OPN contains a conserved calcium binding site and interacts directly with CD44v6- and v7-containing isoforms [44,60], although CD44v3 might indirectly bind OPN through a heparin bridge [52]. This RGD-independent interaction appears to require the presence of β_1 integrins [61]. It has been recently proposed a model for human OPN structure in which a sequence in the C-terminal region forms a β-sheet structure with the RGDSVVYGLR domain in the N-terminus, thus interfering with RGD-integrin interaction [46]. This model might explain the ability of monoclonal antibody against the C-terminus domain to inhibit cell adhesion to OPN, thus suggesting the possibility that CD44/OPN interaction modulates the cells' capacity to recognize the RGD sequence [62].

Although expressed as a $\sim$ 33 kDa nascent protein, extensive posttranslational modifications (PTMs) such as Ser/Thr phosphorylation, O-linked/N-linked glycosylation, sialylation, Tyr sulfation and enzymatic cleavage, increase its apparent molecular weight, thus determining a protein migration in SDS-PAGE gels in the range of 44-80 kDa depending on conditions [24,63]. Polymeric form of OPN has been recently reported which produces a band around 200 kDa that is mediated by transglutaminase [64,65]. Many sites of PTMs are conserved across species; however, the degree of modification of the protein varies depending on the source tissue and cell type or differentiation stage [66-68] and influence OPN function [46]. Phosphorylation of OPN appears necessary for various physiological functions, including migration of cancer cells [69], adhesion and bone resorption by osteoclasts [70], inhibition of smooth muscle cell calcification [71] and regulation of mineralization [72]. The phosphorylation of OPN is usually heterogeneous, and it is not known whether certain specific sites are critical for a given function; furthermore, it is possible that differences in OPN post-translational modification status, together with variations in the target cell receptor repertoire, modulate OPN's functions or the cellular response to OPN [46].

4. OPN SIGNALING

The role of both secreted and intracellular OPN in cell signaling has been recently reviewed in the context of cancer progression and immune response [40,73].

Many of the signaling pathways mediated by secreted OPN are activated by ligation of the integrin and CD44 families of receptors. OPN signaling through

Fig. (1). OPN protein structure. (A) Schematic representation of the human OPN protein. OPN contains a thrombin cleavage site that separates the N-terminus/integrin binding and the C-terminus/CD44v binding domains (amino acid residues 17-168 and 169-314, respectively). Conserved regions involved in receptor interactions are indicated. (B) Amino acid sequence (single letter code) of the human OPN protein (GenBank accession number: J04765). The N-terminus and C-terminus domains are underlined and shown as dotted line, respectively. The signal sequence (amino acid residues 1-16) is in Italics. Arrow indicates the thrombin cleavage site.

In keeping with its ability to associate with different ECM proteins, such as collagen and fibronectin [57,58], a novel functional domain, spanning both the integrins can modulate (via activation of Ras and Src) the phosphorylation of kinases (NIK, IKKβ) involved in NFκB activation [74,75], that regulates expression of many inflammatory cytokines. Also, OPN stimulates NIK-dependent NF-kB-mediated urokinase plasminogen activator (uPA) secretion and MMP-9 activation through both IKKα/β and MAPK-mediated pathways in cancer cells [76,77]. Both OPN/integrin and OPN/CD44 interactions activates PI3K/Akt pathway (via cSrc and PLCγ/PKC activation, respectively), thus promoting cell survival and motility [78,79].

Intracellular OPN exists as an integral component of a CD44-ezrin/radixin/moesin (ERM) attachment complex on the inner surface of the plasma membrane [80]. The interaction of intracellular OPN with CD44 presumably involves a constant intracellular domain of CD44 in contrast with the interaction of secreted OPN with extracellular variant domains of CD44. In association with the CD44 receptor inside migratory cells, intracellular OPN modulates cytoskeletal-related functions including cell motility, cell fusion and survival of different cell types such as embryonic fibroblasts, activated macrophages, metastatic cells and osteoclasts [80-82]. Recent findings have revealed that intracellular OPN also localizes with TLR9/MyD88 complex and activates nuclear translocation of transcription factor IRF7, inducing IFN-α expression in plasmacytoid dendritic cells [10].

5. OPN, ANGIOGENESIS AND TISSUE REPAIR

Cumulative evidence suggests that OPN positively regulates angiogenesis in several experimental models [83]. Supporting this pro-angiogenic role of OPN is the observation that VEGF induces OPN and $\alpha_v\beta_3$ integrin expression in microvascular endothelial cells [9,84]. Indeed, OPN induces neovascularization by up-regulating endothelial cell migration, survival, and lumen formation during angiogenesis [75,84]. In addition, it has been suggested that the SVVYGLR sequence may play a direct role in angiogenesis [85,86]. That OPN promotes angiogenesis by a direct effect on endothelial cells indicates the physiological significance of OPN in cardiovascular remodeling [41]. This hypothesis is corroborated by the fact that OPN is not expressed in healthy cardiac muscle tissue, while its expression is accelerated by mechanical stress including pressure/volume loading and hypoxia [87]. Indeed, OPN, increased in the heart following myocardial infarction (MI), plays an important role in post-MI remodeling and lack of OPN impairs myocardial angiogenic response, leading to adverse remodeling post-MI [88]. Interestingly, other findings support the hypothesis that OPN induces myocardial

fibrosis and remodeling in the process of tissue repair following inflammation [89]. Again, mice lacking OPN grow normally but deposit collagen in an abnormal manner with faulty wound healing [90]. The relevance of OPN in vascular remodeling and tissue repair has been highlighted by a recent report, where OPN was required for estrogen-stimulated endothelial repair, both for bone marrow-derived cell recruitment and for endothelial cell migration and proliferation [91].

It is widely accepted that wound healing and tissue repair are characterized by an hypoxic microenvironment [92]. Interestingly, up-regulation of OPN induced by hypoxia has been previously observed in many cell types, including rat aortic vascular smooth muscle cells [93], human renal proximal tubular epithelial cells [94], head and neck squamous cell carcinoma cell lines and in NIH3T3 cells [95] and mouse osteocytes [96]. More recently, it has been reported that hypoxia affects mesenchymal stromal cell osteogenic differentiation and angiogenic factor expression [97], indicating, again, that OPN plays an important role in bone remodelling and osteoclast recruitment processes. In this context, it is important to underline that the most striking property of OPN may be its ability to promote macrophage infiltration [98,99]. Thus, increased OPN expression by hypoxic mesenchymal stromal cells may therefore culminate in attracting macrophages to the bone defect site and exacerbating the inflammatory process [97]. In bone, this molecule mediates the attachment of several cell types, including osteoblasts, endothelial cells and osteoclasts [47]. More interestingly, OPN facilitates angiogenesis, accumulation of osteoclasts, and resorption in ectopic bone [100].

6. OPN AND TUMOR ANGIOGENESIS

High levels of OPN expression correlate with tumor invasion, progression, or metastasis in breast, gastric, lung, prostate, liver, and colon cancer [22]. It is widely accepted that the progression of tumors is largely dependent on their vascularization [101]. Neovascularization is a fundamental process also in tumor metastasis and several pro-angiogenic molecules, including VEGF, are up-regulated during tumor progression [102,103]. OPN functions as an angiogenic factor by promoting neovascularization through integrin-mediated endothelial cell migration, prevention of endothelial cell apoptosis, and vascular lumen formation [84,104,105]. In addition, the cryptic Arg-Gly-Asp (RGD) site exposed by thrombin-induced proteolysis may guide the path in front of invading host or tumor cells [22]. Thus, OPN appears to be crucially involved in tumor progression and angiogenesis. This hypothesis is supported by several experimental reports. A recent study reveals that reduced OPN production by gastric cancer cells, using the small interference RNA method, would reduce the proliferation, migration, and tube formation of human umbilical vein endothelial cells, and lead to a lower microvessel density, i.e., angiogenesis, in transplanted tumors of mice [106]. A previous report has shown that OPN induces angiogenesis of murine neuroblastoma cells in mice [104] and, more recently, it has been described that OPN expression correlates with angiogenesis and survival in malignant astrocytoma [107]. OPN is also implicated in breast cancer progression, as this molecule promotes VEGF-dependent breast tumor growth and angiogenesis via autocrine and paracrine mechanisms [108]. The role played by OPN in tumor angiogenesis has been extensively described in the physio-pathology of multiple myeloma [109]. Human myeloma cells express the bone regulating gene Runx2/Cbfa1 and produce OPN, that is involved in angiogenesis in multiple myeloma patients [110]. In this study, using an 'in vitro' angiogenesis system, the authors show that OPN production by myeloma cells is critical for the proangiogenic effect of myeloma cells. Furthermore, a more recent report describes that the new tumor-suppressor gene inhibitor of growth family member 4 (ING4) regulates the production of pro-angiogenic molecules (e.g. OPN and IL-8) by myeloma cells and suppresses hypoxia-inducible factor-1 α (HIF-1α) activity [111]. In the same study, the authors show that the inhibition of HIF-1α by siRNA suppresses IL-8 and OPN production by multiple myeloma cells under hypoxia, suggesting a tight relationship between hypoxia and OPN. Indeed, a direct interaction between ING4 and the HIF prolyl hydroxylase 2 (HPH-2) was demonstrated. More interestingly, they show that ING4 suppression in multiple myeloma cells significantly increases vessel formation in vitro, blunted by blocking IL-8 or OPN. The relevant role played by OPN in bone marrow physiopathology has been also underlined by a report showing that OPN is a key component of the hematopoietic stem cell niche and regulator of primitive hematopoietic progenitor cells [112]. In this study the authors unequivocally show that primitive hematopoietic cells demonstrate specific adhesion to OPN in vitro via β_1 integrin. Furthermore, exogenous OPN potently suppresses the proliferation of primitive hematopoietic stem cells in vitro, the physiologic relevance of which was demonstrated by the markedly enhanced cycling of hematopoietic stem cells in Opn-/- mice. Thus, the authors suggest that their data provide strong evidence that OPN is an important component of the hematopoietic stem cell niche which participates in hematopoietic stem cell location and as a physiologic-negative regulator of hematopoietic stem cell proliferation.

7. ROLE OF OPN IN ANGIOGENESIS/ INFLAMMATION CROSS-TALK

Experimental evidence suggests that OPN may affect angiogenesis by acting directly on endothelial cells [75,84,113]. However, the ability of OPN to promote macrophage infiltration indicates that this molecule may promote angiogenesis also indirectly via mononuclear phagocyte engagement and monocyte-derived pro-angiogenic cytokines. We have previously demonstrated the cross-talk among angiogenic growth factors and cytokines during angiogenesis and pointed to OPN upregulation as a monocyte-mediated mechanism of amplification of growth factor-induced neovascularization [98]. In such report, we show that OPN enhances the expression of monocyte-derived pro-angiogenic cytokines, such as TNF-α and IL-8, in endothelial cells. The in vitro findings were confirmed in vivo where OPN elicited a potent angiogenic response by causing the recruitment of proangiogenic monocytes. Monocyte/macrophage functions are deeply affected by OPN [8,9]. OPN is also implicated in Th1 cell-mediated immunity during infection, autoimmune demyelinating disease, rheumatoid arthritis, wound healing, and bone resorption [13,90,114,115]. All these conditions are characterized by mononuclear phagocyte involvement as well as by the presence of proinflammatory cytokines, including IL-1β [116], which plays a pivotal role in angiogenesis [117]. In a recent report, in keeping with a putative role for recruited monocytes in OPN-triggered angiogenesis, we showed that OPN induced the expression and release of IL-1β [99]. This was accompanied by the enhanced production of other proinflammatory/proangiogenic cytokines (e.g. IL-6, IL-8 and TNF-α) and by a reduced production of antiinflammatory/antiangiogenic IL-10 in human monocytes. Thus, our observations are in agreement with the hypothesis that OPN may cause a switch of the angiogenic balance in human monocytes that favors the neovascularization process. Accordingly, in the same study we showed that the conditioned medium from OPN-treated monocytes exerted a chemotactic response for murine aortic endothelial cells significantly higher than that triggered by the conditioned medium of control monocytes. These results were confirmed in vivo in the chorioallantoic membrane (CAM) assay. More interestingly, IL-1β neutralization completely abolished neovascularization triggered by OPN-activated monocytes [99], suggesting that IL-1β is the master regulator of OPN-induced angiogenesis. In agreement with our results, other authors have previously reported that neovascularization is impaired in either IL-1β or OPN null mice [100,117]. Thus, our study supports the hypothesis that OPN promotes angiogenesis indirectly, through monocyte activation and IL-1β. The proinflammatory/proangiogenic response induced by OPN may represent an additional mechanism for promoting neovascularization in different physio-pathological conditions, including wound healing, and tumor growth.

8. CONCLUSIONS

In the scenario described above, it is clear that OPN is emerging as a key regulator of angiogenesis. Most of the evidence indicates that OPN functions as an angiogenic factor by promoting neovascularization through integrin-mediated endothelial cell migration, prevention of endothelial cell apoptosis, and vascular lumen formation. Furthermore, in vitro and in vivo studies show that increased OPN expression is associated with tumor invasion, progression and metastasis in numerous human cancers. Therefore, we would like to propose that OPN may be critically involved in tumor angiogenesis.

Recent evidence also suggests that OPN elicits a potent angiogenic response indirectly, by causing the recruitment of proangiogenic monocytes, associated with the enhancement of monocyte-derived pro-angiogenic cytokine expression. Thus, the proinflammatory/proangiogenic response induced by OPN may represent an additional mechanism for promoting neovascularization in different physio-pathological conditions, including wound healing, and tumor growth.

9. ACKNOWLEDGEMENTS

This work was supported by grants from MIUR (PRIN 2007) and PAR Università di Siena (Progetti 2006) to A.N.

10. REFERENCES

1. Fisher LW, Torchia DA, Fohr B, Young MF, Fedarko NS. Flexible structures of SIBLING proteins, bone sialoprotein, and osteopontin. Biochem Biophys Res Commun 2001; 280(2): 460-465.
2. Senger DR, Wirth DF, Hynes RO. Transformed mammalian cells secrete specific proteins and phosphoproteins. Cell 1979; 16(4): 885-893.
3. Fisher LW, Hawkins GR, Tuross N, Termine JD. Purification and partial characterization of small proteoglycans I and II, bone sialoproteins I and II, and osteonectin from the mineral compartment of developing human bone. J Biol Chem 1987; 262(20): 9702-9708.
4. Craig AM, Nemir M, Mukherjee BB, Chambers AF, Denhardt DT. Identification of the major phosphoprotein secreted by many rodent cell lines as 2ar/osteopontin: enhanced expression in H-ras-transformed 3T3 cells. Biochem Biophys Res Commun 1988; 157(1): 166-173.
5. Patarca R, Freeman GJ, Singh RP, Wei FY, Durfee T, Blattner F, Regnier DC, Kozak CA, Mock BA, Morse HC, III, . Structural and functional studies of

the early T lymphocyte activation 1 (Eta-1) gene. Definition of a novel T cell-dependent response associated with genetic resistance to bacterial infection. J Exp Med 1989; 170(1): 145-161.
6. Wrana JL, Zhang Q, Sodek J. Full length cDNA sequence of porcine secreted phosphoprotein-I (SPP-I, osteopontin). Nucleic Acids Res 1989; 17(23): 10119.
7. Shiraga H, Min W, VanDusen WJ, Clayman MD, Miner D, Terrell CH, Sherbotie JR, Foreman JW, Przysiecki C, Neilson EG, . Inhibition of calcium oxalate crystal growth in vitro by uropontin: another member of the aspartic acid-rich protein superfamily. Proc Natl Acad Sci U S A 1992; 89(1): 426-430.
8. O'Regan AW, Nau GJ, Chupp GL, Berman JS. Osteopontin (Eta-1) in cell-mediated immunity: teaching an old dog new tricks. Immunol Today 2000; 21(10): 475-478.
9. Denhardt DT, Noda M, O'Regan AW, Pavlin D, Berman JS. Osteopontin as a means to cope with environmental insults: regulation of inflammation, tissue remodeling, and cell survival. J Clin Invest 2001; 107(9): 1055-1061.
10. Shinohara ML, Lu L, Bu J, Werneck MB, Kobayashi KS, Glimcher LH, Cantor H. Osteopontin expression is essential for interferon-alpha production by plasmacytoid dendritic cells. Nat Immunol 2006; 7(5): 498-506.
11. Chabas D, Baranzini SE, Mitchell D, Bernard CC, Rittling SR, Denhardt DT, Sobel RA, Lock C, Karpuj M, Pedotti R, Heller R, Oksenberg JR, Steinman L. The influence of the proinflammatory cytokine, osteopontin, on autoimmune demyelinating disease. Science 2001; 294(5547): 1731-1735.
12. Ishijima M, Tsuji K, Rittling SR, Yamashita T, Kurosawa H, Denhardt DT, Nifuji A, Noda M. Resistance to unloading-induced three-dimensional bone loss in osteopontin-deficient mice. J Bone Miner Res 2002; 17(4): 661-667.
13. Yumoto K, Ishijima M, Rittling SR, Tsuji K, Tsuchiya Y, Kon S, Nifuji A, Uede T, Denhardt DT, Noda M. Osteopontin deficiency protects joints against destruction in anti-type II collagen antibody-induced arthritis in mice. Proc Natl Acad Sci U S A 2002; 99(7): 4556-4561.
14. Gravallese EM . Osteopontin: a bridge between bone and the immune system. J Clin Invest 2003; 112(2): 147-149.
15. O'Regan AW, Hayden JM, Berman JS. Osteopontin augments CD3-mediated interferon-gamma and CD40 ligand expression by T cells, which results in IL-12 production from peripheral blood mononuclear cells. J Leukoc Biol 2000; 68(4): 495-502.
16. Kerbel R, Folkman J. Clinical translation of angiogenesis inhibitors. Nat Rev Cancer 2002; 2(10): 727-739.
17. Lingen MW . Role of leukocytes and endothelial cells in the development of angiogenesis in inflammation and wound healing. Arch Pathol Lab Med 2001; 125(1): 67-71.
18. Romagnani P, Annunziato F, Piccinni MP, Maggi E, Romagnani S. Th1/Th2 cells, their associated molecules and role in pathophysiology. Eur Cytokine Netw 2000; 11(3): 510-511.

19.   El Awad B, Kreft B, Wolber EM, Hellwig-Burgel T, Metzen E, Fandrey J, Jelkmann W. Hypoxia and interleukin-1beta stimulate vascular endothelial growth factor production in human proximal tubular cells. Kidney Int 2000; 58(1): 43-50.

20.   O'Reilly MS, Boehm T, Shing Y, Fukai N, Vasios G, Lane WS, Flynn E, Birkhead JR, Olsen BR, Folkman J. Endostatin: an endogenous inhibitor of angiogenesis and tumor growth. Cell 1997; 88277-285.

21.   Chambers AF, Groom AC, MacDonald IC. Dissemination and growth of cancer cells in metastatic sites. Nat Rev Cancer 2002; 2(8): 563-572.

22.   Furger KA, Menon RK, Tuckl AB, Bramwelll VH, Chambers AF. The functional and clinical roles of osteopontin in cancer and metastasis. Curr Mol Med 2001; 1(5): 621-632.

23.   Denhardt DT, Guo X. Osteopontin: a protein with diverse functions. FASEB J 1993; 7(15): 1475-1482.

24.   Sodek J, Ganss B, McKee MD. Osteopontin. Crit Rev Oral Biol Med 2000; 11(3): 279-303.

25.   Suzuki K . [Osteopontin-gene, structure and biosynthesis]. Nippon Rinsho 2005; 63 Suppl 10608-612.

26.   Korber B, Mermod N, Hood L, Stroynowski I. Regulation of gene expression by interferons: control of H-2 promoter responses. Science 1988; 239(4845): 1302-1306.

27.   El-Tanani MK, Campbell FC, Kurisetty V, Jin D, McCann M, Rudland PS. The regulation and role of osteopontin in malignant transformation and cancer. Cytokine Growth Factor Rev 2006; 17(6): 463-474.

28.   O'Regan A, Berman JS. Osteopontin: a key cytokine in cell-mediated and granulomatous inflammation. Int J Exp Pathol 2000; 81(6): 373-390.

29.   He B, Mirza M, Weber GF. An osteopontin splice variant induces anchorage independence in human breast cancer cells. Oncogene 2006; 25(15): 2192-2202.

30.   Mirza M, Shaughnessy E, Hurley JK, Vanpatten KA, Pestano GA, He B, Weber GF. Osteopontin-c is a selective marker of breast cancer. Int J Cancer 2008; 122(4): 889-897.

31.   Shinohara ML, Kim HJ, Kim JH, Garcia VA, Cantor H. Alternative translation of osteopontin generates intracellular and secreted isoforms that mediate distinct biological activities in dendritic cells. Proc Natl Acad Sci U S A 2008; 105(20): 7235-7239.

32.   Craig AM, Denhardt DT. The murine gene encoding secreted phosphoprotein 1 (osteopontin): promoter structure, activity, and induction in vivo by estrogen and progesterone. Gene 1991; 100163-171.

33.   Denhardt DT, Noda M. Osteopontin expression and function: role in bone remodeling. J Cell Biochem Suppl 1998; 30-3192-102.

34.   Weber GF . The metastasis gene osteopontin: a candidate target for cancer therapy. Biochim Biophys Acta 2001; 1552(2): 61-85.

35.   Pollack SB, Linnemeyer PA, Gill S. Induction of osteopontin mRNA expression during activation of murine NK cells. J Leukoc Biol 1994; 55(3): 398-400.

36.   Bulfone-Paus S, Paus R. Osteopontin as a new player in mast cell biology. Eur J Immunol 2008; 38(2): 338-341.

37.   Guo B, Tumang JR, Rothstein TL. B cell receptor crosstalk: B cells express osteopontin through the combined action of the alternate and classical BCR signaling pathways. Mol Immunol 2008.

38.   Nagasaka A, Matsue H, Matsushima H, Aoki R, Nakamura Y, Kambe N, Kon S, Uede T, Shimada S. Osteopontin is produced by mast cells and affects IgE-mediated degranulation and migration of mast cells. Eur J Immunol 2008; 38(2): 489-499.

39.   Ramaiah SK, Rittling S. Pathophysiological role of osteopontin in hepatic inflammation, toxicity, and cancer. Toxicol Sci 2008; 103(1): 4-13.

40.   Wang KX, Denhardt DT. Osteopontin: Role in immune regulation and stress responses. Cytokine Growth Factor Rev 2008.

41.   Okamoto H . Osteopontin and cardiovascular system. Mol Cell Biochem 2007; 300(1-2): 1-7.

42.   Scatena M, Liaw L, Giachelli CM. Osteopontin: a multifunctional molecule regulating chronic inflammation and vascular disease. Arterioscler Thromb Vasc Biol 2007; 27(11): 2302-2309.

43.   Bellahcene A, Castronovo V, Ogbureke KU, Fisher LW, Fedarko NS. Small integrin-binding ligand N-linked glycoproteins (SIBLINGs): multifunctional proteins in cancer. Nat Rev Cancer 2008; 8(3): 212-226.

44.   Wai PY, Kuo PC. Osteopontin: regulation in tumor metastasis. Cancer Metastasis Rev 2008; 27(1): 103-118.

45.   Hijiya N, Setoguchi M, Matsuura K, Higuchi Y, Akizuki S, Yamamoto S. Cloning and characterization of the human osteopontin gene and its promoter. Biochem J 1994; 303 (Pt 1)255-262.

46.   Kazanecki CC, Uzwiak DJ, Denhardt DT. Control of osteopontin signaling and function by post-translational phosphorylation and protein folding. J Cell Biochem 2007; 102(4): 912-924.

47.   Denhardt DT, Giachelli CM, Rittling SR. Role of osteopontin in cellular signaling and toxicant injury. Annu Rev Pharmacol Toxicol 2001; 41723-749.

48.   Senger DR, Perruzzi CA, Papadopoulos-Sergiou A, Van de WL. Adhesive properties of osteopontin: regulation by a naturally occurring thrombin-cleavage in close proximity to the GRGDS cell-binding domain. Mol Biol Cell 1994; 5(5): 565-574.

49.   Denda S, Reichardt LF, Muller U. Identification of osteopontin as a novel ligand for the integrin alpha8 beta1 and potential roles for this integrin-ligand interaction in kidney morphogenesis. Mol Biol Cell 1998; 9(6): 1425-1435.

50.   Helluin O, Chan C, Vilaire G, Mousa S, DeGrado WF, Bennett JS. The activation state of alphavbeta 3 regulates platelet and lymphocyte adhesion to intact and thrombin-cleaved osteopontin. J Biol Chem 2000; 275(24): 18337-18343.

51.   Yokosaki Y, Tanaka K, Higashikawa F, Yamashita K, Eboshida A. Distinct structural requirements for binding of the integrins alphavbeta6, alphavbeta3, alphavbeta5, alpha5beta1 and alpha9beta1 to osteopontin. Matrix Biol 2005; 24(6): 418-427.

52. Salih E, Ashkar S, Gerstenfeld LC, Glimcher MJ. Identification of the phosphorylated sites of metabolically 32P-labeled osteopontin from cultured chicken osteoblasts. J Biol Chem 1997; 272(21): 13966-13973.

53. Barry ST, Ludbrook SB, Murrison E, Horgan CM. Analysis of the alpha4beta1 integrin-osteopontin interaction. Exp Cell Res 2000; 258(2): 342-351.

54. Agnihotri R, Crawford HC, Haro H, Matrisian LM, Havrda MC, Liaw L. Osteopontin, a novel substrate for matrix metalloproteinase-3 (stromelysin-1) and matrix metalloproteinase-7 (matrilysin). J Biol Chem 2001; 276(30): 28261-28267.

55. Bayless KJ, Davis GE. Identification of dual alpha 4beta1 integrin binding sites within a 38 amino acid domain in the N-terminal thrombin fragment of human osteopontin. J Biol Chem 2001; 276(16): 13483-13489.

56. Cao Z, Dai J, Fan K, Wang H, Ji G, Li B, Zhang D, Hou S, Qian W, Zhao J, Wang H, Guo Y. A novel functional motif of osteopontin for human lymphocyte migration and survival. Mol Immunol 2008; 45(14): 3683-3692.

57. Singh K, DeVouge MW, Mukherjee BB. Physiological properties and differential glycosylation of phosphorylated and nonphosphorylated forms of osteopontin secreted by normal rat kidney cells. J Biol Chem 1990; 265(30): 18696-18701.

58. Kaartinen MT, Pirhonen A, Linnala-Kankkunen A, Maenpaa PH. Cross-linking of osteopontin by tissue transglutaminase increases its collagen binding properties. J Biol Chem 1999; 274(3): 1729-1735.

59. Lee JY, Choo JE, Park HJ, Park JB, Lee SC, Jo I, Lee SJ, Chung CP, Park YJ. Injectable gel with synthetic collagen-binding peptide for enhanced osteogenesis in vitro and in vivo. Biochem Biophys Res Commun 2007; 357(1): 68-74.

60. Weber GF, Ashkar S, Glimcher MJ, Cantor H. Receptor-ligand interaction between CD44 and osteopontin (Eta-1). Science 1996; 271(5248): 509-512.

61. Katagiri YU, Sleeman J, Fujii H, Herrlich P, Hotta H, Tanaka K, Chikuma S, Yagita H, Okumura K, Murakami M, Saiki I, Chambers AF, Uede T. CD44 variants but not CD44s cooperate with beta1-containing integrins to permit cells to bind to osteopontin independently of arginine-glycine-aspartic acid, thereby stimulating cell motility and chemotaxis. Cancer Res 1999; 59(1): 219-226.

62. Kazanecki CC, Kowalski AJ, Ding T, Rittling SR, Denhardt DT. Characterization of anti-osteopontin monoclonal antibodies: Binding sensitivity to post-translational modifications. J Cell Biochem 2007; 102(4): 925-935.

63. Prince CW, Oosawa T, Butler WT, Tomana M, Bhown AS, Bhown M, Schrohenloher RE. Isolation, characterization, and biosynthesis of a phosphorylated glycoprotein from rat bone. J Biol Chem 1987; 262(6): 2900-2907.

64. Prince CW, Dickie D, Krumdieck CL. Osteopontin, a substrate for transglutaminase and factor XIII activity. Biochem Biophys Res Commun 1991; 177(3): 1205-1210.

65. Higashikawa F, Eboshida A, Yokosaki Y. Enhanced biological activity of polymeric osteopontin. FEBS Lett 2007; 581(14): 2697-2701.

66. Christensen B, Nielsen MS, Haselmann KF, Petersen TE, Sorensen ES. Post-translationally modified residues of native human osteopontin are located in clusters: identification of 36 phosphorylation and five O-glycosylation sites and their biological implications. Biochem J 2005; 390(Pt 1): 285-292.

67. Keykhosravani M, Doherty-Kirby A, Zhang C, Brewer D, Goldberg HA, Hunter GK, Lajoie G. Comprehensive identification of post-translational modifications of rat bone osteopontin by mass spectrometry. Biochemistry 2005; 44(18): 6990-7003.

68. Christensen B, Kazanecki CC, Petersen TE, Rittling SR, Denhardt DT, Sorensen ES. Cell type-specific post-translational modifications of mouse osteopontin are associated with different adhesive properties. J Biol Chem 2007; 282(27): 19463-19472.

69. Al-Shami R, Sorensen ES, Ek-Rylander B, Andersson G, Carson DD, Farach-Carson MC. Phosphorylated osteopontin promotes migration of human choriocarcinoma cells via a p70 S6 kinase-dependent pathway. J Cell Biochem 2005; 94(6): 1218-1233.

70. Razzouk S, Brunn JC, Qin C, Tye CE, Goldberg HA, Butler WT. Osteopontin posttranslational modifications, possibly phosphorylation, are required for in vitro bone resorption but not osteoclast adhesion. Bone 2002; 30(1): 40-47.

71. Jono S, Peinado C, Giachelli CM. Phosphorylation of osteopontin is required for inhibition of vascular smooth muscle cell calcification. J Biol Chem 2000; 275(26): 20197-20203.

72. Gericke A, Qin C, Spevak L, Fujimoto Y, Butler WT, Sorensen ES, Boskey AL. Importance of phosphorylation for osteopontin regulation of biomineralization. Calcif Tissue Int 2005; 77(1): 45-54.

73. Rangaswami H, Bulbule A, Kundu GC. Osteopontin: role in cell signaling and cancer progression. Trends Cell Biol 2006; 16(2): 79-87.

74. Rice J, Courter DL, Giachelli CM, Scatena M. Molecular mediators of alphavbeta3-induced endothelial cell survival. J Vasc Res 2006; 43(5): 422-436.

75. Scatena M, Almeida M, Chaisson ML, Fausto N, Nicosia RF, Giachelli CM. NF-kappaB mediates alphavbeta3 integrin-induced endothelial cell survival. J Cell Biol 1998; 141(4): 1083-1093.

76. Rangaswami H, Bulbule A, Kundu GC. Nuclear factor-inducing kinase plays a crucial role in osteopontin-induced MAPK/IkappaBalpha kinase-dependent nuclear factor kappaB-mediated promatrix metalloproteinase-9 activation. J Biol Chem 2004; 279(37): 38921-38935.

77. Rittling SR, Chambers AF. Role of osteopontin in tumour progression. Br J Cancer 2004; 90(10): 1877-1881.

78. Lin YH, Yang-Yen HF. The osteopontin-CD44 survival signal involves activation of the

phosphatidylinositol 3-kinase/Akt signaling pathway. J Biol Chem 2001; 276(49): 46024-46030.

79.   Das R, Mahabeleshwar GH, Kundu GC. Osteopontin stimulates cell motility and nuclear factor kappaB-mediated secretion of urokinase type plasminogen activator through phosphatidylinositol 3-kinase/Akt signaling pathways in breast cancer cells. J Biol Chem 2003; 278(31): 28593-28606.

80.   Zohar R, Suzuki N, Suzuki K, Arora P, Glogauer M, McCulloch CA, Sodek J. Intracellular osteopontin is an integral component of the CD44-ERM complex involved in cell migration. J Cell Physiol 2000; 184(1): 118-130.

81.   Suzuki K, Zhu B, Rittling SR, Denhardt DT, Goldberg HA, McCulloch CA, Sodek J. Colocalization of intracellular osteopontin with CD44 is associated with migration, cell fusion, and resorption in osteoclasts. J Bone Miner Res 2002; 17(8): 1486-1497.

82.   Zohar R, Zhu B, Liu P, Sodek J, McCulloch CA. Increased cell death in osteopontin-deficient cardiac fibroblasts occurs by a caspase-3-independent pathway. Am J Physiol Heart Circ Physiol 2004; 287(4): H1730-H1739.

83.   Chakraborty G, Jain S, Behera R, Ahmed M, Sharma P, Kumar V, Kundu GC. The multifaceted roles of osteopontin in cell signaling, tumor progression and angiogenesis. Curr Mol Med 2006; 6(8): 819-830.

84.   Senger DR, Ledbetter SR, Claffey KP, Papadopoulos-Sergiou A, Peruzzi CA, Detmar M. Stimulation of endothelial cell migration by vascular permeability factor/vascular endothelial growth factor through cooperative mechanisms involving the alphavbeta3 integrin, osteopontin, and thrombin. Am J Pathol 1996; 149(1): 293-305.

85.   Hamada Y, Nokihara K, Okazaki M, Fujitani W, Matsumoto T, Matsuo M, Umakoshi Y, Takahashi J, Matsuura N. Angiogenic activity of osteopontin-derived peptide SVVYGLR. Biochem Biophys Res Commun 2003; 310(1): 153-157.

86.   Hamada Y, Yuki K, Okazaki M, Fujitani W, Matsumoto T, Hashida MK, Harutsugu K, Nokihara K, Daito M, Matsuura N, Takahashi J. Osteopontin-derived peptide SVVYGLR induces angiogenesis in vivo. Dent Mater J 2004; 23(4): 650-655.

87.   Xie Z, Singh M, Singh K. Osteopontin modulates myocardial hypertrophy in response to chronic pressure overload in mice. Hypertension 2004; 44(6): 826-831.

88.   Zhao X, Johnson JN, Singh K, Singh M. Impairment of myocardial angiogenic response in the absence of osteopontin. Microcirculation 2007; 14(3): 233-240.

89.   Trueblood NA, Xie Z, Communal C, Sam F, Ngoy S, Liaw L, Jenkins AW, Wang J, Sawyer DB, Bing OH, Apstein CS, Colucci WS, Singh K. Exaggerated left ventricular dilation and reduced collagen deposition after myocardial infarction in mice lacking osteopontin. Circ Res 2001; 88(10): 1080-1087.

90.   Liaw L, Birk DE, Ballas CB, Whitsitt JS, Davidson JM, Hogan BL. Altered wound healing in mice lacking a functional osteopontin gene (spp1). J Clin Invest 1998; 101(7): 1468-1478.

91.   Leen LL, Filipe C, Billon A, Garmy-Susini B, Jalvy S, Robbesyn F, Daret D, Allieres C, Rittling SR, Werner N, Nickenig G, Deutsch U, Duplaa C, Dufourcq P, Lenfant F, Desgranges C, Arnal JF, Gadeau AP. Estrogen-stimulated endothelial repair requires osteopontin. Arterioscler Thromb Vasc Biol 2008; 28(12): 2131-2136.

92.   Albina JE, Reichner JS. Oxygen and the regulation of gene expression in wounds. Wound Repair Regen 2003; 11(6): 445-451.

93.   Sodhi CP, Phadke SA, Batlle D, Sahai A. Hypoxia stimulates osteopontin expression and proliferation of cultured vascular smooth muscle cells: potentiation by high glucose. Diabetes 2001; 50(6): 1482-1490.

94.   Hampel DJ, Sansome C, Romanov VI, Kowalski AJ, Denhardt DT, Goligorsky MS. Osteopontin traffic in hypoxic renal epithelial cells. Nephron Exp Nephrol 2003; 94(2): e66-e76.

95.   Zhu Y, Denhardt DT, Cao H, Sutphin PD, Koong AC, Giaccia AJ, Le QT. Hypoxia upregulates osteopontin expression in NIH-3T3 cells via a Ras-activated enhancer. Oncogene 2005; 24(43): 6555-6563.

96.   Gross TS, King KA, Rabaia NA, Pathare P, Srinivasan S. Upregulation of osteopontin by osteocytes deprived of mechanical loading or oxygen. J Bone Miner Res 2005; 20(2): 250-256.

97.   Potier E, Ferreira E, Andriamanalijaona R, Pujol JP, Oudina K, Logeart-Avramoglou D, Petite H. Hypoxia affects mesenchymal stromal cell osteogenic differentiation and angiogenic factor expression. Bone 2007; 40(4): 1078-1087.

98.   Leali D, Dell'Era P, Stabile H, Sennino B, Chambers AF, Naldini A, Sozzani S, Nico B, Ribatti D, Presta M. Osteopontin (Eta-1) and fibroblast growth factor-2 cross-talk in angiogenesis. J Immunol 2003; 171(2): 1085-1093.

99.   Naldini A, Leali D, Pucci A, Morena E, Carraro F, Nico B, Ribatti D, Presta M. Cutting edge: IL-1beta mediates the proangiogenic activity of osteopontin-activated human monocytes. J Immunol 2006; 177(7): 4267-4270.

100. Asou Y, Rittling SR, Yoshitake H, Tsuji K, Shinomiya K, Nifuji A, Denhardt DT, Noda M. Osteopontin facilitates angiogenesis, accumulation of osteoclasts, and resorption in ectopic bone. Endocrinology 2001; 142(3): 1325-1332.

101. Carmeliet P, Jain RK. Angiogenesis in cancer and other diseases. Nature 2000; 407(6801): 249-257.

102. Folkman J . Role of angiogenesis in tumor growth and metastasis. Semin Oncol 2002; 29(6 Suppl 16): 15-18.

103. Hanrahan V, Currie MJ, Gunningham SP, Morrin HR, Scott PA, Robinson BA, Fox SB. The angiogenic switch for vascular endothelial growth factor (VEGF)-A, VEGF-B, VEGF-C, and VEGF-D in the adenoma-carcinoma sequence during colorectal cancer progression. J Pathol 2003; 200(2): 183-194.

104. Hirama M, Takahashi F, Takahashi K, Akutagawa S, Shimizu K, Soma S, Shimanuki Y, Nishio K, Fukuchi Y. Osteopontin overproduced by tumor cells

acts as a potent angiogenic factor contributing to tumor growth. Cancer Lett 2003; 198(1): 107-117.

105. Khan SA, Lopez-Chua CA, Zhang J, Fisher LW, Sorensen ES, Denhardt DT. Soluble osteopontin inhibits apoptosis of adherent endothelial cells deprived of growth factors. J Cell Biochem 2002; 85(4): 728-736.

106. Tang H, Wang J, Bai F, Hong L, Liang J, Gao J, Zhai H, Lan M, Zhang F, Wu K, Fan D. Inhibition of osteopontin would suppress angiogenesis in gastric cancer. Biochem Cell Biol 2007; 85(1): 103-110.

107. Matusan-Ilijas K, Behrem S, Jonjic N, Zarkovic K, Lucin K. Osteopontin expression correlates with angiogenesis and survival in malignant astrocytoma. Pathol Oncol Res 2008; 14(3): 293-298.

108. Chakraborty G, Jain S, Kundu GC. Osteopontin promotes vascular endothelial growth factor-dependent breast tumor growth and angiogenesis via autocrine and paracrine mechanisms. Cancer Res 2008; 68(1): 152-161.

109. Cheriyath V, Hussein MA. Osteopontin, angiogenesis and multiple myeloma. Leukemia 2005; 19(12): 2203-2205.

110. Colla S, Morandi F, Lazzaretti M, Rizzato R, Lunghi P, Bonomini S, Mancini C, Pedrazzoni M, Crugnola M, Rizzoli V, Giuliani N. Human myeloma cells express the bone regulating gene Runx2/Cbfa1 and produce osteopontin that is involved in angiogenesis in multiple myeloma patients. Leukemia 2005; 19(12): 2166-2176.

111. Colla S, Tagliaferri S, Morandi F, Lunghi P, Donofrio G, Martorana D, Mancini C, Lazzaretti M, Mazzera L, Ravanetti L, Bonomini S, Ferrari L, Miranda C, Ladetto M, Neri TM, Neri A, Greco A, Mangoni M, Bonati A, Rizzoli V, Giuliani N. The new tumor-suppressor gene inhibitor of growth family member 4 (ING4) regulates the production of proangiogenic molecules by myeloma cells and suppresses hypoxia-inducible factor-1 alpha (HIF-1alpha) activity: involvement in myeloma-induced angiogenesis. Blood 2007; 110(13): 4464-4475.

112. Nilsson SK, Johnston HM, Whitty GA, Williams B, Webb RJ, Denhardt DT, Bertoncello I, Bendall LJ, Simmons PJ, Haylock DN. Osteopontin, a key component of the hematopoietic stem cell niche and regulator of primitive hematopoietic progenitor cells. Blood 2005; 106(4): 1232-1239.

113. Liaw L, Lindner V, Schwartz SM, Chambers AF, Giachelli CM. Osteopontin and beta 3 integrin are coordinately expressed in regenerating endothelium in vivo and stimulate Arg-Gly-Asp-dependent endothelial migration in vitro. Circ Res 1995; 77(4): 665-672.

114. Yoshitake H, Rittling SR, Denhardt DT, Noda M. Osteopontin-deficient mice are resistant to ovariectomy-induced bone resorption. Proc Natl Acad Sci U S A 1999; 96(14): 8156-8160.

115. Ashkar S, Weber GF, Panoutsakopoulou V, Sanchirico ME, Jansson M, Zawaideh S, Rittling SR, Denhardt DT, Glimcher MJ, Cantor H. Eta-1 (osteopontin): an early component of type-1 (cell-mediated) immunity. Science 2000; 287(5454): 860-864.

116. Dinarello CA . Proinflammatory cytokines. Chest 2000; 118(2): 503-508.

117. Voronov E, Shouval DS, Krelin Y, Cagnano E, Benharroch D, Iwakura Y, Dinarello CA, Apte RN. IL-1 is required for tumor invasiveness and angiogenesis. Proc Natl Acad Sci U S A 2003; 100(5): 2645-2650.

The Role of Mesenchymal Stem Cells in Angiogenesis

Lizzia Raffaghello and Vito Pistoia

Laboratory of Oncology, G. Gaslini Children Hospital, Genova, Italy

Address correspondence to:Lizzia Raffaghello, Ph.D; Laboratory of Oncology, G. Gaslini Institute, Largo G. Gaslini 5, 16148 Genova, Italy; Phone and fax: +39-010-3779820; e-mail: lizziaraffaghello@ospedale-gaslini.ge.it

Abstract: Mesenchymal stem cells (MSC) are a heterogeneous subset of stromal stem cells that can be isolated from many adult tissues. They can differentiate into cells of the mesodermal lineage, such as adipocytes, osteocytes and chondrocytes, providing a promising tool for tissue repair. MSC can interact with cells of both the innate and adaptive immune systems, leading to the modulation of several effector functions. The immunoregulatory functions of human MSC, coupled with their low immunogenicity, provide a rationale for the use of allogeneic MSC to treat severe graft-versus-host disease (GvHD) and, possibly, autoimmune disorders. In addition, MSC exhibit tropism for sites of tissue damage as well as for the tumor microenvironment, where they integrate into the tumor-associated stroma supporting cancer growth. However, studies investigating the *in vivo* and *in vitro* effects mediated by MSC on tumor growth provided conflicting results, depending on the experimental model tested. This chapter reviews the role of MSC in different angiogenic processes and underlying mechanisms. In particular, we discuss the involvement of MSC in angiogenesis in ischemic brain and heart after stroke, wound healing, tumor angiogenesis and maintenance of hematopoietic stem cell niche.

1. MESENCHYMAL STEM CELLS: FEATURES AND FUNCTIONS

About 40 years ago Friedestein first identified multipotent stromal cells in the bone marrow. These cells were spindle shaped, adhered to plastic, and proliferated to form colonies representing the progenies of single colony forming units-fibroblastic (CFU-F) [1]. CFU-F derived stromal cells differentiated under defined *in vitro* conditions into multiple cell types including osteoblasts, chondrocytes, and adipocytes [1]. Later on, the definition of bone marrow-derived stromal cells as mesenchymal stem cells (MSC) was proposed [2]. Although the bone marrow represents the most common site from which MSC are isolated, these cells have also been found in many other human tissues (Fig. **1A**) [3]. MSC are able to self renew and to differentiate towards mesodermal lineages *in vivo*, representing a promising tool for tissue repair. Moreover, MSC can differentiate into cells of other lineages *in vitro* (muscle cells, hepatocytes, endothelial cells, and neurons), through a process called trans-differentiation (Fig. **1B**) [4].

MSC cultured *in vitro* lack specific and unique markers. There is now consensus agreement MSC express variable levels of CD105 (endoglin), CD73 (ecto-5'-nucleotidase), CD44, CD90, CD71 (transferring receptor), the ganglioside GD_2 and CD271 (low affinity nerve growth factor receptor), and lack expression of hematopoietic markers

CD45, CD34, CD14 or costimulatory molecules CD40, CD80, CD86 [as reviewed in 1].

One of most the most intriguing features of MSC is their ability to escape immune recognition and inhibit immune responses [1,5,6].

Specifically, MSC mediate immunoregulatory activities by inhibiting the functions of different immune cells including T and B lymphocytes, Natural Killer (NK) cells and dendritic cells (DC) [7-17]. MSC were found to inhibit CD4[+] and CD8[+] T-cell proliferation and functions, induce anergy in naïve T cells, and promote expansion of immunosuppressive regulatory T cells [6-8]. Inhibition of T cell proliferation by MSC appears to depend on both cell-to-cell interaction and the release of soluble factors. In this respect, transforming growth factor-β1 (TGF-β1) and hepatocyte growth factor (HGF), indoleamine 2,3-dioxygenase (IDO) and prostaglandin E-2 (PGE-2) represent the main MSC-derived molecules that have been proposed to exert immunomodulatory activity on CD4[+] T cells [6, 8,18]. Inhibition of CD8[+] T-cell cytotoxicity and induction of T regulatory cell differentiation are partly related to the release of soluble (s) HLA-G [19].

The second cell type involved in adaptive immune responses is the B cell, whose proliferation and differentiation are inhibited by MSC [17]. These effects seem to be related to cell-cell contact and soluble factors, but the exact mechanism is still not

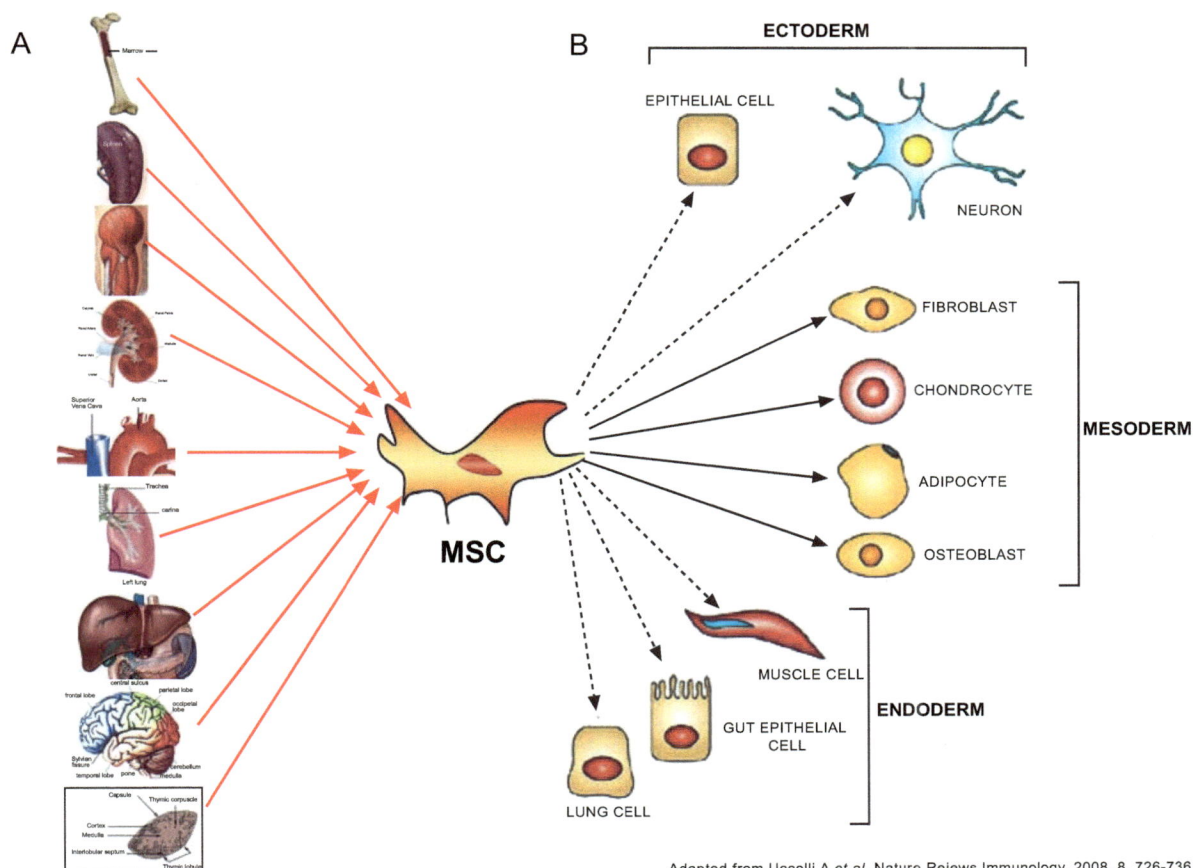

Adapted from Uccelli A *et al.* Nature Reiews Immunology, 2008, 8, 726-736

Fig. (1). Origin and differentiation of mesenchymal stem cells. Panel A shows the main anatomical sites from which MSC can be isolated. Panel B shows the ability of MSC to differentiate into mesodermal cell lineages and the trans-differentiation process, through which MSC can differentiate *in vitro* into endodermal and ectodermal cell types. Dashed arrows indicate that trans-differentiation *in vivo* is still controversial.

elucidated [17]. Other studies showed that MSC stimulated B cell proliferation and differentiation, possible as result of the different experimental conditions used [20].

MSC can also interact with cells of the innate immune system, including NK cells and DC [12-16]. Specifically, MSC inhibit the proliferation and cytotoxicity of resting NK cells and their cytokine production *in vitro* [12]. These effects are mediated by PGE-2, IDO and sHLA-G5 released by MSC [19,21,22]. Interestingly, MSC can be lysed by activated NK cells through the interaction of NKG2D (natural-killer group 2 , member D) expressed by NK cells and its ligands ULBP3 (UL16 binding protein 3) or MICA (MHC class I polypeptide-related sequence A) expressed by MSC, and of NK-associated DNAM1 (DNAX accessory molecule 1) with MSC-associated ligand PVR (poliovirus receptor) or nectin-2 [12, 13].

MSC down-regulate expression of costimulatory molecules on DC, inhibit their *in vitro* differentiation from monocytes and CD34[+] progenitors, reduce proinflammatory cytokine secretion (IL-12 and tumor necrosis factor-α) by myeloid DC and increase IL-10 secretion by plasmacytoid DC (pDC) [8,14-16]. The main factor involved in these latter effects is PGE-2.

Human MSC are poorly immunogenic, in spite of constitutive human leukocyte antigen (HLA)-class I expressionand Interferon-γ(IFN-γ) inducible HLA-class II expression [23].

It has been reported that, in a narrow window of IFN-γ concentration, human MSC can exert antigen-presenting cell (APC) functions for HLA-class II-restricted recall antigens, such as Candida albicans and Tetanus toxoid. MSC up-regulate their HLA-class II antigen expression by autocrine secretion of low IFN-γ levels; however, when IFN-γ concentration in culture increases, HLA-class II antigen expression is down-regulated and the APC function is inhibited [24]. Moreover, MSC do not trigger effector functions in activated cytotoxic T lymphocytes (CTL), inducing an abortive activation program in the latter cells [25]. A recent report showed that human MSC can process and present HLA class I-restricted viral or tumor antigens to specific CTL with a limited efficiency, likely because of some defects in the antigen processing machinery (APM) components. However, MSC are protected from CTL-mediated lysis through a mechanism that is partly sHLA-G-dependent [26].

The immunoregulatory functions of human MSC, coupled with their low immunogenicity, provide a rationale for the use of allogeneic MSC to treat severe graft-versus-host disease (GvHD) and, possibly, autoimmune disorders [27-29]. In this connection, encouraging results have been obtained in patients with GvHD, in which the effect mediated by MSC was probably due to the inhibition of donor T-cell reactivity to histocompatibility antigens of the normal tissues of the recipient [30].

On the other hand, MSC have been used to treat children with severe osteogenesis imperfecta, resulting in increased growth velocity and total body mineral content, and fewer fractures, and cancer patients who underwent high-dose chemotherapy, accelerating bone-marrow recovery [31, 32]. The immunomodulatory potential of MSC is currently being tested for the treatment of Crohn's disease, in which these cells could also contribute to the regeneration of gastrointestinal epithelial cells [33].

MSC exhibit tropism for sites of tissue damage as well as for the tumor microenvironment [34]. A tumor has been defined as a "wound that never heals" and many of the same inflammatory mediators that are secreted by wounds are also released in the tumor microenvironment and are thought to be involved in attracting MSC to the tumor site [35]. Cell migration is dependent on a multitude of signals ranging from growth factors to chemokines secreted by injured cells. MSC are likely to have chemotactic properties similarly to other immune cells that respond to signals originating from injured and inflamed tissues [34]. Thus, the well-described model of leukocyte migration can serve as a reasonable example to facilitate the identification of factors involved in MSC migration [34].

Once MSC reach the tumor microenvironment, they integrate into the tumor-associated stroma supporting cancer growth [35]. However, studies investigating the *in vivo* and *in vitro* effects mediated by MSC on tumor growth provided conflicting results [36-40]. Depending on the experimental model tested, either inhibition or stimulation of tumor cell proliferation *in vitro* and/or tumor growth *in vivo* have been reported.

Many different receptors have been implicated in the homing of MSC: (1) up-regulation of chemokine (CXC and CC) receptors (R) on the surface MSC promoted by tissue-derived growth factors; (2) activation of MSC associated Toll like receptors (TLR) that target downstream expression of CXCR and CCR; (3) up-regulation of MSC associated adhesion molecules and integrins possibly involved in paracrine cell movement [34]. The key players implicated in MSC migration to date include the chemokines CCL2, CXCL8, CCL5; LL-37, integrin β1, receptors CD44, CCR2, CCR3, and the receptor tyrosine kinases for insulin growth factor (IGF)-1, platelet derived growth factor (PDGF)-bb, HGF, and vascular endothelial growth factor (VEGF) [34].

In this respect, an elegant paper showed that MSC induce breast cancer cells to increase their metastatic potential by secreting CCL5, which then acts in a paracrine fashion on the tumor cells to enhance their motility, invasion and metastasis [40].

The cancer tropism of MSC after systemic injection provided a rationale for their development as vehicles for tumor-specific delivery of genes encoding antineoplastic molecules. Most studies have demonstrated that MSC transfected with the antineoplastic IFN-β gene inhibit tumor growth and angiogenesis in melanoma, breast cancer and glioma models [41-44].

In conclusion, different data clearly support the clinical use of MSC but some opportune cautions about their uncontrolled use should also be used.

2. THE ROLE OF MESENCHYMAL STEM CELLS IN THE HEMATOPOIE-TIC-STEM-CELL NICHE

The bone marrow (BM) is the major site of adult hematopoiesis, a process that is maintained by specific interactions between hematopoietic and non hematopoietic cells [45]. Hematopoietic stem cells (HSCs) are self renewing multipotent progenitors able to give rise to all types of mature blood cells, whereas the non hematopoietic component is comprised of stromal cells including osteoblasts, endothelial cells, fibroblasts, reticular cells and MSC. Stromal cells play a pivotal role in supporting hematopoiesis [45]. An elegant work showed that human MSC transplanted into the BM of immunodeficient mice engraft, integrate in the hematopoietic microenvironment and differentiate into pericytes, myofibroblasts, osteocytes, osteoblasts and endothelial cells [46]. All of these cells constitute a specialized microenvironment of the BM, known as HSC niche [45,47]. Two types of HSC niches have been identified so far, the endosteal niche composed of quiescent and proliferating HSC, osteoblasts and stromal progenitor cells, and the vascular niche formed by endothelial cells, stromal cells and mobilized HSC that have migrated to sinusoids following an appropriate stimulus [1,45]. BM stromal cells participate in the HSC maintenance, by regulating the quiescence of the latter cells in the endosteal niche and by controlling HSC proliferation, differentiation and migration in the vascular compartment [1, 45].

A recent study identified a new cell population of stromal progenitors that localize in perivascular areas of the BM, and are able to regenerate bone and stroma and establish hematopoiesis *in vivo* [48]. These cells have the putative immunophenotype of MSC together with high expression of melanoma-associated cell adhesion molecule MCAM/CD146, angiopoietin-1 (Ang-1), and CXC-chemokine ligand 12 (CXCL12) [48]. Ang-1, the ligand of the Tie-2 tyrosine kinase receptor, is produced by osteoblasts and appears to promote HSC quiescence [49]. Similarly, CXCL12 is produced by osteoblasts and perivascular reticular BM cells and regulates HSC migration and localization in the BM. After subcutaneous transplantation into immunocompromised mice, CD146$^+$ clonogenic cells give rise to a developmental sequence of structures in which bone formation preceded the appearance of sinusoids and finally of hematopoiesis [48].

These observations reveal new functional relationships between the *in vivo* hematopoiesis, the role of skeletal progenitors in BM sinusoids and angiogenesis.

3. MESENCHYMAL STEM CELLS AND ANGIOGENESIS IN STROKE

MSC secrete significant amounts of different growth factors and cytokines with pro-angiogenic activity. Among them, VEGF represents the most relevant player involved in the promotion of angiogenesis [50]. VEGF exerts its biological activity upon binding to VEGF receptor 2 (VEGFR2) which has been shown to be essential for endothelial progenitor cell proliferation and differentiation [51-52]. Angiogenesis has been associated with improved neurological recovery from stroke [53-54]. Different reports showed that stroke patients with higher cerebral blood vessel density present more favorable clinical course and higher survival than patients with lower vascular density [55]. Moreover, new vessels improve tissue perfusion around the ischemic area and enhancement of angiogenesis promotes the recovery of rats after stroke [53-54]. In this connection, MSC, administered intravenously in rats after stroke, have been shown to promote angiogenesis in the ischemic brain by increasing the endogenous levels of VEGF, VEGFR2, and basic-Fibroblast Growth Factors (bFGF) [55]. An additional axis involved in MSC-mediated angiogenesis is represented by Ang-1 and its receptor Tie2 [56]. Specifically, after injection into rats subjected to middle cerebral artery occlusion, MSC promote vascular stabilization and decrease in the blood-brain barrier leakage by increasing the endogeneous levels of Ang-1/Tie2 and VEGF/VEGFR2 in the ischemic border [56].

MSC have also shown to induce myocardial regeneration and improve cardiac functions after direct injection into the infarcted heart [57]. Similarly, MSC, injected intravenously in rats with acute myocardial infarction, are able to engraft in the ischemic myocardium, and differentiate into cardiomiocytes and vascular endothelial cells, resulting in a enhancement of myogenesis and angiogenesis [57]. In addition, in a canine chronic ischemia model, MSC differentiate into smooth and endothelial cells, resulting in increased vascular density and improved cardiac function [58].

Taken together, these observations suggest that MSC contribute to neovascularization in ischemic organs through their ability to differentiate into an endothelial phenotype and through secretion of growth factors with angiogenic activity.

4. THE EFFECT MEDIATED BY MESENCHYMAL STEM CELLS IN THE ANGIOGENESIS OF WOUND REPAIR

Neovascularization is a crucial step in the wound healing process [59-60]. Specifically, the generation of new blood vessels is necessary to sustain the formation of granular tissue and the survival of keratinocytes. Using an excisional wound splinting model in mice, MSC, injected around the wound, enhance wound healing by promoting re-epithelization and angiogenesis [61].

In particular, MSC-treated wounds showed a rich network of vessels, that extended into the wound and expressed the typical endothelial marker CD31 [61]. In addition, MSC induce enhancement of the capillary density. Interestingly, MSC are not found in the walls of blood vessels but in close proximity, suggesting that a pro-angiogenic paracrine effect mediated by MSC could occur [61]. In this regard, MSC conditioned medium show to induce endothelial tube formation, and real-time PCR and western blot reveal high expression of VEGF and Ang-1 in MSC [61]. In conclusion, a beneficial effect mediated by MSC has been observed in cutaneous regeneration and wound healing in mice through induction of differentiation and angiogenesis.

5. THE ROLE OF MESENCHYMAL STEM CELLS IN TUMOR ANGIOGE-NESIS

There is striking evidence that supports the involvement of MSC in tumor angiogenesis, through different mechanisms.

- MSC as progenitors of tumor pericytes

In angiogenesis, new blood vessels originate from preexisting ones through proliferation of endothelial cells as well as recruitment of vascular mural cells [62]. BM represents an important source of cells that contribute to tumor angiogenesis. The BM-derived cells are mobilized in response to different stimuli, including tumor growth, circulate and home to sites of new blood-vessel formation where they stimulate or amplify the angiogenic process [63]. Different BM-derived cell populations have been identified so far, and among them, tumor stroma-derived mesenchymal progenitors attracted vivid interest [64]. These latter cells specifically express Tie2, together with typical mesodermal markers such as CD13 and Sca-1, and are negative for CD31 and

CD45 [64]. Tie2 is a receptor tyrosine kinase, whose ligand is Ang-1. Tie2 expression is restricted to endothelial cells and Tie2 expressing monocytes (TEMs) in tumors. Interestingly, Tie2$^+$ MSC, after isolation, are capable of long-term self-renewal and differentiation into different mesodermal lineages *in vitro*, supporting their multipotency [64]. *In vivo* transplantation experiments showed that, after subcutaneous injection of tumor cells together with Tie2$^+$ MSC, the latter cells are found in tumor stroma, and generate tumor pericytes [64]. Consistently with these observations, other studies showed that MSC are triggered by the tumor microenvironment to differentiate first into myofibroblasts, and then into pericytes, and proposed a BM origin of tumor pericytes in the adult [65].

Tie2$^+$ MSC express VEGF and bFGF, confirming that these cells contribute to the angiogenic process [64]. Furthemore, Ang-1 has been proposed as a crucial factor promoting the recruitment of Tie2$^+$ expressing pericyte precursors to newly formed vessels [64]. In this connection, brain tumors over expressing Ang-1 exhibit abnormal infiltration with MSC and pericytes [66].

A recent study demonstrates that intratumorally injected MSC integrate into tumor vessel walls and express the pericyte markers alpha-smooth muscle actin, neuron-glia 2, and platelet-derived growth factor receptor-beta but not endothelial cell markers [67]. The pericyte marker expression profile and perivascular location of grafted MSC indicate that these cells act as pericytes within tumors. Intratumorally grafted pericyte-like MSC might represent a suitable vector system for delivering molecules inhibiting tumor angiogenesis and for targeting cancer stem cells within the perivascular niche.

• MSC as source of pro-angiogenic factors

It is has been suggested that the MSC-mediated pro-angiogenic effects can be attributed to biologically active factors released by MSC themselves at the target sites.

A recent study demonstrated that MSC support angiogenesis of pancreatic carcinoma *in vivo*, through VEGF release, which could be enhanced by hypoxia [68]. Specifically, MSC-secreted VEGF is capable to induce sprouting of endothelial cells *in vitro* as well as to increase the vessel density *in vivo* [68]. In contrast, MSC do not differentiate into endothelial cells upon culture in endothelial cell culture medium containing VEGF. The VEGF-dependent neo-angiogenic effect mediated by MSC is also confirmed using an in vivo murine Matrigel model [68].

Similarly, the pro-angiogenic effect mediated by MSC is also observed in an *in vivo* model of melanoma, where, MSC are intravenously injected into immunodepressed mice previously inoculated

with B16 melanoma cells [69]. The interaction between B16 melanoma cells and MSC *in vitro* demonstrates that the latter cells acquire an endothelial phenotype after co-culture with B16 melanoma cells, and at the same time, up-regulate the expression of VEGF, VEGFR1, VEGFR2 and Factor VIII [69].

A recent study demonstrated that MSC exposed to tumor-conditioned medium assume a carcinoma-associated fibroblast (CAF)-like phenotype, and exhibit functional properties of CAF including expression and high secretion of stromal-derived factor-1 (SDF-1), a well known chemokine with pro-angiogenic activity [70].

Taken together, these studies indicate that MSC contribute to angiogenesis by secreting pro-angiogenic paracrine factors and, in some models, trans-differentiating into endothelial cells.

• The role of bone-morphogenetic protein-2 in angiogenesis promotion by MSC

The bone morphogenetic protein-2 (BMP-2) promotes vascularisation, inhibits hypoxic tumor cell apoptosis and is involved in tumor angiogenesis [71]. Furthemore, BMP-2 plays an important role in the regulation of differentiation, function, and angiogenic activity of MSC [72]. Specifically, treatment of MSC with recombinant (rh) BMP-2 induce the production of paracrine angiogenic growth factors including VEGF and placental growth factor (PlGF) [73]. The latter molecule is a well known gene of VEGF family member, able to recruit endothelial and hematopoietic stem cells in pathological angiogenesis such as cancer [74]. Moreover, PlGF has been shown to amplify the responsiveness of endothelial cells to VEGF during the angiogenic switch in different pathological conditions [75].

• Hypoxia elicits a pro-angiogenic program in mesenchymal stem cells.

There is striking evidence that hypoxia, a typical feature of tumor microenvironment, promotes an angiogenic switch in MSC, by induction of migration and capillary-like structure formation of these latter cells [76]. Both these effects are partially due to the functional expression of membrane-type (MT)1-metallo proteinase (MMP) [76]. In this connection, the hypoxia-regulated factor erythropoietin (EPO), a glycoprotein hormone that stimulates the formation and differentiation of erythroid precursor cells in the BM, has been shown to drive an angiogenic program in MSC [77]. Specifically, MSC express EPO receptor and are capable of proliferating and secreting pro-angiogenic factors following EPO treatment. Notably, VEGF secretion and MMP2 activation in MSC induced by EPO treatment of MSC occurred in the early phase of angiogenesis [77]. Furthermore, EPO treatment of MSC leads to *in vitro* capillary-like formation, and to a greater vessel density in an *in vivo* Matrigel plug assay [77]. Taken together, confirm that MSC promote angiogenesis by secreting pro-angiogenic factors after specific stimulation and, to a lower extent, by differentiating into endothelial like cells.

- Epidermal growth factor (EGF) pathway in mesenchymal stem cells.

EGF receptor-1 (EGFR-1/HER-1/ErbB-1) and its ligand epidermal growth factor-like growth factor (HB-EGF) are involved in tissue repair, tumor growth, and angiogenesis [78]. A recent report demonstrated that MSC express HER-1but not HB-EGF itself. Interestingly, following HB-EGF treatment, MSC proliferate more rapidly without undergoing differentiation. So far, there are no data indicating the implication of EGF pathway in MSC-induced angiogenesis [78]. However, it is conceivable that HB-EGF/HER-1 signaling may contribute *in vivo* to maintain a proliferating pool of undifferentiated MSC. This might ensure an efficient angiogenesis for tumor growth.

6. NEW FINDINGS

A recent study demonstrated that MSC can differentiate into arterial- or venous-specific endothelial cells depending on VEGF concentration, through regulation by the Notch pathway [79]. Specifically, low concentration of VEGF (50 ng/mL) up regulates the typical venous markers ephrinB4, whereas a higher concentration (100 ng/mL) induce the expression of arterial markers genes including ephrinB2, Dll4 and Notch4 [79]. The VEGF-induced MSC differentation into arterial endothelial cells is attenuated by inhibition of Notch signaling.

CD34 is a sialomucin expressed by hematopoietic stem/progenitor cells and, more in general, a marker

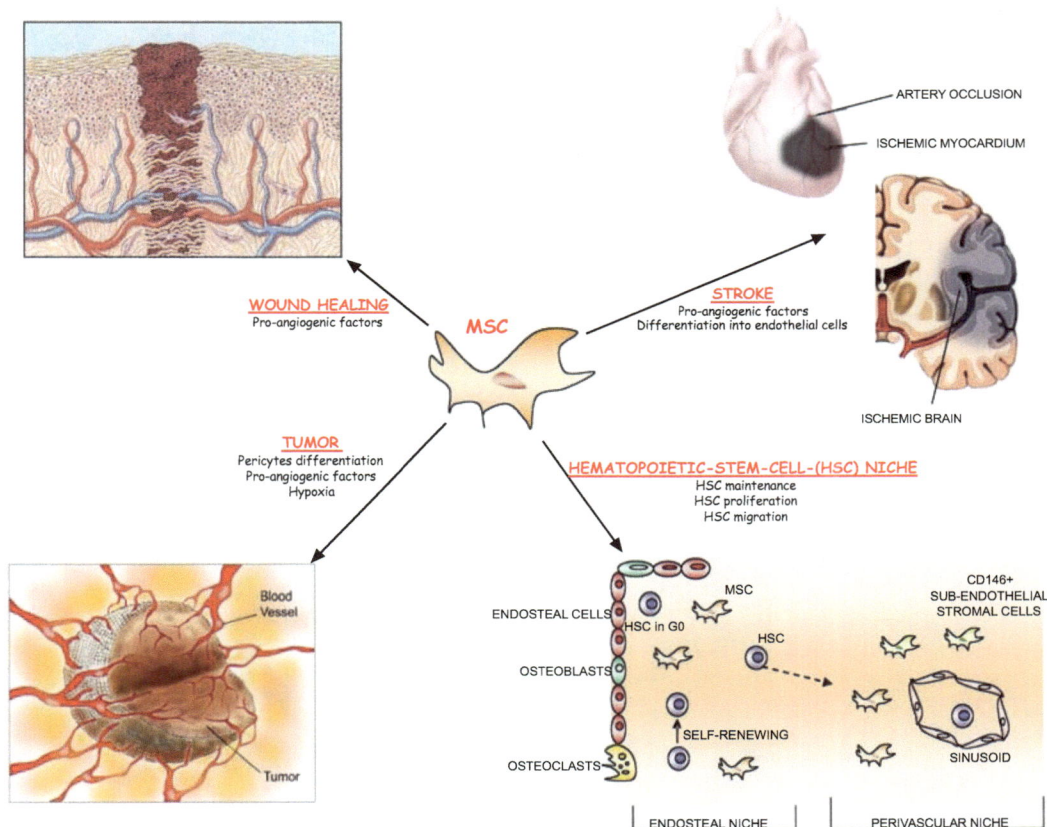

Fig. (2). The role of mesenchymal stem cells in different angiogenic processes and underlying mechanisms. The figure shows the involvement of MSC in different angiogenic processes including angiogenesis in ischemic brain and heart after stroke, wound healing, tumor angiogenesis and maintenance of hematopoietic stem cell niche. In the bone marrow, MSC participate in the hematopoietic stem cell (HSC) niche. In the endosteal niche, MSC contribute to the maintenance of HSC in a quiescent state (G0 phase), as well as to their self-renewal. Upon an appropriate stimulus, HSC acquire migratory capabilities to the vascular niche, where Ang-1$^+$CXCL12$^+$CD146$^+$ sub-endothelial stromal cells and MSC regulate HSC proliferation, differentiation and recruitment. Among the mechanisms underlying MSC-mediated angiogenesis the more frequent include production of pro-angiogenic factors, and MSC differentiation into endothelial like cells. MSC have a pivotal role in angiogenesis occurring in ischemic heart and brain after stroke, through the production of pro-angiogenic factors and differentiation into endothelial cells. Similarly, MSC participate in the angiogenic processes during wound healing by secretion of pro-angiogenic factors. Tumor angiogenesis is finely regulated by MSC. The more frequent mechanisms involved in MSC-mediated tumor angogenesis include: i) MSC differentiation into pericytes, ii) pro-angiogenic paracrine mechanisms mediated by factors released by MSC, and iii) hypoxia as inducer of a MSC pro-angiogenic switch.

of staminality [80]. Recently, a fraction of MSC positive for the expression of CD34 has been identified. Interestingly, CD34$^+$ MSC up regulate different angiogenesis-associated genes, and display higher expression of genes related to vascular differentiation, compared to CD34$^-$MSC [80]. Taken together, these observations demonstrate a clear correlation between CD34 expression in MSC and enhanced vasculogenesis and angiogenesis potential.

7. CONCLUSIONS

MSC are multipotent stromal progenitors that have an important role in angiogenesis. In order to recapitulate all the information mentioned in the previous paragraphs, (Fig. **2**) shows the central role of MSC in different angiogenic processes occurring in ischemic brain and heart after stroke, in wound healing, inside a tumor, and in the hematopoietic stem cell niche. As shown in (Fig. **2**), different mechanisms are involved in MSC-mediated angiogenesis, among which paracrine factors with pro-angiogenic activity, and trans-differentiation into endothelial-like structures are the more representative ones.

8. ACKNOWLEDGEMENTS

Lizzia Raffaghello was supported by a fellowship from Fondazione Italiana Lotta al Neuroblastoma.

9. REFERENCES

1. Uccelli A, Moretta L, Pistoia V. Mesenchymal stem cells in health and disease. Nat Rev Immunol 2008; 8(9): 726-36..
2. Caplan AI. Mesenchymal stem cells. J Orthop Res 1999; 9(6): 641-650.
3. da Silva Meirelles L, Chagastelles PC, Nardi NB. Mesenchymal stem cells reside in virtually all post-natal organs and tissues. J Cell Sci 2006; 119(Pt11): 2204-13.
4. Pittenger MF, Mackay AM, Beck SC, Jaiswal RK, Douglas R, Mosca JD, Moorman MA, Simonetti DW, Craig S, Marshak DR. Multilineage potential of adult human mesenchymal stem cells. Science 1999; 284(5411): 143-7.
5. Uccelli A, Moretta L, Pistoia V. Immunoregulatory function of mesenchymal stem cells. Eur J Immunol 2006; 36(10): 2566-73.
6. Nauta AJ, Fibbe WE. Immunomodulatory properties of mesenchymal stromal cells. Blood 2007; 110(10): 3499-506.
7. Di Nicola M, Carlo-Stella C, Magni M, Milanesi M, Longoni PD, Matteucci P, Grisanti S, Gianni AM. Human bone marrow stromal cells suppress T-lymphocyte proliferation induced by cellular or nonspecific mitogenic stimuli. Blood 2002; 99(10): 3838-43.
8. Aggarwal S, Pittenger MF. Human mesenchymal stem cells modulate allogeneic immune cell responses. Blood 2005; 105(4): 1815-22.
9. Krampera M, Glennie S, Dyson J, Scott D, Laylor R, Simpson E, Dazzi F. Bone marrow mesenchymal stem cells inhibit the response of naive and memory antigen-specific T cells to their cognate peptide. Blood 2003; 101(9): 3722-9.
10. Maccario R, Podestà M, Moretta A, Cometa A, Comoli P, Montagna D, Daudt L, Ibatici A, Piaggio G, Pozzi S, Frassoni F, Locatelli F. Interaction of human mesenchymal stem cells with cells involved in alloantigen-specific immune response favors the differentiation of CD4+ T-cell subsets expressing a regulatory/suppressive phenotype. Haematologica 2005; 90(4): 516-25.
11. Potian JA, Aviv H, Ponzio NM, Harrison JS Rameshwar P. Veto-like activity of mesenchymal stem cells: functional discrimination between cellular responses to alloantigens and recall antigens. J Immunol 2003; 17(7): 3426-34.
12. Spaggiari GM, Capobianco A, Becchetti S, Mingari MC, Moretta L. Mesenchymal stem cell-natural killer cell interactions: evidence that activated NK cells are capable of killing MSCs, whereas MSCs can inhibit IL-2-induced NK-cell proliferation. Blood 2006; 107(4): 1484-90.
13. Poggi A, Prevosto C, Massaro AM, Negrini S, Urbani S, Pierri I, Saccardi R, Gobbi M, Zocchi MR. Interaction between human NK cells and bone marrow stromal cells induces NK cell triggering: role of NKp30 and NKG2D receptors. J Immunol 2005; 175(10): 6352-60.
14. Zhang W, Ge W, Li C, You S, Liao L, Han Q, Deng W, Zhao RC. Effects of mesenchymal stem cells on differentiation, maturation, and function of human monocyte-derived dendritic cells. Stem Cells Dev 2004; 13(3): 263-71.
15. Jiang XX, Zhang Y, Liu B, Zhang SX, Wu Y, Yu XD, Mao N. Human mesenchymal stem cells inhibit differentiation and function of monocyte-derived dendritic cells. Blood 2005; 105(10): 4120-6.
16. Nauta AJ, Kruisselbrink AB, Lurvink E, Willemze R, Fibbe WE. Mesenchymal stem cells inhibit generation and function of both CD34+-derived and monocyte-derived dendritic cells. J Immunol 2006; 177(4): 2080-7.
17. Concione A, Benvenuto F, Ferretti E Giunti D Cappiello V, Cazzanti F, Risso M Gualandi, F, Mancardi GL, Pistoia V, Uccelli A. Human mesenchymal stem cells modulate B-cell functions. Blood 2006; 107(1): 367-72.
18. Meisel R, Zibert A, Laryea M, Göbel U, Däubener W, Dilloo D. Human bone marrow stromal cells inhibit allogeneic T-cell responses by indoleamine 2,3-dioxygenase-mediated tryptophan degradation. Blood 2004; 103(12): 4619-21.
19. Selmani Z, Naji A, Zidi I, Favier B, Gaiffe E, Obert L, Borg C, Saas P, Tiberghien P, Rouas-Freiss N, Carosella ED, Deschaseaux F. Human leukocyte antigen-G5 secretion by human mesenchymal stem cells is required to suppress T lymphocyte and natural killer function and to induce CD4+CD25highFOXP3+ regulatory T cells. Stem Cells 2008; 26(1): 212-22.
20. Traggiai E, Volpi S, Schena F, Gattorno M, Ferlito F, Moretta L, Martini A. Bone marrow-derived mesenchymal stem cells induce both polyclonal expansion and differentiation of B cells isolated from healthy donors and systemic lupus erythematosus patients. Stem Cells 2008; 26(2): 562-9.

21. Spaggiari GM, Capobianco A, Abdelrazik H, Becchetti F, Mingari MC, Moretta L. Mesenchymal stem cells inhibit natural killer-cell proliferation, cytotoxicity, and cytokine production: role of indoleamine 2,3-dioxygenase and prostaglandin E2. Blood 2008; 111(3): 1327-33.

22. Sotiropoulou PA, Perez SA, Gritzapis AD, Baxevanis CN, Papamichail M. Interactions between human mesenchymal stem cells and natural killer cells. Stem Cells 2006; 24(1): 74-85.

23. Le Blanc K, Tammik C, Rosendahl K, Zetterberg E, Ringdén O. HLA expression and immunologic properties of differentiated and undifferentiated mesenchymal stem cells. Exp Hematol 2003; 31(10): 890-6.

24. Chan JL, Tang KC, Patel AP, Bonilla LM, Pierobon N, Ponzio NM, Rameshwar P. Antigen-presenting property of mesenchymal stem cells occurs during a narrow window at low levels of interferon-gamma. Blood 2006; 107(12): 4817-24.

25. Rasmusson I, Uhlin M, Le Blanc K, Levitsky V. Mesenchymal stem cells fail to trigger effector functions of cytotoxic T lymphocytes. J Leukoc Biol 2007; 82(4): 887-93.

26. Morandi F, Raffaghello L, Bianchi G, Meloni F, Salis A, Millo E, Ferrone S, Barnaba V, Pistoia V. Immunogenicity of human mesenchymal stem cells in HLA-class I-restricted T-cell responses against viral or tumor-associated antigens. Stem Cells 2008; 26(5): 1275-87.

27. Le Blanc K, Rasmusson I, Sundberg B, Götherström C, Hassan M, Uzunel M, Ringdén O. Treatment of severe acute graft-versus-host disease with third party haploidentical mesenchymal stem cells. Lancet 2004; 363(9419): 1439-41.

28. Zappia E, Casazza S, Pedemonte E, Benvenuto F, Bonanni I, Gerdoni E, Giunti D, Ceravolo A, Cazzanti F, Frassoni F, Mancardi G, Uccelli A. Mesenchymal stem cells ameliorate experimental autoimmune encephalomyelitis inducing T-cell anergy. Blood 2005; 106(5): 1755-61.

29. Uccelli A, Zappia E, Benvenuto F, Frassoni F, Mancardi G. Stem cells in inflammatory demyelinating disorders: a dual role for immunosuppression and neuroprotection. Expert Opin Biol Ther 2006; 6(1): 17-22.

30. Ringdén O Uzunel M, Rasmusson I, Remberger M, Sundberg B, Lönnies H, Marschall HU, Dlugosz A, Szakos A, Hassan Z, Omazic B, Aschan J, Barkholt L, Le Blanc K. Mesenchymal stem cells for treatment of therapy-resistant graft-versus-host disease. Transplantation 2006; 81(10): 1390-7.

31. Horwitz EM, Prockop DJ, Fitzpatrick LA, Koo WW, Gordon PL, Neel M, Sussman M, Orchard P, Marx JC, Pyeritz RE, Brenner MK. Transplantability and therapeutic effects of bone marrow-derived mesenchymal cells in children with osteogenesis imperfecta. Nat Med 1999; 5(3): 309-13.

32. Koç ON, Gerson SL, Cooper BW, Dyhouse SM, Haynesworth SE Caplan AI, Lazarus HM. Rapid hematopoietic recovery after coinfusion of autologous-blood stem cells and culture-expanded marrow mesenchymal stem cells in advanced breast cancer patients receiving high-dose chemotherapy. J Clin Oncol 2000; 18(2): 307-16.

33. Prockop DJ, Olson SD. Clinical trials with adult stem/progenitor cells for tissue repair: let's not overlook some essential precautions. Blood 2007; 109(8): 3147-51.

34. Spaeth E, Klopp A, Dembinski J, Andreeff M, Marini F. Inflammation and tumor microenvironments: defining the migratory itinerary of mesenchymal stem cells. Gene Ther 2008; 15(10): 730-8.

35. Dvorak HF. Tumors: wounds that do not heal. Similarities between tumor stroma generation and wound healing. N Engl J Med 1986; 315(26): 1650-9.

36. Ramasamy R, Lam EW, Soeiro I, Tisato V, Bonnet D, Dazzi F. Mesenchymal stem cells inhibit proliferation and apoptosis of tumor cells: impact on in vivo tumor growth. Leukemia 2007; 21(2): 304-10.

37. Djouad F, Plence P, Bony C, Tropel P, Apparailly F, Sany J, Noël D, Jorgensen C. Immunosuppressive effect of mesenchymal stem cells favors tumor growth in allogeneic animals. Blood 2003; 102(10): 3837-44.

38. Amé-Thomas P, Maby-El Hajjami H, Monvoisin C, Jean R, Monnier D, Caulet-Maugendre S, Guillaudeux T, Lamy T, Fest T, Tarte K. Human mesenchymal stem cells isolated from bone marrow and lymphoid organs support tumor B-cell growth: role of stromal cells in follicular lymphoma pathogenesis. Blood 2007; 109(2): 693-702.

39. Khakoo AY, Pati S, Anderson SA, Reid W, Elshal MF, Rovira II, Nguyen AT, Malide D, Combs CA, Hall G, Zhang J, Raffeld M, Rogers TB, Stetler-Stevenson W, Frank JA, Reitz M, Finkel T. Human mesenchymal stem cells exert potent antitumorigenic effects in a model of Kaposi's sarcoma. J Exp Med 2006; 203(5): 1235-47.

40. Karnoub AE, Dash AB, Vo AP, Sullivan A, Brooks MW, Bell GW, Richardson AL, Polyak K, Tubo R, Weinberg RA. Mesenchymal stem cells within tumour stroma promote breast cancer metastasis. Nature 2007; 449(7162): 557-63.

41. Studeny M, Marini FC, Dembinski JL, Zompetta C, Cabreira-Hansen M, Bekele BN, Champlin RE Andreeff M. Mesenchymal stem cells: potential precursors for tumor stroma and targeted-delivery vehicles for anticancer agents. J Natl Cancer Inst 2004; 96(21): 1593-603.

42. Kanehira M, Xin H, Hoshino K, Maemondo M, Mizuguchi H, Hayakawa T, Matsumoto K, Nakamura T, Nukiwa T, Saijo Y. Targeted delivery of NK4 to multiple lung tumors by bone marrow-derived mesenchymal stem cells. Cancer Gene Ther 2007; 14(11): 894-903.

43. Hall B, Dembinski J, Sasser AK, Studeny M, Andreeff M, Marini F. Mesenchymal stem cells in cancer: tumor-associated fibroblasts and cell-based delivery vehicles. Int J Hematol 2007; 86(1): 8-16.

44. Nakamizo A, Marini F, Amano T, Khan A, Studeny M, Gumin J, Chen J, Hentschel S, Vecil G, Dembinski J, Andreeff M, Lang FF. Human bone marrow-derived mesenchymal stem cells in the treatment of gliomas. Cancer Res 2005; 65(8): 3307-18.

45. Kiel MJ, Morrison SJ. Uncertainty in the niches that maintain haematopoietic stem cells. Nat Rev Immunol 2008; 8(4): 290-301.

46. Muguruma Y, Yahata T, Miyatake H, Sato T, Uno T, Itoh J, Kato S, Ito M, Hotta T, Ando K. Reconstitution of the functional human hematopoietic microenvironment derived from human mesenchymal stem cells in the murine bone marrow compartment. Blood 2006; 107(5): 1878-87.

47. Wilson A, Trumpp A. Bone-marrow haematopoietic-stem-cell niches. Nat Rev Immunol 2006; 6(2): 93-106.

48. Sacchetti B, Funari A, Michienzi S, Di Cesare S, Piersanti S, Saggio I, Tagliafico E, Ferrari S, Robey PG, Riminucci M, Bianco P. Self-renewing osteoprogenitors in bone marrow sinusoids can organize a hematopoietic microenvironment. Cell 2007; 131(2): 324-36.

49. Arai F, Hirao A, Ohmura M, Sato H, Matsuoka S, Takubo K, Ito K, Koh GY, Suda T. Tie2/angiopoietin-1 signaling regulates hematopoietic stem cell quiescence in the bone marrow niche. Cell 2004; 118(2): 149-61.

50. Kögler G, Radke TF, Lefort A, Sensken S, Fischer J, Sorg RV, Wernet P. Cytokine production and hematopoiesis supporting activity of cord blood-derived unrestricted somatic stem cells. Exp Hematol 2005; 33(5): 573-83.

51. Gille H, Kowalski J, Li B, LeCouter J, Moffat B, Zioncheck TF, Pelletier N, Ferrara N. Analysis of biological effects and signaling properties of Flt-1 (VEGFR-1) and KDR (VEGFR-2). A reassessment using novel receptor-specific vascular endothelial growth factor mutants. J Biol Chem 2001; 276(5): 3222-30.

52. Tille JC, Wood J, Mandriota SJ, Schnell C, Ferrari S, Mestan J, Zhu Z, Witte L, Pepper MS. Vascular endothelial growth factor (VEGF) receptor-2 antagonists inhibit VEGF- and basic fibroblast growth factor-induced angiogenesis in vivo and in vitro. J Pharmacol Exp Ther 2001; 299(3): 1073-85.

53. Zhang ZG, Zhang L, Jiang Q, Zhang R, Davies K, Powers C, Bruggen N, Chopp M. VEGF enhances angiogenesis and promotes blood-brain barrier leakage in the ischemic brain. J Clin Invest 2000; 106(7): 829-38.

54. Zhang ZG, Zhang L, Jiang Q, Chopp M. Bone marrow-derived endothelial progenitor cells participate in cerebral neovascularization after focal cerebral ischemia in the adult mouse. Circ Res 2002; 90(3): 284-8.

55. Chen J, Zhang ZG, Li Y, Wang L, Xu YX, Gautam SC, Lu M, Zhu Z, Chopp M. Intravenous administration of human bone marrow stromal cells induces angiogenesis in the ischemic boundary zone after stroke in rats. Circ Res 2003; 92(6): 692-9.

56. Zacharek A, Chen J, Cui X, Li A, Li Y, Roberts C, Feng Y, Gao Q, Chopp M. Angiopoietin1/Tie2 and VEGF/Flk1 induced by MSC treatment amplifies angiogenesis and vascular stabilization after stroke. J Cereb Blood Flow Metab 2007; 27(10): 1684-91.

57. Nagaya N, Fujii T, Iwase T, Ohgushi H, Itoh T, Uematsu M, Yamagishi M, Mori H, Kangawa K, Kitamura S. Intravenous administration of mesenchymal stem cells improves cardiac function in rats with acute myocardial infarction through angiogenesis and myogenesis. Am J Physiol. Heart Circ Physiol 2004; 287(6): H2670-6.

58. Silva GV, Litovsky S, Assad JA, Sousa AL, Martin BJ, Vela D, Coulter SC, Lin J, Ober J, Vaughn WK, Branco RV, Oliveira EM, He R, Geng YJ, Willerson JT, Perin EC. Mesenchymal stem cells differentiate into an endothelial phenotype, enhance vascular density, and improve heart function in a canine chronic ischemia model. Circulation 2005; 111(2): 150-6.

59. Singer AJ, Clark RA. Cutaneous wound healing. N Engl J Med 1999; 341(10): 738-46.

60. Arnold F, West DC. Angiogenesis in wound healing. Pharmacol Ther 1991; 52(3): 407-22.

61. Wu Y, Chen L, Scott PG, Tredget EE. Mesenchymal stem cells enhance wound healing through differentiation and angiogenesis. Stem Cells 2007; 25(10): 2648-59.

62. Jain RK. Molecular regulation of vessel maturation. Nat Med 2003; 9(6): 685-93.

63. Jain RK, Duda DG. Role of bone marrow-derived cells in tumor angiogenesis and treatment. Cancer Cell 2003; 3(6): 515-6.

64. De Palma M, Venneri MA, Galli R, Sergi L, Politi LS, Sampaolesi M, Naldini L. Tie2 identifies a hematopoietic lineage of proangiogenic monocytes required for tumor vessel formation and a mesenchymal population of pericyte progenitors. Cancer Cell 2005; 8(3): 211-26.

65. Rajantie I, Ilmonen M, Alminaite A, Ozerdem U, Alitalo K, Salven P. Adult bone marrow-derived cells recruited during angiogenesis comprise precursors for periendothelial vascular mural cells. Blood 2004; 104(7): 2084-6.

66. Winkler F, Kozin SV, Tong RT, Chae SS, Booth MF, Garkavtsev I, Xu L, Hicklin DJ, Fukumura D, di Tomaso E, Munn LL, Jain RK. Kinetics of vascular normalization by VEGFR2 blockade governs brain tumor response to radiation: role of oxygenation, angiopoietin-1, and matrix metalloproteinases. Cancer Cell 2004; 6(6): 553-63.

67. Bexell D, Gunnarsson S, Tormin A, Darabi A, Gisselsson D, Roybon L, Scheding S, Bengzon J. Bone Marrow Multipotent Mesenchymal Stroma Cells Act as Pericyte-like Migratory Vehicles in Experimental Gliomas. Mol Ther 2008; 17(1): 183-90.

68. Beckermann BM, Kallifatidis G, Groth A, Frommhold D, Apel A, Mattern J, Salnikov AV, Moldenhauer G, Wagner W, Diehlmann A, Saffrich R, Schubert M, Ho AD, Giese N, Büchler MW, Friess H, Büchler P, Herr I. VEGF expression by mesenchymal stem cells contributes to angiogenesis in pancreatic carcinoma. Br J Cancer 2008; 99(4): 622-31.

69. Sun T, Sun BC, Ni CS, Zhao XL, Wang XH, Qie S, Zhang DF, Gu Q, Qi H, Zhao N. Pilot study on the interaction between B16 melanoma cell-line and bone-marrow derived mesenchymal stem cells. Cancer Lett 2008; 263(1): 35-43.

70. Mishra PJ, Humeniuk R, Medina DJ, Alexe G, Mesirov JP, Ganesan S, Glod JW, Banerjee D. Carcinoma-associated fibroblast-like differentiation of human mesenchymal stem cells. Cancer Res 2008; 68(11): 4331-9.

71. Langenfeld EM, Kong Y, Langenfeld J. Bone morphogenetic protein 2 stimulation of tumor growth involves the activation of Smad-1/5. Oncogene 2006; 25(5): 685-92.

72.   Date T, Doiguchi Y, Nobuta M, Shindo H. Bone morphogenetic protein-2 induces differentiation of multipotent C3H10T1/2 cells into osteoblasts, chondrocytes, and adipocytes in vivo and in vitro. J Orthop Sci 2004; 9(5): 503-8.

73.   Raida M, Heymann AC, Günther C, Niederwieser D. Role of bone morphogenetic protein 2 in the crosstalk between endothelial progenitor cells and mesenchymal stem cells. Int J Mol Med 2006; 18(4): 735-9.

74.   Hattori K, Heissig B, Wu Y, Dias S, Tejada R, Ferris B, Hicklin DJ, Zhu Z, Bohlen P, Witte L, Hendrikx J, Hackett NR, Crystal RG, Moore MA, Werb Z, Lyden D, Rafii S. Placental growth factor reconstitutes hematopoiesis by recruiting VEGFR1(+) stem cells from bone-marrow microenvironment. Nat Med 2002; 8(8): 841-9.

75.   Carmeliet P, Moons L, Luttun A, Vincenti V, Compernolle V, De Mol M, Wu Y, Bono F, Devy L, Beck H, Scholz D, Acker T, DiPalma T, Dewerchin M, Noel A, Stalmans I, Barra A, Blacher S, Vandendriessche T, Ponten A, Eriksson U, Plate KH, Foidart JM, Schaper W, Charnock-Jones DS, Hicklin DJ, Herbert JM. Collen D, Persico MG. Synergism between vascular endothelial growth factor and placental growth factor contributes to angiogenesis and plasma extravasation in pathological conditions. Nat Med 2001; 7(9): 575-83.

76.   Annabi B, Lee YT, Turcotte S, Naud E, Desrosiers RR, Champagne M, Eliopoulos N, Galipeau J, Béliveau R. Hypoxia promotes murine bone-marrow-derived stromal cell migration and tube formation. Stem Cells 2003; 21(3): 337-47.

77.   Zwezdaryk KJ, Coffelt SB, Figueroa YG, Liu J, Phinney DG, LaMarca HL, Florez L, Morris CB, Hoyle GW, Scandurro AB. Erythropoietin, a hypoxia-regulated factor, elicits a pro-angiogenic program in human mesenchymal stem cells. Exp Hematol 2007 35(7): 1153-61.

78.   Krampera M, Pasini A, Rigo A, Scupoli MT, Tecchio C, Malpeli G, Scarpa A, Dazzi F, Pizzolo G, Vinante F. HB-EGF/HER-1 signaling in bone marrow mesenchymal stem cells: inducing cell expansion and reversibly preventing multilineage differentiation. Blood 2005; 106(1): 59-66

79.   Zhang G, Zhou J, Fan Q, Zheng Z, Zhang F, Liu X , Hu S. Arterial-venous endothelial cell fate is related to vascular endothelial growth factor and Notch status during human bone mesenchymal stem cell differentiation. FEBS Lett 2008; 582(19): 2957-64.

80.   Copland I, Sharma K, Lejeune L, Eliopoulos N, Stewart D, Liu P, Lachapelle K, Galipeau J. CD34 expression on murine marrow-derived mesenchymal stromal cells: impact on neovascularization. Exp Hematol 2008; 36(1): 93-103.

CHAPTER 4

Cross-Link Between Inflammation and Angiogenesis

Enrico Crivellato[1] and Domenico Ribatti[2]

[1]Department of Medical and Morphological Researches, Anatomy Section, University of Udine Medical School, Udine, Italy and [2]Department of Human Anatomy and Histology, University of Bari Medical School, Bari, Italy

Correspondence to: Prof. Enrico Crivellato, Department of Medical and Morphological Researches, Anatomy Section, Piazzale Kolbe, 3, 33100 Udine, Italy. Tel: 0039.0432.494221; Fax: 0039.0432.494201; Email: enrico.crivellato@uniud.it

Abstract: Angiogenesis refers to the formation of new blood vessels from pre-existing vascular structures, i.e. capillaries and post-capillary venules. This process occurs in different conditions, such as embryo development and post-natal tissue growth, inflammation like wound healing and chronic allergies, and cancer. Both structural cells and inflammatory cells in the different tissues are involved in the mechanisms of endothelial cell proliferation, migration and activation, through the production and release of a large spectrum of pro-angiogenic mediators. These may create the specific micro-environment that favours an increased rate of tissue vascularization. In this review, we will present the most recent findings on the contribution of inflammatory cells to the development and progression of inflammation-associated angiogenesis. We will also provide some insight of the complex signaling network, which links each inflammatory cell to the surrounding scenario.

1. INTRODUCTION

Angiogenesis is a complex and highly orchestrated process leading to the formation of new blood vessels from pre-existing capillaries and venules [1]. This process is fundamental for organ development. During the later stages of embryogenesis, the vascularization of many tissues occurs by angiogenesis. This mechanism of vessel production consists in a multistep and highly orchestrated process, which is under control of different genetic and epigenetic mechanisms [2]. There are at least two types of angiogenesis: (a) the so-called "sprouting" angiogenesis, which is characterized by the proliferation and migration of endothelial cells into avascular sites; (b) the "non-sprouting" angiogenesis or intussusceptive microvascular growth, which occurs by splitting of the existing vasculature by transluminal pillars or transendothelial bridges [1, 3]. In the adult life, angiogenesis accompanies various physiological and pathophysiological conditions, such as ovulation, endometrial vascularization in menstrual cycle and pregnancy, and wound healing.

There is increasing evidence to support the view that angiogenesis is an integral component of a diverse range of chronic inflammatory and autoimmune diseases, including atherosclerosis, rheumatoid arthritis, diabetic retinopathy, psoriasis, airway inflammation, peptic ulcers, and Alzheimer's disease [4]. Indeed, angiogenesis is intrinsic to chronic inflammation and is associated with structural changes, including activation and proliferation of endothelial cells, capillary and venule remodeling, all of which result in expansion of the tissue microvascular bed. Chronic inflammation in the airways, for instance, is associated with dramatic architectural changes in the walls of the airways and in the vasculature they contain. Therefore, it seems that an imbalance in favour of pro-angiogenic factors leads to the abnormal growth of new blood vessels in asthma. Inflammatory diseases, such as rheumatoid arthritis and psoriasis, are characterized by proliferating tissue containing an abundance of inflammatory cells and newly formed blood vessels. During prolonged inflammatory reactions, many structural and resident cells, such as fibroblasts, epithelial cells, smooth muscle cells, mast cells, and/or infiltrating cells, such as monocytes/macrophages, neutrophils, lymphocytes and eosinophils, synthesize and secrete pro-angiogenic factors that promote neovascularization. The anatomic expansion of the microvascular bed combined with its increased functional activation can therefore foster further recruitment of inflammatory cells, and angiogenesis and inflammation become chronically codependent processes. In addition, many of the mediators that are fundamental players in angiogenesis are also inflammatory molecules. Inflammation-associated angiogenesis also occurs during pathophysiological reactions, like wound healing and scar formation. The process of extracellular matrix remodeling that accompanies this kind of tissue responses is strictly dependent upon angiogenic events. Inflammatory cells contribute even to angiogenesis concomitant with physiological processes, such as ovulation and endometrial vascularization during the reconstructive phase of the menstrual cycle and in pregnancy.

2. VASCULAR ENDOTHELIAL GROWTH FACTOR AND INFLAMMATORY ANGIOGENESIS

Vascular endothelial growth factor (VEGF) is a secreted mitogen highly specific for endothelial cells. In vivo VEGF induces microvascular permeability and plays a central role in both angiogenesis and vasculogenesis [5]. Through alternative mRNA splicing, a single gene gives rise to several distinct isoforms of VEGF, which differ in their expression patterns as well as their biochemical and biological properties. Two VEGF receptor tyrosine kinases (VEGFRs) have been identified, VEGFR-1 (Flt-1) and VEGFR-2 (KDR/Flk-1). VEGFR-2 seems to mediate almost all observed endothelial cell responses to VEGF, whereas roles for VEGFR-1 are more elusive. VEGFR-1 might act predominantly as a ligand-binding molecule, sequestering VEGF from VEGFR-2 signaling. Several isoform-specific VEGF receptors exist that modulate VEGF activity. Neuropilin-1 acts as a co-receptor for VEGF(165), enhancing its binding to VEGFR-2 and its bioactivity. Heparan sulphate proteoglycans (HSPGs), as well as binding certain VEGF isoforms, interact with both VEGFR-1 and VEGFR-2. HSPGs have a wide variety of functions, such as the ability to partially restore lost function to damaged VEGF(165) and thereby prolonging its biological activity.

Increasing evidence suggests that VEGF-A is one of the major proangiogenic molecules involved in both normal and pathologic angiogenesis. The expression of VEGF-A and its receptor VEGFR-2 is elevated in patients with inflammatory skin diseases that are associated with enhanced vascularity such as psoriasis. Recently, transgenic mice expressing VEGF have been described to develop a psoriasis-like inflammation characterized by increased angiogenesis, acanthosis, and immune cell infiltration [6].

Similarly in human and experimental rheumatoid arthritis, the VEGF-A pathway is strongly overexpressed and activated, and its blockade is clinically beneficial. Indeed, the vasculature plays a crucial role in inflammation, angiogenesis, and atherosclerosis associated with the pathogenesis of inflammatory rheumatic diseases [7]. The endothelium lining the blood vessels becomes activated during the inflammatory process, resulting in the production of several mediators, the expression of endothelial adhesion molecules, and increased vascular permeability (leakage). All of this enables the extravasation of inflammatory cells into the interstitial matrix. The endothelial adhesion and transendothelial migration of leukocytes is a well-regulated sequence of events that involves many adhesion molecules and chemokines. Primarily selectins, integrins, and members of the immunoglobulin family of adhesion receptors are involved in leukocyte 'tethering', 'rolling', activation, and transmigration. There is a perpetuation of angiogenesis, the formation of new capillaries from pre-existing vessels, as well as that of vasculogenesis, the generation of new blood vessels in arthritis and connective tissue diseases. Several soluble and cell-bound angiogenic mediators produced mainly by monocytes/macrophages and endothelial cells stimulate neovascularization. On the other hand, endogenous angiogenesis inhibitors and exogenously administered angiostatic compounds may downregulate the process of capillary formation. Thus, the formation of new vessels appears to be an early and fundamental process for the evolution of the inflammatory response in synovial joints affected by arthritis. The propagation of new vessels in the synovial membrane allows the invasion of this tissue over the intraarticular cartilage in an adherent fashion. This process appears to support the active infiltration of synovial membrane into cartilage and results in erosion and destruction of the cartilage. This process results in joint damage and ultimately in deformity, as the normal joint architecture and balance of tendons becomes disrupted.

Activation of the VEGF-A pathway has been demonstrated also in the actively inflamed mucosa of patients with inflammatory bowel disease. Expression of both VEGF-A and its receptor VEGFR-2 are enhanced in tissue biopsy specimens from inflamed bowel segments. Interestingly, besides its classical angiogenic activity, VEGF-A can exert proinflammatory effects on intestinal endothelium, both in vitro and in vivo. Indeed, recent evidence shows that angiogenesis is crucial during inflammatory bowel disease and in experimental models of colitis [8]. Examination of the relationship between angiogenesis and inflammation in experimental colitis shows that initiating factors for these responses simultaneously increase as disease progresses and correlate in magnitude. Recent studies show that inhibition of the inflammatory response attenuates angiogenesis to a similar degree and, importantly, that inhibition of angiogenesis does the same to inflammation. Recent data provide evidence that differential regulation of the angiogenic mediators involved in inflammatory bowel disease-associated chronic inflammation is the root of this pathological angiogenesis [9]. Many factors are involved in this phenomenon, including growth factors/cytokines, chemokines, adhesion molecules, integrins, matrix-associated molecules, and signaling targets. These factors are produced by various vascular, inflammatory, and immune cell types that are involved in inflammatory bowel disease pathology. Moreover, recent studies provide evidence that antiangiogenic therapy is a novel and effective approach for inflammatory bowel disease treatment.

The VEGF family of growth factors control pathological angiogenesis and increased vascular permeability in important eye diseases such as diabetic retinopathy and age-related macular degeneration. Recent findings suggest a role of VEGFR-1 as a functional receptor for placenta growth factor (PlGF) and VEGF-A in pericytes and vascular smooth muscle cells in vivo rather than in endothelial cells [10]. In addition, VEGFs secreted by epithelia, including the retinal pigment epithelium, are likely to mediate paracrine vascular survival signals for adjacent endothelia. In the choroid, derailment of this paracrine relation and overexpression of VEGF-A by the retinal pigment epithelium may explain the pathogenesis of subretinal neovascularisation in age-related macular degeneration. On the other hand, this paracrine relation and other physiological functions of VEGFs may be endangered by therapeutic VEGF inhibition, as is currently used in several clinical trials in diabetic retinopathy and age-related macular degeneration.

In addition to this, the VEGF family of growth factors appears to stimulate neuroprotection after stroke. Recent findings from experiments performed on animals with experimentally evoked focal cerebral ischemia suggest that the neuroprotective activity of VEGF runs in parallel with its ability to promote neurogenesis and angiogenesis and that these effects may operate independently through multiple mechanisms [11]. The above-mentioned three major features characterizing the neurobiological activity of VEGF, i.e. neuroprotection, neurogenesis, and angiogenesis, together with their possible functional link(s), provide the rationale for considering VEGF-based therapy as a promising future avenue for a more effective treatment of at least some neurodegenerative disorders and stroke. Moreover, the possibility of using neutralizing factors of VEGF or VEGF receptor antagonists may reveal a way of preventing many dangerous pathologies, including post-ischemic disturbances in cardiac and neurological disorders, or hypervascularization in avascular structures of the eye.

3. NEUTROPHILS

Neutrophils, or polymorphonuclear granulocytes, are blood cell leukocytes which play a basic role in host defence and inflammation. During the acute inflammatory response, neutrophils extravasate from the circulation into the tissue, where they exert their defence functions. Increasing evidence supports the concept that these immune cells also contribute to inflammation-mediated angiogenesis in different flogistic conditions. Neutrophils indeed are a source of soluble mediators which, besides proinflammatory activity, exert important angiogenic functions. VEGF, interleukin (IL)-8, tumor necrosis factor (TNF)-α, hepatocyte growth factor (HGF) and matrix

metalloproteinases (MMPs) are the most important activators of angiogenesis produced by these cells [12-14]. In this perspective, microarray technique has recently revealed about thirty angiogenesis-relevant genes in human polymorphonuclear granulocytes [15]. Interestingly, neutrophil-derived VEGF can stimulate neutrophil migration [16]. Thus neutrophil contribution to both normal and pathological angiogenesis may be sustained by an autocrine amplification mechanism that allows persistent VEGF release to occur at sites of neutrophil accumulation. Production and release of VEGF from neutrophils has been shown to depend from the granulocyte-colony stimulating factor (G-CSF) [17]. Evidence for the possible role of polymorphonuclear granulocytes in inflammation-mediated angiogenesis and tissue remodeling was initially provided by the finding that CXC receptor 2 (CXCR2)-deficient mice, which lacks neutrophil infiltration in thioglycollate-induced peritonitis [18], showed delayed angiogenesis and impaired cutaneous wound healing [19]. More recently, human polymorphonuclear granulocytes have demonstrated the ability to directly induce the sprouting of capillary-like structures in in vitro angiogenesis assay. This angiogenic capacity appears to be mediated by secretion of both preformed VEGF from cell stores and de novo synthesized IL-8 [15].

Angiogenesis is a hallmark of the synovium in chronic septic arthritis. Analysis of the synovium in patients with chronic pyogenic arthritis identified dramatic neovascularization and cell proliferation, accompanied by persistent bacterial colonization and heterogeneous inflammatory infiltrates rich in CD15+ neutrophils, as histopathologic hallmarks [20]. By using a modified angiogenic model, allowing for a direct analysis of exogenously added cells and their products in collagen onplants grafted on the chorioallantoic membrane of the chicken embryo, it has recently been demonstrated that intact human neutrophils and their granule contents are highly angiogenic [21]. Furthermore, purified neutrophil MMP-9, isolated from the released granules as a zymogen (proMMP-9), constitutes a distinctly potent proangiogenic moiety inducing angiogenesis at subnanogram levels. The angiogenic response induced by neutrophil proMMP-9 requires activation of the tissue inhibitor of metalloproteinases (TIMP)-free zymogen and the catalytic activity of the activated enzyme.

Neutrophils not only activate but also modulate the angiogenic process. Neutrophil elastase, a serine protease released from the azurophil granules of activated neutrophil, proteolytically cleaves angiogenic growth factors such as basic-fibroblast growth factor (FGF)-2 and VEGF [22]. Neutrophil elastase degrades FGF-2 and VEGF in a time- and concentration-dependent manner, and these degradations are suppressed by sivelestat, a synthetic inhibitor of neutrophil elastase. The FGF-2- or VEGF-mediated proliferative activity of human umbilical vein endothelial cells is inhibited by neutrophil elastase, and the activity is recovered by sivelestat. Furthermore, neutrophil elastase reduces the FGF-2- or VEGF-induced tubulogenic response of the mice aortas, ex vivo angiogenesis assay, and these effects are also recovered by sivelestat. Neutrophil-derived elastase degrades potent angiogenic factors, resulting in loss of their angiogenic activity. These findings provide additional insight into the role played by neutrophils in the angiogenesis process at sites of inflammation.

4. LYMPHOCYTES

Lymphocytes have important pro-angiogenic functions in the course of pregnancy. In particular, natural killer (NK) cells are the most abundant leukocytes in preimplantation endometrium. These cells have been shown to accumulate and actively proliferate in the endometrium of murine, porcine and human developing placenta [23].

In pathological conditions, lymphocytes have been shown to be essential for the airway remodeling that occurs during prolonged infections. In such perspective, studies have been performed in mice chronically infected with the respiratory pathogen Mycoplasma pneumoniae. Mice lacking B cells have been shown to express a great reduction of angiogenesis when infected with this micro organism [24]. The humoral response, indeed, causes deposition of immune complexes on the airway wall, followed by recruitment of inflammatory cells at sites of infected airways which, in turn, are responsible for local production of remodeling factors. In asthma, key cells of allergy such as mast cells, produce significant amounts of IL-1 that contributes to lymphocyte infiltration [25] and IL-4, essential for the triggering of Th2 lymphocytes that themselves produce IL-4 to initiate inflammatory cell accumulation and B lymphocytes immunoglobulin class switching to IgE [26].

Angiogenesis is a hallmark of chronic inflammation such as psoriasis. Unraveling the pathogenesis of psoriasis shows that several proangiogenic mediators are activated and highly expressed during this cutaneous disease [27]. VEGF, hypoxia- inducible factor, TNF-α, IL-8 and angiopoietins are considered to be the main players responsible for the strong vessel formation in psoriasis. The proangiogenic milieu in the skin seems to result from a proinflammatory immune response initiated by T helper cells. Interestingly, several small molecules as well as modern biologics used for systemic therapy of psoriasis have been shown to provide not only immune regulatory effects but also influence endothelial cell biology. Thus, direct targeting of angiogenesis may not only help to understand psoriasis pathogenesis but also to develop new strategies to treat psoriasis with therapeutics that halt the angiogenesis required for the inflammatory disease. It has recently been demonstrated that transgenic mice expressing VEGF under the keratin 14 promoter develop a psoriasis-like inflammation characterized by increased angiogenesis, acanthosis, and immune cell infiltration. It has also been shown that application of 12-O-tetradecanoylphorbol-13-acetate (TPA) in these mice induces a severe and long-lasting skin inflammation with a Th17 cell signature. Lymphocytes isolated from inflamed ears show a significantly higher number of activated T cells, in contrast to the primarily naive lymphocytes isolated from blood. In addition, there is an increase in regulatory T cells (CD4(+)CD25(+)CD127(-/low)) within the skin. Interestingly, CD4 depletion results in augmented ear thickness and proinflammatory cytokine levels, indicating that CD4(+) T cells have a suppressive rather than a proinflammatory function in this model. Subsequently, sorted regulatory CD4(+)CD25(+) T cells are transferred to naive K14/VEGF transgenic mice before TPA challenge. CD4(+)CD25(+) T-cell transfer significantly reduces ear thickness and proinflammatory cytokine production compared to controls, indicating that a persistent skin inflammation with similarities to psoriasis can be controlled by a single injection of few regulatory T cells [28].

5. MAST CELLS

Mast cells are common components of inflammatory infiltrates and exert basic functions in the cross-talk between immunological, inflammatory and reparative tissue reactions [29]. Mast cells produce a large spectrum of pro-angiogenic factors such as FGF-2 and VEGF [30, 31]. Human cord blood-derived mast cells release VEGF upon stimulation through FcεRI and c-kit. Human mast cells are a potent source of VEGF in the absence of degranulation through activation of the EP(2) receptor by prostaglandin E2 (PGE2) [32]. It has also been demonstrated that rat peritoneal mast cells contain angiogenic factors stored in their secretory granules. Granulated mast cells and their granules, but not degranulated mast cells, are able indeed to stimulate an intense angiogenic reaction in the chick embryo chorioallantoic membrane (CAM) assay. This angiogenic activity is partly inhibited by anti-FGF-2 and -VEGF antibodies, suggesting that these cytokines are involved in the angiogenic reaction [33].

Mast cells store large amounts of preformed active serine proteases, such as tryptase and chymase [29], which have important roles in the angiogenic process. Tryptase, in particular, stimulates the proliferation of human vascular endothelial cells, promotes vascular tube formation in culture and also degrades connective tissue matrix to provide space for neovascular growth. Mast cell-derived chymase degrades extracellular matrix components and therefore matrix-bound VEGF could be potentially released.

Other mast cell specific mediators with angiogenic properties include histamine and heparin [34]. Both molecules have been shown to stimulate proliferation of endothelial cells and to induce the formation of new blood vessels in the CAM-assay [35]. In addition, other cytokines produced by mast cells, such as IL-8 [36], TNF-α [37], transforming growth factor (TGF)-β, nerve growth factor (NGF) [38] and urokinase-type PA have been implicated in normal and tumor-associated angiogenesis [39]. Lastly, mast cells also contain preformed MMPs, such as MMP-2 and MMP-9, and TIMPs, which enable mast cells to directly modulate extracellular matrix degradation. This, in turn, allows for tissue release of extracellular matrix-bound angiogenic factors.

Interestingly, PGE2 dose-dependently induces primary mast cells to release the proangiogenic chemokine monocyte chemoattractant protein-1 (MCP-1) [40]. This release of MCP-1 is complete by 2 h after PGE2 exposure, reaches levels of MCP-1 at least 15-fold higher than background, and is not accompanied by degranulation or increased MCP-1 gene expression. By immunoelectron microscopy, MCP-1 is detected within mast cells at a cytoplasmic location distinct from the secretory granules. Dexamethasone and cyclosporine A inhibit PGE2-induced MCP-1 secretion by approximately 60%. Agonists of PGE2 receptor subtypes revealed that the EP1 and EP3 receptors can independently mediate MCP-1 release from mast cells. These observations identify PGE2-induced MCP-1 release from mast cells as a pathway underlying inflammation-associated angiogenesis and extend current understanding of the activities of PGE2.

Mast cells appear to be actively involved in postinfarction inflammation. Myocardial infarction is associated with an acute inflammatory response, leading to replacement of injured cardiomyocytes with granulation tissue [41]. Myocardial necrosis is associated with complement activation and free radical generation, triggering a cytokine cascade and chemokine upregulation. IL-8 and C5a are released in the ischemic myocardium, and may have a crucial role in neutrophil recruitment. Extravasated neutrophils may induce potent cytotoxic effects through the release of proteolytic enzymes and the adhesion with intercellular adhesion molecule (ICAM)-1 expressing cardiomyocytes. MCP-1 is induced in the infarcted area and may regulate mononuclear cell recruitment. Accumulation of monocyte-derived macrophages, and mast cells may increase expression of growth factors inducing angiogenesis and fibroblast accumulation in the infarct. In addition, expression of cytokines inhibiting the inflammatory response, such as IL-10 may suppress injury. MMPs and their inhibitors regulate extracellular matrix deposition and play an important role in mediating ventricular remodeling. Mast cells are actively involved in postinfarction

inflammation by releasing histamine and TNF-α, triggering a cytokine cascade. During the proliferative phase of healing, mast cells accumulate in the infarct and may regulate fibrous tissue deposition and angiogenesis by releasing growth factors, angiogenic mediators, and proteases. In the healing infarct, mast cells are associated with other cell types that are important for granulation tissue formation. Inflammatory mediators may induce recruitment of blood-derived primitive stem cells in the healing infarct, which may differentiate into endothelial cells and even lead to limited myocardial regeneration.

Mast cells have been implied in the neovascularization associated with rosacea. Indeed, angiogenesis seems to play an important role in the pathogenesis especially of the more severe clinical form of rosacea. Mast cells seem to participate in evolution to disease chronicity by contributing to inflammation, angiogenesis and tissue fibrosis [42].

Atopic dermatitis skin lesions are characterized by inflammatory changes and epithelial hyperplasia requiring angiogenesis. Mast cells may participate in this process via bidirectional secretion of tissue-damaging enzymes and pro-angiogenic factors. It has been shown that mast cells are abundantly localized in the papillary dermis and migrate through the basal lamina into the epidermis of atopic dermatitis lesions [43]. Approximately 80% were chymase positive. A high number of mast cells express c-kit. Most papillary and epidermal mast cells localize close to endothelial cells. Vascular expression of endoglin (CD105) demonstrates neoangiogenic processes. Mast cells stimulation leads to the expression of proangiogenic factors and tissue-damaging factors such MMPs. These data suggest that in atopic dermatitis, mast cells close to papillary vessels and within the epidermis may be implicated in stimulation of neoangiogenesis.

Increasing evidence suggests that mast cells are involved in the pathogenesis of chronic inflammatory diseases and in particular in rheumatoid arthritis. Mast cells reside in connective tissues and in synovial tissue of joints. As already shown, they produce an array of proinflammatory mediators, tissue destructive proteases, and cytokines, most prominently TNF-α, which is one of the key cytokines in the pathogenesis of rheumatoid arthritis [44]. Mast cells may also participate in the development of secondary or amyloid A amyloidosis, as the partial degradation of the serum amyloid A protein by mast cells leads to the generation of a highly amyloidogenic N-terminal fragment of serum amyloid A. Mast cells may contribute to the pathogenesis of connective tissue diseases, scleroderma, vasculitic syndromes, and systemic lupus erythematosus, although the data available are limited. Inhibition of the most important growth factor receptor of human mast cells, c-Kit, by the selective tyrosine kinase inhibitor imatinib mesylate, induces apoptosis of synovial tissue mast cells. As mast cells are long-lived cells, induction of their apoptosis could be a feasible approach to inhibit their functions.

Mast cells have recently been implicated in the vascular inflammation leading to aneurism formation. Abdominal aortic aneurysm is histologically characterized by medial degeneration and various degrees of chronic adventitial inflammation, although the mechanisms for progression of aneurysm are poorly understood. Remarkably, the number of mast cells was found to increase in the outer media or adventitia of human abdominal aortic aneurysm, showing a positive correlation between the cell number and the aneurism diameter [45]. Aneurysmal dilatation of the aorta was seen in the control (+/+) rats following periaortic application of calcium chloride (CaCl2) treatment but not in the mast cell-deficient mutant Ws/Ws rats. The aneurism formation was accompanied by accumulation of mast cells, T lymphocytes and by activated MMP-9, reduced elastin levels and augmented angiogenesis in the aortic tissue, but these changes were much less in the Ws/Ws rats than in the controls. Similarly, mast cells were accumulated and activated at the adventitia of aneurysmal aorta in the apolipoprotein E-deficient mice. The pharmacological intervention with the tranilast, an inhibitor of mast cell degranulation, attenuated aneurism development in these rodent models. In the cell culture experiment, a mast cell directly augmented MMP-9 activity produced by the monocyte/macrophage. Collectively, these data suggest that adventitial mast cells play a critical role in the progression of abdominal aortic aneurysm.

6. EOSINOPHILS

Eosinophils are blood circulating granulocytes that have an important role both in the development of allergic inflammation and in the pathophysiology of tissue remodeling [46]. They are key cells in the late stages of allergic inflammation. In several conditions such as asthma, rhinitis, vernal keratoconjunctivitis and atopic dermatitis these cells contribute to the perpetuation of inflammatory process and to the development of tissue remodeling. Eosinophils synthesize and store in their granules several pro-angiogenic mediators such as VEGF [47], FGF-2 [48], TNF-α [49], granulocyte/monocyte-colony stimulating factor (GM-CSF) [50], NGF [51], IL-8 [52], angiogenin [53], and are positively stained for VEGF and FGF-2 in the airways of asthmatic patients [54]. Eosinophils have been shown to release VEGF following stimulation with GM-CSF and IL-5 [50]. In vitro experiments have shown that eosinophils promote endothelial cells proliferation and induce new vessel formation in the aorta rings and in the chick embryo CAM models [54]. Because eosinophils, like mast cells, are a rich source of preformed MMP-9, it is reasonable to believe that they may promote angiogenesis also by acting on matrix degradation.

In the majority of nasal polyps, eosinophils comprise more than 60% of the cell population [55]. Besides eosinophils, mast cells and activated T cells are also increased. An increased production of cytokines/chemokines like GM-CSF, IL-5, RANTES and eotaxin contribute to eosinophil migration and survival. Increased levels of IL-8 can induce neutrophil infiltration. Again, increased expression of VEGF and its upregulation by TGF-β can contribute to the edema and increased angiogenesis in nasal polyps.

Although mouse models of inflammatory skin diseases such as psoriasis and atopic dermatitis fail to completely phenocopy disease in humans, they provide invaluable tools to examine the molecular and cellular mechanisms responsible for the epidermal hyperplasia, inflammation, and excess angiogenesis observed in human disease. Interestingly, treatment of Tie-2 transgenic mice with anti-CD4 antibody appeared to resolve aspects of inflammation but did not resolve epidermal hyperplasia, suggesting an important role for eosinophils in mediating the inflammatory skin disease observed in these mice [56]. Indeed, there were an increased numbers of CD3-positive T lymphocytes in the blood and increased infiltration of eosinophils in the skin associated with a deregulated expression of cytokines associated with Th1 and eosinophil immune responses.

Recently, the 33-amino acid peptide secretoneurin has been shown to potently and specifically attract eosinophils towards a concentration gradient and acts as an angiogenic cytokine comparable in potency to VEGF [57]. Thus, secretoneurin contributes to neurogenic inflammation and might play a role in the (hypoxia-driven) induction of neo-vascularisation in ischemic diseases like peripheral or coronary artery disease, diabetic retinopathia, cerebral ischemia or in solid tumors.

7. MONOCYTES

Sarcoidosis is a systemic granulomatous inflammatory disease characterized by recruitment and activation of peripheral blood mononuclear cells to the sites of disease. Neovascularisation is a principal vascular response in chronic inflammation and hypoxia. It has been shown that sera from sarcoidosis patients enhance angiogenic capability of normal peripheral human mononuclear cells significantly stronger than sera from healthy donors [58]. Angiogenic activity of sera in sarcoidosis depends on the stage of disease and appears most pronounced in stage II. In addition, sera from patients with extrapulmonary changes exert stronger effect on angiogenesis than sera from patients with thoracic changes only. IL-6 and IL-8 serum level correlates with each other, but no correlation is observable between IL-6 and IL-8 serum level and angiogenic activity of the examined sera. Removal of monocytes from peripheral human mononuclear cells eliminates the effect of sera from sarcoidosis patients on angiogenesis compared with the effect of these sera on intact peripheral human mononuclear cells. Sera from sarcoidosis patients and from healthy people constitute a source of mediators participating in angiogenesis. Sera from sarcoidosis patients prime monocytes for production of proangiogenic factors.

There is accumulating evidence that delivery of bone marrow cells to sites of ischemia by direct local injection or mobilization into the blood can stimulate angiogenesis. This has stimulated tremendous interest in the translational potential of angiogenic cell population(s) in the bone marrow to mediate therapeutic angiogenesis. However, the mechanisms by which these cells stimulate angiogenesis are unclear. It has been recently shown that the inflammatory subset of monocytes is selectively mobilized into blood after surgical induction of hindlimb ischemia in mice and is selectively recruited to ischemic muscle [59]. Adoptive-transfer studies show that delivery of a small number of inflammatory monocytes early (within 48 h) of induction of ischemia results in a marked increase in the local production of MCP-1, which in turn, is associated with a secondary, more robust wave of monocyte recruitment. Studies of mice genetically deficient in MCP-1 or CCR2 indicate that although not required for the early recruitment of monocytes, the secondary wave of monocyte recruitment and subsequent stimulation of angiogenesis are dependent on CCR2 signaling. Collectively, these data suggest a novel role for MCP-1 in the inflammatory, angiogenic response to ischemia.

It has recently been demonstrated that healing of myocardial infarction requires monocytes/macrophages. These mononuclear phagocytes likely degrade released macromolecules and aid in scavenging of dead cardiomyocytes, while mediating aspects of granulation tissue formation and remodeling. It has also been recognized that distinct monocyte subsets contribute in specific ways to myocardial ischemic injury in mouse myocardial infarction. Two distinct phases of monocyte participation after myocardial infarction have been identified [60]. Infarcted hearts modulate their chemokine expression profile over time, and they sequentially and actively recruit Ly-6C(hi) and -6C(lo) monocytes via CCR2 and CX(3)CR1, respectively. Ly-6C(hi) monocytes dominate early (phase I) and exhibit phagocytic, proteolytic, and inflammatory functions. Ly-6C(lo) monocytes dominate later (phase II), have attenuated inflammatory properties, and express vascular-endothelial growth factor. Consequently, Ly-6C(hi) monocytes digest damaged tissue, whereas Ly-6C(lo) monocytes promote healing via myofibroblast accumulation, angiogenesis, and deposition of collagen. Myocardial infarction in atherosclerotic mice with chronic Ly-6C(hi) monocytosis results in impaired healing, underscoring the need for a balanced and coordinated response.

A role for inflammation in modulating the extent of angiogenesis has been shown for systemic angiogenesis of the lung after left pulmonary artery ligation in a mouse model of chronic pulmonary thromboembolism. Depletion of neutrophils do not alter the angiogenic outcome, but blood flow to the left lung is significantly reduced after dexamethasone (general anti-inflammatory) treatment compared with untreated control left pulmonary artery ligation mice and significantly increased in T/B lymphocyte-deficient mice [61]. Adoptive transfer of splenocytes (T/B lymphocytes) significantly reverses the degree of angiogenesis observed in the Rag-1(-/-) (T/B lymphocyte deficient) mice back to the level of control left pulmonary artery ligation. These findings indicate that inflammatory cells modulate the degree of angiogenesis in this lung model where lymphocytes appear to limit the degree of neovascularization, whereas monocytes/macrophages likely promote angiogenesis.

It has also shown that shear stress regulates the angiogenic potential of endothelial cells in vitro by an Angiopoietin-2 (Ang-2)-dependent mechanism [62]. The pathophysiological significance of this mechanism in vivo has been clarified in that Ang-2 plays an important role in blood flow recovery after arterial occlusion by regulating angiogenesis and arteriogenesis. In fact, C57Bl/6J mice subjected to femoral artery ligation and injected with a specific Ang-2 inhibitor, L1-10, show a blunted blood flow recovery. L1-10, indeed, decreases smooth muscle cell coverage of neovessels without affecting capillary density, suggesting a specific role for Ang-2 in arteriogenesis. Ang-2 likely operates through monocyte activation. L1-10 decreases expression of intercellular and vascular cell adhesion molecules as well as infiltrating monocytes/macrophages in the ischemic tissue. Although L1-10 has no effect on the number of CD11b+ cells (monocytes/macrophages) mobilized in the bone marrow, it maintains elevated numbers of circulating CD11b+ cells in the peripheral blood. Thus, these results suggest that Ang-2 induces in ischemic tissue plays a critical role in blood flow recovery by stimulating inflammation and arteriogenesis.

Monocytes are one of the initial cell types to be recruited to a wound, in the context of fibrin clot invasion. Recent evidence has indicated additional involvement of Ang-2 in vascular homeostatic responses such as coagulation and inflammation, which are central to wound healing. Ang-2 significantly increased monocyte invasion of fibrin in the presence of serum. In the absence of serum, it required a combination of Ang-2 and platelet-derived growth factor BB (PDGF-BB) to increase invasion by threefold. Furthermore, it was shown that the heightened invasion was dependent on serine proteases and MMPs and that the combination of Ang-2 and PDGF-BB increased urokinase plasminogen-activator receptor expression, as well as MMP-9 and membrane type 1 MMP expression. These data give further credence to the concept of Ang-2 as a key regulator of several essential phases of wound healing [63].

Monocyte-macrophage activation by interferon (IFN)-γ is a key initiating event in inflammation. Usually, the macrophage response is self-limiting and inflammation resolves. A mechanism has been described by which IFN-γ contributes to inflammation resolution by suppressing expression of VEGF-A [64]. Although IFN-γ induced persistent VEGF-A mRNA expression, translation is suppressed by delayed binding of the IFN-γ-activated inhibitor of translation complex to a specific element delineated in the 3'UTR. Translational silencing results in decreased VEGF-A synthesis and angiogenic activity. In addition, it contributes to inflammation resolution.

Angiogenesis and inflammation are important features in atherosclerotic plaque destabilization. In this context, the transcription factor hypoxia-inducible factor (HIF)-1α is a key regulator of angiogenesis and is also involved in inflammatory reactions. It has recently been shown that in atherosclerotic plaque, the transcription factor HIF-1α is associated with an atheromatous inflammatory plaque phenotype and with VEGF expression [65]. Remarkably, HIF-1α expression is upregulated in activated macrophages under normoxic conditions.

Another study directly demonstrates hypoxia in advanced human atherosclerosis and its correlation with the presence of macrophages and the expression of HIF and VEGF [66]. Also, the HIF pathway was associated with lesion progression and angiogenesis, suggesting its involvement in the response to hypoxia and the regulation of human intraplaque angiogenesis.

8. CONCLUSIONS

This review summarizes the most recent experimental and clinical data providing evidence for the involvement of inflammatory cells in flogistic angiogenesis. The cross-talk between the different inflammatory cells and the structural tissue cells establishes a definite micro-environment, which promote the growth, migration and activation of endothelial cells leading to expansion of the pre-existing vascular supply. This process is the result of a complex balance between pro- and anti-angiogenic stimuli generated locally in the tissue milieu. Manipulating this mediators' puzzle by potentiating the local production of anti-angiogenic cytokines would allow to modulate and even inhibit the angiogenic process. Given the detrimental effects pro-angiogenic molecules may exert in chronic inflammation and cancer, it seems of primary importance to understand the contribution of inflammatory cells to normal and pathological angiogenesis.

9. ACKNOWLEDGMENTS

This work has been supported by local funds and PRIN 2007 from Ministero dell'Istruzione, dell'Università e della Ricerca, Rome to the Department of Medical and Morphological Research, Anatomy Section, University of Udine to EC and DR, and by Fondazione Cassa di Risparmio di Puglia, Bari, Italy, to DR .

10. REFERENCES

1. Risau W. Mechanisms of angiogenesis. Nature 1997; 386(6626): 671-674.
2. Ribatti D. Genetic and epigenetic mechanisms in the early development of the vascular system. J Anat 2006; 208(2): 139-152.
3. Kurz H, Burri PH, Djonov D. Angiogenesis and vascular remodeling by intussusception: from form to function. News Physiol Sci 2002; 18: 65-70.
4. Puxeddu I, Ribatti D, Crivellato E, Levi-Schaffer F. Mast cells and eosinophils: a novel link between inflammation and angiogenesis in allergic diseases. J Allergy Clin Immunol 2005; 116(3): 531-536.
5. Robinson CJ, Stringer SE. The splice variants of vascular endothelial growth factor (VEGF) and their receptors. J Cell Sci 2001; 114(5): 853-865.
6. Teige I, Hvid H, Svensson L, Kvist PH, Kemp K. Regulatory T Cells Control VEGF-Dependent Skin Inflammation. J Invest Dermatol 2008 (in press).
7. Szekanecz Z, Koch AE. Vascular involvement in rheumatic diseases: 'vascular rheumatology'. Arthritis Res Ther 2008; 10(5): 224.
8. Chidlow JH, Shukla D, Grisham MB, Kevil CG. Pathogenic angiogenesis in IBD and experimental colitis: new ideas and therapeutic avenues. Am J Physiol Gastrointest Liver Physiol 2007; 293(1): 5-18.
9. Scaldaferri F, Vetrano S, Sans M, Arena V, Straface G, Stigliano E, Repici A, Sturm A, Malesi A, Panes J, Yla-Herttuala S, Fiocchi C, Silvio D. VEGF-A links angiogenesis and inflammation in inflammatory bowel disease pathogenesis. Gastroenterology 2009; 136(2): 585-595.
10. Witmer AN, Vrensen GF, Van Noorden CJ, Schlingemann RO. Vascular endothelial growth factors and angiogenesis in eye disease. Prog Retin Eye Res 2003; 22(1): 1-29.
11. Vezzani A. VEGF as a target for neuroprotection. Epilepsy Curr 2008; 8(5); 135-137.
12. Dubravec DB, Spriggs DR, Mannick JA, Rodrick ML. Circulating human peripheral blood granulocytes synthesize and secrete tumor necrosis factor alpha. Proc Natl Acad Sci USA 1990; 87(17); 6758-6761.
13. Bazzoni F, Cassatella MA, Rossi F, Ceska M, Dewald B., Baggiolini M. Phagocytosing neutrophils produce and release high amounts of the neutrophil-activating peptide 1/interleukin 8. J Exp Med 1991; 173(3): 771-774.
14. Grenier A, Chollet-Martin S, Crestani B, Izumi H, Ishibashi T, Suzuki H, Kuwano M. Presence of a mobilizable intracellular pool of hepatocyte growth

factor in human polymorphonuclear neutrophils. Blood 2002; 99(8): 2997-3004.

15.   Schruefer R, Sulyok S, Schymeinsky J, Peters T, Scharffetter-Kochanek K, Walzog B. The proangiogenic capacity of polymorphonuclear neutrophils delineated by microarray technique and by measurement of neovascularization in wounded skin of CD18-deficient mice. J Vasc Res 2006; 43(1): 1-11.

16.   Ancelin M, Chollet-Martin S, Herve MA, Legrand C, El Benna J, Perrot-Applant M. Vascular endothelial growth factor VEGF189 induces human neutrophil chemotaxis in extravascular tissue via an autocrine amplification mechanism. Lab Invest 2004; 84(4)502-512.

17.   Ohki Y, Heissig B, Sato Y, Akiyama H, Zhu Z, Hicklin DJ, Shimada K, Ogawa H, Daida H, Hattori K, Ohsaka A. Granulocyte colony-stimulating factor promotes neovascularization by releasing vascular endothelial growth factor from neutrophils. FASEB J 2005; 19(14): 2005-2007.

18.   Calcalano G, Lee J, Kikly K, Ryan AM, Pitts-Meek S, Hultgren B, Wood WI, Moore MW. Neutrophil and B cell expansion in mice that lack the murine IL-8 receptor homolog. Science 1994; 265(5172): 682-684.

19.   Devalaraja RM, Nanney LB, Qian Q, Du J, Yu Y, Devalaraja MN, Richmond A. Delayed wound healing in CXCR2 knockout mice. J Invest Dermatol 2000; 115(2): 234-244.

20.   Pessler F, Dai L, Diaz-Torne C, Ogdie A, Gomez-Vaquero C, Paessler ME, Einhorn E, Chen LX, Schumacher HR. Increased angiogenesis and cellular proliferation as hallmarks of the synovium in chronic septic arthritis. Arthritis Rheum 2008; 59(8): 1137-1146.

21.   Ardi VC, Kuptiyanova TA, Deryugina EI, Quigley JP. Human neutrophils uniquely release TIMP-free MMP-9 to provide a potent catalytic stimulator of angiogenesis. Proc Natl Acad Sci USA 2007; 104(51): 20262-20267.

22.   Ai S, Cheng XW, Inoue A, Nakamura K, Okumura K, Iguchi A, Murohara T, Kuzuya M. Angiogenic activity of bFGF and VEGF suppressed by proteolytic cleavage by neutrophil elastase. Biochem Biophys Res Commmun 2008; 364(2): 395-401.

23.   Leonard S, Murrant C, Tayade C, van den Heuvel M, Watering R, Croy BA. Mechanisms regulating immune cell contributions to spiral artery modification - facts and hypotheses. Placenta 2006; 27(Suppl A): S40-46.

24.   Aurora AB, Baluk P, Zhang D, Sidhu SS, Dolganov GM, Basbaum C, McDonald DM, Killen N. Immune complex-dependent remodeling of the airway vasculature in response to a chronic bacterial infection. J Immunol 2005; 175(10): 6319-6326.

25.   Bochner BS, Charlesworth EN, Lichtenstein LM, Derse CP, Gillis S, Dinarello CA, Schleimer RP. Interleukin-1 is released at sites of human cutaneous allergic reactions. J Allergy Clin Immunol 1990: 86(6): 830-839.

26.   Bradding P, Feather IH, Wilson S, Bardin PG, Heusser CH, Holgate ST, Howard PH. Immunolocalization of cytokines in the nasal mucosa of normal and perennial rhinitic subjects. The mast cell as a source of IL-4, IL-5, and IL-6 in human allergic mucosal inflammation. J Immunol 1993; 151(7): 3853-3865.

27.   Heidenreich R, Röcken M, Ghoreschi K. Angiogenesis: the new potential target for the therapy of psoriasis? Drug News Perspect 2008; 21(2): 97-105.

28.   Teige I, Hvid H, Svensson L, Kvist PH, Kemp K. Regulatory T Cells Control VEGF-Dependent Skin Inflammation. J Invest Dermatol 2008 (in press).

29.   Metcalfe DD, Baram D, Mekori YA. Mast cells. Physiol Rev 1997; 77(4): 1033-1079.

30.   Qu Z, Liebler JM, Powers MR, Galey T, Ahmadi P, Huang XN, Ansel JC, Butterfield JH, Planck SR, Rosenbaum JT. Mast cells are a major source of basic fibroblast growth factor in chronic inflammation and cutaneous hemangioma. Am J Pathol 1995; 147(3): 547-573.

31.   Grutzkau A, Kruger-Krasagakes S, Baumesteir H, Schwarz C, Kogel H, Welker P, Lippert U, Henz BM, Moller A. Synthesis, storage, and release of vascular endothelial growth factor/vascular permeability factor (VEGF/VPF) by human mast cells: implications for the biological significance of VEGF206. Mol Biol Cell 1998; 9(4): 875-884.

32.   Abdel-Majid RM, Marshall JS. Prostaglandin E2 induces degranulation-independent production of vascular endothelial growth factor by human mast cells. J Immunol 2004; 172(2): 1227-1236.

33.   Ribatti D, Crivellato E, Candussio L, Nico B, Vacca A, Roncali L, Dammacco F. Mast cells and their secretory granules are angiogenic in the chick embryo chorioallantoic membrane. Clin Exp Allergy 2001; 31(4): 602-608.

34.   Norrby K. Angiogenesis: new aspects relating to its initiation and control. APMIS 1997; 105(6): 417-437.

35.   Ribatti D, Roncali L, Nico B, Bertossi M. Effects of exogenous heparin on the vasculogenesis of the chorioallantoic membrane. Acta Anat (Basel) 1987; 130(3): 257-263.

36.   Möller A, Lippert U, Lessmann D, Kolde G, Hamann K, Welker P, Schadendorf D, Rosenbach T, Luger T, Czarnetzki BM. Human mast cells produce IL-8. J Immunol 1993; 151(6): 3261-3266.

37.   Walsh LJ, Trinchieri G, Waldorf HA, Whiraker D, Murphy GF. Human dermal mast cells contain and release tumor necrosis factor alpha, which induces endothelial leukocyte adhesion molecule 1. Proc Natl Acad Sci USA 1991; 88(10): 4220-4224.

38.   Nilsson G, Forsberg-Nilsson K, Xiang Z, Hallbook F, Nilsson K, Metcalfe DD. Human mast cells express functional TrkA and are a source of nerve growth factor. Eur J Immunol 1997; 27(9): 2295-2301.

39.   Aoki M, Pawankar R, Niimi Y, Kawana S. Mast cells in basal cell carcinoma express VEGF, IL-8 and RANTES. Int Arch Allergy Immunol 2003; 130(3): 216-223.

40.   Nakayama T, Mutsuga N, Yao L, Tosato G. Prostaglandin E2 promotes degranulation-independent release of MCP-1 from mast cells. J Leukoc Biol 2006; 79(1): 95-104.

41. Ren G, Dewald O, Frangogiannis NG. Inflammatory mechanisms in myocardial infarction. Curr Drug Targets Inflamm Allergy 2003; 2(3): 242-256.

42. Aroni K, Tsagroni E, Kavantzas N, Patsouris E, Ioannidis E. A study of the pathogenesis of rosacea: how angiogenesis and mast cells may participate in a complex multifactorial process. Arch Dermatol Res 2008; 300(3): 125-131.

43. Groneberg DA, Bester C, Grützkau A, Serowka F, Fischer A, Henz BM, Welker P. Mast cells and vasculature in atopic dermatitis--potential stimulus of neoangiogenesis. Allergy 2005; 60(1): 90-97.

44. Eklund KK. Mast cells in the pathogenesis of rheumatic diseases and as potential targets for anti-rheumatic therapy. Immunol Rev 2007; 217: 38-52.

45. Tsuruda T, Kato J, Hatakeyama K, Kojima K, Yano M, Nakamura K, Nakamura-Uchiyama F, MatsushimaY, Imamura T, Onitsuka T, Asada Y, Nawa Y, Eto T, Kitamuta K. Adventitial mast cells contribute to pathogenesis in the progression of abdominal aortic aneurysm. Cric Res 2008; 102(11): 1368-1377.

46. Munitz A, Levi-Schaffer F. Eosinophils: 'new' roles for 'old' cells. Allergy 2004; 59(3): 268-275.

47. Horiuchi T, Weller PF. Expression of vascular endothelial growth factor by human eosinophils: upregulation by granulocyte macrophage colony-stimulating factor and interleukin-5. Am J Respir Cell Mol Biol 1997; 17(1): 70-77.

48. Hoshino M, Takahashi M, Aoike N. Expression of vascular endothelial growth factor, basic fibroblast growth factor, and angiogenin immunoreactivity in asthmatic airways and its relationship to angiogenesis. J Allergy Clin Immunol 2001; 107(2): 295-301.

49. Wong DT, Weller PF, Galli SJ, Elovic A, Rand TH, Gallagher GT, Chiang T, Chou MY, Matossian K, McBride J, Todd R. Human eosinophils express transforming growth factor alpha. J Exp Med 1990; 172(3): 673-681.

50. Kita H, Ohnishi T, Okubo Y, Weiler D, Abrams JS, Gleich GJ. Granulocyte/macrophage colony-stimulating factor and interleukin 3 release from human peripheral blood eosinophils and neutrophils. J Exp Med 1991; 174(3): 745-748.

51. Solomon A, Aloe L, Pe'er J, Frucht-Pery J, Bonini S, Levi-Schaffer F. Nerve growth factor is preformed in and activates human peripheral blood eosinophils. J Allergy Clin Immunol 1998; 102(3): 454-460.

52. Yousefi S, Hemmann S, Weber M, Holzer C, Hartung K, Blaser K, Simon HU. IL-8 is expressed by human peripheral blood eosinophils. Evidence for increased secretion in asthma. J Immunol 1995; 154(10): 5481-5490.

53. Barry Kay A, Phipps S, Robinson DS. A role for eosinophils in airway remodelling in asthma. Trends Immunol 2004; 25(9): 477-482.

54. Puxeddu I, Alian A, Piliponsky AM, Ribatti D, Panet A, Levi-Schaffer F. Human peripheral blood eosinophils induce angiogenesis. Int J Biochem Cell Biol 2005; 37(3): 628-636.

55. Pawankar R. Nasal polyposis: an update. Curr Opin Allergy Clin Immunol 2003; 3(1): 1-6.

56. Voskas D, Babichev Y, Ling LS, Alami J, Shaked Y, Kerbel RS, Ciruna B, Dumont DJ. An eosinophil immune response characterizes the inflammatory skin disease observed in Tie-2 transgenic mice. J Leukoc Biol 2008; 84(1): 59-67.

57. Fischer-Colbrie R, Kirchmair R, Kähler CM, Wiedermann CJ, Saria A. Secretoneurin: a new player in angiogenesis and chemotaxis linking nerves, blood vessels and the immune system. Curr Protein Pept Sci 2005; 6(4): 373-385.

58. Zielonka TM, Demkow U, Bialas B, Filewska M, Zycinska K, Radzikowska E, Szopinski J, Skopinska-Rozewska E. Modulatory effect of sera from sarcoidosis patients on mononuclear cell-induced angiogenesis. J Physiol Pharmacol 2007; 58(Suppl 5): 753-766.

59. Capoccia BJ, Gregory AD, Link DC. Recruitment of the inflammatory subset of monocytes to sites of ischemia induces angiogenesis in a monocyte chemoattractant protein-1-dependent fashion. J Leukoc Biol 2008; 84(3): 760-768.

60. Nahrendorf M, Swirski FK, Aikawa E, Stangenberg L, Wurdinger T, Figueiredo JL, Libby P, Weissleder R, Pittet MJ. The healing myocardium sequentially mobilizes two monocyte subsets with divergent and complementary functions. J Exp Med 2007; 204(12): 3037-3047.

61. Wagner EM, Sanchez J, McClintock JY, Jenkins J, Moldobaeva A. Inflammation and ischemia-induced lung angiogenesis. Am J Physiol Cell. Mol Physiol 2008; 294(2): L351-L357.

62. Tressel SL, Kim H, Ni CW, Chang K, Velasquez-Castano JC, Taylor WR, Yoon YS, Jo H. Angiopoietin-2 stimulates blood flow recovery after femoral artery occlusion by inducing inflammation and arteriogenesis. Arterioscler Thromb Vasc Biol 2008; 28(11): 1989-1995.

63. Bezuidenhout L, Bracher M, Davison G, Zilla P, Davies N. Ang-2 and PDGF-BB cooperatively stimulate human peripheral blood monocyte fibrinolysis. J Leukoc Biol 2007; 81(6): 1496-1503.

64. Ray PS, Fox PL. A post-transcriptional pathway represses monocyte VEGF-A expression and angiogenic activity. EMBO J 2007; 26(14): 3360-3372.

65. Vink A, Schoneveld AH, Lamers D, Houben AJ, van der Groep P, van Diest PJ, Pasterkamp G. HIF-1 alpha expression is associated with an atheromatous inflammatory plaque phenotype and upregulated in activated macrophages. Atherosclerosis 2007; 195(2): e69-e75.

66. Sluimer JC, Gasc JM, van Wanroij JL, Kisters N, Groeneweg G, Sollewijn Gelpke MD, Cleutjens JP, van den Akker LH, Corvol P, Wouters BG, Daemen MJ, Bijnens AP. Hypoxia, hypoxia-inducible transcription factor, and macrophages in human atherosclerotic plaques are correlated with intraplaque angiogenesis. J Am Coll Card 2008; 51(13): 1258-1265.

CHAPTER 5

Thymus and Angiogenesis

Marius Raica and Anca Maria Cimpean

Department of Histology and Molecular Pathology, "Victor Babes" University of Medicine and Pharmacy, 2 Eftimie Murgu Square, Tmisoara, 300041, Romania

Address correspondence to: Dr. Marius Raica, Department of Histology and Molecular Pathology, "Victor Babes" University of Medicine and Pharmacy, 2 Eftimie Murgu Square, Tmisoara, 300041, Romania; Tel: 004-0256204476; E-mail: raica@umft.ro

Abstract: Thymus plays a key role in the development of the immune system of the organism and vasculature seems to be involved in some steps of its development. Few data are available about vasculogenesis/angiogenesis in the thymus in normal and pathological conditions, despite the architecture of the vascular tree being relatively well known. There are some particular models of expression of endothelial cell (EC) markers in the thymus. In normal conditions, CD31 and CD105 are less expressed, opposite to CD34 and factor VIII that stain almost all vessels. The aspect is different in thymoma, where both CD31 and CD105 stain intratumoral blood vessels. Microvessel density significantly increases from normal thymus to thymic involution, myasthenia gravis and thymoma. In the tumor area, most of the vessels are immature or intermediate, and their number and type correlate with progression of thymoma. Proliferative ECs, defined by the co-expression of CD34 and Ki67, were found in high number mainly in high-grade advanced-stage thymoma. Progenitor ECs were not found in the prenatal and normal postnatal thymus, but isolated ECs that co-express AC133 and Tie2 were found in high grade thymoma. Besides ECs and perivascular cells, mast cells seem to be involved in thymus angiogenesis. A strong correlation was found between mast cell number and MVD. Few data are available about the expression of angiogenic factors and their receptors in the thymus. Vascular endothelial growth factor (VEGF) is expressed by epithelial cells of the normal thymus and overexpressed by tumor cells in thymoma B3 and thymic carcinoma. The expression of VEGF correlates with the presence of immature blood vessels and Masaoka clinical stage. VEGF receptors 1 and 2 are also expressed in normal and tumoral thymus. A divergent expression of VEGFR1 and 2 is found during thymoma progression. Other growth factors, like fibroblast growth factor and platelet derived growth factor and their receptors may contribute to angiogenesis in the thymus as they are expressed with different patterns in normal and pathological conditions. Lymphatic vessels seem to be better developed than previously thought, and they were also found in the thymic medulla. On the other hand, D2-40/podoplanin stains a subset of stromal epithelial cells and the corresponding thymoma. Thymus is not only a site for angiogenesis, but also a source for angiogenic factors. From these, it was shown that thymosins are involved not only in thymus but also in systemic angiogenesis.

1. INTRODUCTION

The thymus is a unique organ in the human body that initiates and maintains the normal functioning immune system. Since its development from the endoderm of the third pharyngeal pouch [1] till the late postnatal life, the thymus suffers some significant changes that are globally referred to as physiological involution or atrophy. These changes are more evident after puberty, and after 20-25 years, the general microscopic aspect maybe described as atrophy. An initial depletion in lymphocytes and changes in the arrangement of epithelial cells characterize this process [2].

The general microscopic appearance of the postnatal thymus is characterized by the parenchyma with cortex, containing densely packed lymphocytes, and

medulla with less lymphocytes and more heterogeneous cell population (Fig. **1**). In the medulla reside the typical structures of the thymus known as Hassall's bodies that consist of epithelial cells and scattered S100 positive cells. Hassall's corpuscles are not residual structures because it was demonstrated that epithelial cells secrete thymic stromal lymphopoietin that is crucial for B and T lymphocytes development in the medulla [3, 4]. Interestingly, the thymus medulla seems to arise as a series of clonal islets that aggregate as the thymus matures [5]. The close association of the adult medullary compartment with the vasculature could indicate that blood vessels may have a role in the initial organization of the mature medulla. Medullary epithelium was associated with intermediate size blood vessels, but not with capillaries or large vessels [6]. This effect might be direct by vascular endothelium-derived factors or indirect, in the form of factors carried through the circulation [1].

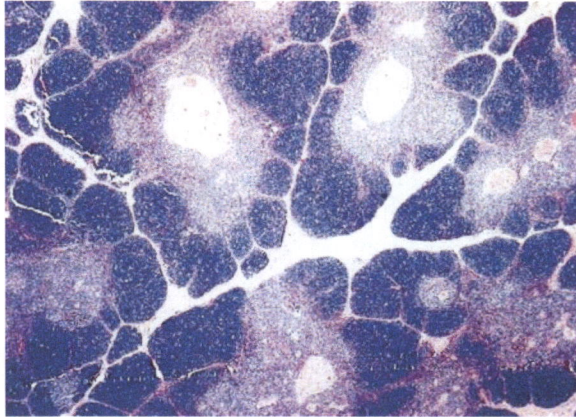

Fig. (1). Architecture of the human postnatal thymus (H&E, x4).

A rich network of epithelial cells is found throughout the cortex and medulla (Fig. **2**) and based on their structure and functions there six different subtypes were described. These cells express mainly basal cytokeratin and were used to propose a histogenetic classification of thymoma [7]. Therefore, the thymus is unique not only in terms of its functions and dramatic changes during physiological involution but also in structure, because it is the only organ in the human body that has an epithelial stroma.

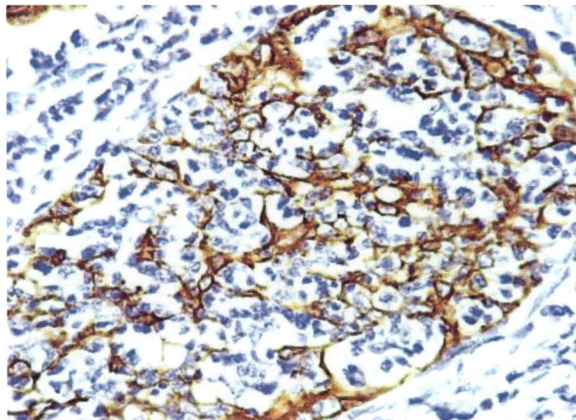

Fig. (2). The network of epithelial cells (cytokeratin, high molecular weight, x400).

Besides lymphocytes and epithelial cells, the medulla consists of a mixture of macrophages, antigen-presenting cells, mast cells, eosinophils (mainly in the interlobular septa in children), scattered myoid and neuroendocrine cells. The functions and behavior of all these cells that form the thymus parenchyma were largely investigated but for some of them, there are still uncertain aspects in human.

The particular development and structure of the thymus is the base for some specific diseases, as developmental abnormalities with associated immunodeficiency, myasthenia gravis and tumors. A broad spectrum of tumors was described in the thymus. Among them, thymoma is the only specific neoplastic proliferation of the organ and consists of proliferating epithelial cells of the stroma. Thymomas are relatively rare tumors with the most elusive histological classification presently and unpredictable behavior. In all the normal and pathologic conditions of the thymus, angiogenesis was significantly less investigated than in other organs. Angiogenesis, the formation of new blood vessels from preexisting, seems to be directly involved in the development and involution of the normal thymus, and in different pathologic conditions. Moreover, the thymus can be considered as a source for proangiogenic molecules.

Of particular interest, mainly in pathology, is the perivascular space (PVS), defined as the tissue found within the capsule but outside the thymic epithelial network [8]. PVS is a virtual space containing only blood vessels in the infant thymus. It becomes more prominent with aging and does not contain developing thymocytes [9]. High endothelial venules can be frequently identified in lymphocyte-rich PVS in both normal thymus and in patients with myasthenia gravis. The recirculation of peripheral lymphocytes was hypothesized through a MECA-79 and L-selectin dependent mechanism [9].

The formation of the blood and efferent lymphatic vessels of the thymus is largely unknown and few data are available about vasculogenesis and angiogenesis in the normal human thymus and its pathologic conditions.

2. BLOOD VESSELS

Arteries of the thymus derive from the internal mammary, superior and inferior thyroid arteries and to a lesser degree the pericardiophrenic arteries [10]. Arterial branches enter the interlobular connective tissue and then in the parenchyma, near the corticomedullary junction. This is why on histological sections, the vessels with the largest lumen of the parenchyma are found at the corticomedullary junction (Fig. **3**). On occasion, in the interlobular area can be found pillow arterioles that regulate the blood flow. Blood vessels of the parenchyma are surrounded by a sheath of connective tissue that gradually becomes thinner in small vessels [11]. Capillaries are found in both cortex and medulla. Capillaries of the cortex descend into the medulla and give rise to postcapillary venules and then interlobular veins. Finally, the venous system drains into the left brachiocephalic, internal thoracic and inferior thyroid veins [10]. Vascular endothelial growth factor (VEGF) secretion by thymic epithelial cells is required for normal vascular architecture of the thymus [12].

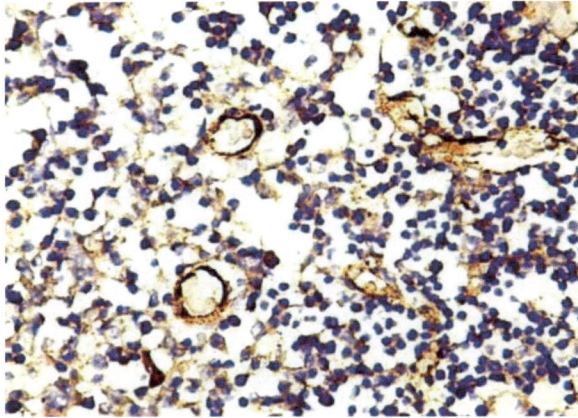

Fig. (3). Normal human thymus. Blood vessels with large lumen near the corticomedullary junction, x200. Immunoreaction for factor VIII.

Endothelial cell (EC) markers: It is difficult to identify blood vessels in the thymus parenchyma on slides stained with haematoxylin-eosin because of the closely packed lymphocytes. In order to evaluate the microvasculature it is necessary to perform immunohistochemistry, using a specific EC marker. Factor VIII seems to be the most specific marker of the ECs in the normal and pathologic thymus (Fig. **4**).

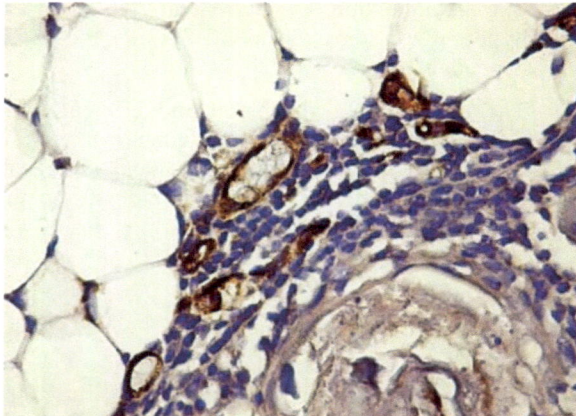

Fig. (4). Involution of the normal human thymus, anti-factor VIII, x400.

CD34 is highly sensitive but less specific. CD31, because of unknown reasons, shows only a weak expression in the interlobular vessels and almost does not stain intralobular blood vessels of the normal thymus (fetal and postnatal, including physiological involution). On the other hand, CD31 strongly stains blood vessels in thymoma, and therefore, it can be used to count vessels (Fig. **5**). CD105 (endoglin) does not stain blood vessels of the fetal and postnatal thymus but becomes positive in scattered vessels in thymoma B3 and thymic carcinoma. Initially, CD105

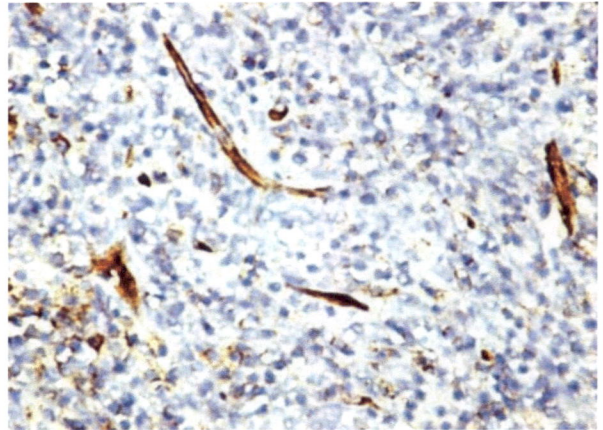

Fig. (5). Thymoma, CD31 expression in ECs, x400.

was thought to identify some tumor blood vessels with activated ECs. This is not completely true, because CD105-positive ECs may be found also in most mature vessels containing a relatively thick sheath of perivascular cells (Fig. **6**). Therefore, CD105 should be used to identify activated ECs but not to perform microvessel density.

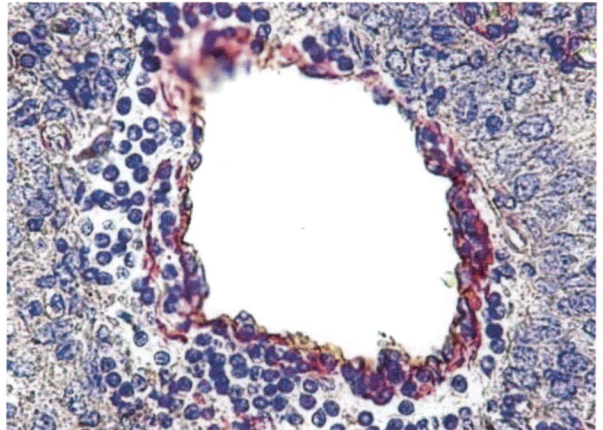

Fig. (6). Mature blood vessels with ECs stained for CD105 (brown) and smooth muscle cell actin (red), x400.

Microvessel density (MVD): MVD was introduced many years ago by *Weidner et al* [13] to evaluate tumor angiogenesis. There were accumulated many data that showed a correlation between MVD, invasion and lymph node and systemic metastasis in many human tumors [14]. On the other hand, MVD reflects the intercapillary distance and present data do not support the use of this parameter as predictor of the response to antiangiogenic therapy. Despite the large interest in this evaluation, few data are available about MVD in the normal counterpart of malignant tumors. In the normal fetal and postnatal thymus till puberty, on slides stained for factor VIII, we found an average of 21.4 blood vessels / x200. MVD significantly increases during thymus involution, and numerous large vessels can be seen at the interface between the remaining thymic tissue and surrounding fat. MVD increases to an average of 33.5 in patients with myasthenia gravis and to 31.8 in patients with thymoma [15]. These results are in contrast with data published by *Tomita et al* [16], which found a decreased MVD in patients with myasthenia gravis. In the tumor area of thymoma, blood vessels are smaller and more irregular than in the normal thymus and many of them lack perivascular cells. In thymoma, MVD does not correlate with the histological type because we found more vessels in type AB and B1 than in B3 but correlates with stage of the tumor, as it also has been shown by others [16]. Very few data are available about MVD in thymoma, and present data showed that in non-invasive thymoma, small blood vessels are predominantly found in the periphery of the tumor, and in invasive thymoma and thymic carcinoma, they are also present in the tumor area [16]. On the other hand, MVD alone is not enough to characterize the angiogenic phenotype of thymoma and thymic carcinoma, and this implies the expression of angiogenic factors and their receptors.

The relationship between MVD and thymoma/thymic carcinoma seems to be a more complex process. In an experimental model on malignant thymic tumor in SV12 transgenic mice expressing SV40 T and t antigens, an extensive development was shown of the vascular network even from the early phase of thymic hyperplasia [17]. A significant increase in the number of CD34/CD31-positive blood vessels and isolated cells was found in the thymic carcinoma and a correlation with VEGFR-2 was found. Based on these data, it was concluded that tumor development is associated with extensive angiogenesis. Unfortunately, this model does not overlap with findings in human tissues, in which VEGF and its receptors are expressed not only by tumor cells, but also by the normal counterpart [18]. The expression of VEGF correlates with previous findings, which showed that VEGF is spatial and temporally related with the remodeling of the large vessels derived from the posterior pharyngeal arches [19]. Moreover, the mice expressing only the 120 amino acid VEGF isoform display athymia, hypoplastic thymus or ectopically located thymus [20]. Additional evidences were found by *Park et al* [21], which showed that high level of VEGF is concomitant with reparative angiogenesis during regeneration that follows acute involution induced by cyclophosphamide in the rat thymus. Other players are also involved in this process, because it was shown that nerve growth factor mediated thymic epithelial induction of VEGF expression *in vivo* and *in vitro*.

Types of vessels in thymoma: Blood vessels in the area of malignant tumors are significantly different from those found in their normal counterpart. According to the structure of their wall, these vessels are classified as immature, intermediate and mature, based on the presence of the lumen, proliferation on

ECs, and perivascular cells [22]. The evaluation of the vessels' type is mainly based on the double immunostaining for EC marker with smooth muscle cell actin and EC marker with Ki67. In the human fetus, few actin-positive vessels were found in the medulla and none in the cortex. In the postnatal thymus the large majority of vessels exhibit covering perivascular cells. We found CD105 positive/smooth muscle cell actin negative blood vessels in the tumor area in invasive thymomas and this reflects in part the active angiogenesis during tumor progression (Fig. **7** and Fig. **8**) *(unpublished)*. On the other hand, immature and intermediate blood vessels are less frequent than mature vessels that correlate with low progression rate of thymoma in the majority of the cases.

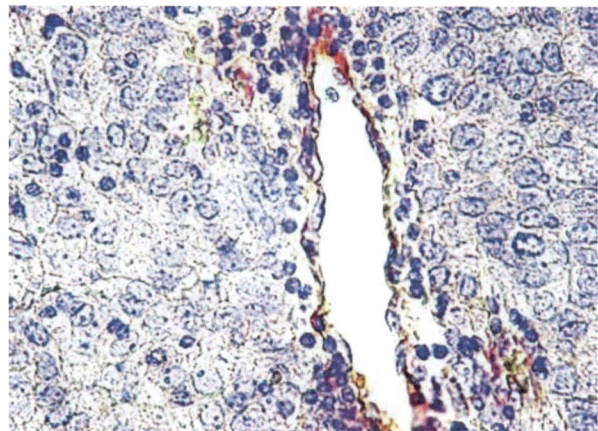

Fig. (7). Intermediate vessel with focal perivascular cells. Double immunostaining CD105 (brown) - smooth muscle actin (red). (x400).

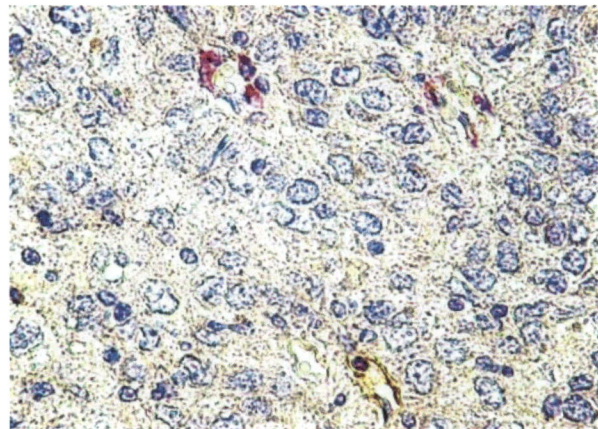

Fig. (8). Small mature vessel positive for smooth muscle actin and immature, positive for CD105. Double immunostaining CD105 (brown)/smooth muscle actin (red). (x400).

Proliferation of endothelial cells: In normal conditions, ECs are quiescent cells with long lifespan and divisions are very rarely seen in usual stained section. During normal and pathological angiogenesis, a significant increase in the rate of proliferation is noticed in ECs mainly of immature and intermediate type. The assessment of the proliferation rate is usually performed using double immunostaining based on an EC marker associated with the expression of the proliferation marker Ki67, but at present, data regarding the application of this method to the normal and pathologic conditions of the thymus have not been published. In a study based on the proliferating cell nuclear antigen (PCNA) performed on other tumors, a high proliferation rate of ECs was found in immature vessels (39 to 69%) and low in mature vessels (12 to 18%) [22], but. PCNA usually overestimates the rate of proliferation. This is why we used double immunostaining with CD34/Ki67, and we found no co-expression of these markers in ECs in the fetal and postnatal normal thymus (Fig. **9**). In high grade advanced-stage thymoma, many vessels in the tumor area showed proliferative activity of ECs (Fig. **10**).

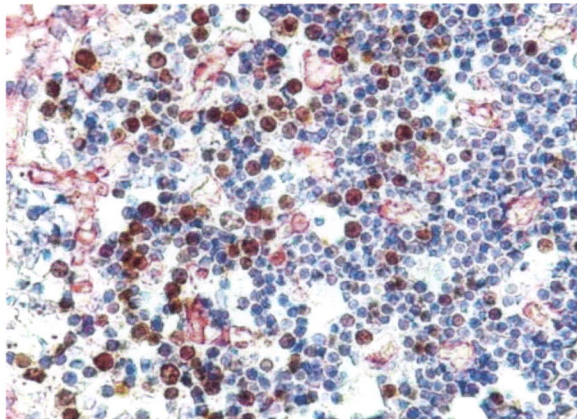

Fig. (9). Double immunostaining Ki67 (brown)/CD34 (red). Normal fetal thymus. Capillaries of the cortex, Ki67 negative ECs, x400.

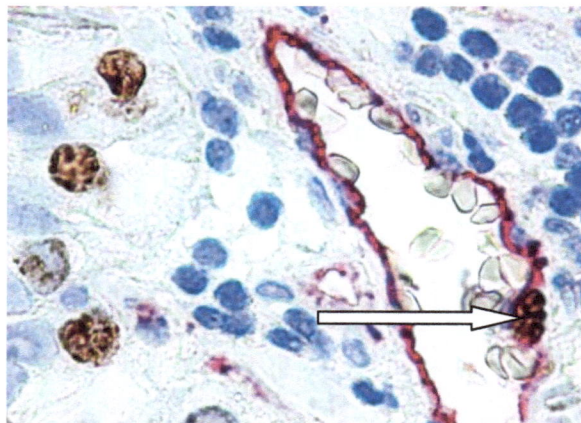

Fig. (10). Thymoma type B2, intermediate vessel with single Ki67-positive EC (arrow), x900.

Ki67 co-expressed with CD34 was found mainly in immature vessels (Fig. **11**), with a lesser degree in intermediate and no co-expression was noticed in mature blood vessels. The high MVD found in low grade thymoma (type A, AB, B1) was not correlated with ECs proliferation. Moreover, we found Ki67 positive ECs only in the tumor area and not in the fibrous connective tissue and perivascular spaces *(unpublished)*.

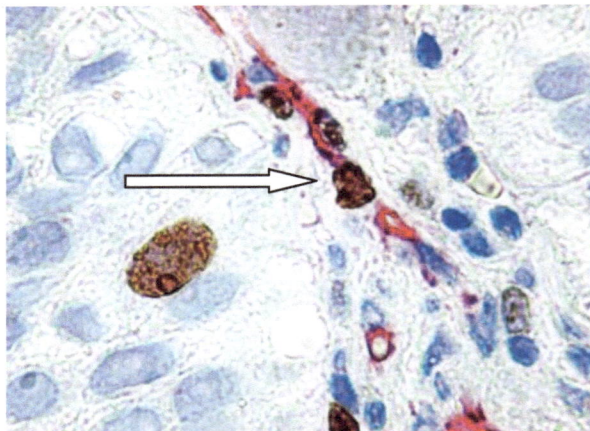

Fig. (11). Immature vessel (arrow) in thymoma B3 with multiple positive nuclei, x900.

Endothelial cell progenitors (EPCs): More than 100 years, it was thought that mesenchymal cells differentiate into angioblasts and then in ECs, exclusively during the prenatal life. In 1997, it was shown that CD34 positive adult hematopoietic progenitor cells can differentiate *ex vivo* in cells with endothelial phenotype [23]. These cells were called endothelial progenitor cells (EPCs), are of bone marrow origin and can be incorporated in the endothelium of newly formed blood vessels [24]. The rate of EPCs' incorporation was investigated in ischemic and tumoral conditions but at present results are still controversial. Moreover, it was shown that circulating mononuclear cells can differentiate into ECs, the existence can be suspected of multiple EPCs [25]. EPCs can be defined based on the co-expression of CD34, AC133, VEGFR2 and Tie2. AC133 seems to be the most specific, because it is expressed in hematopoietic stem cells but not by mature ECs [26]. Controversial data were published about the incorporation of EPCs in tumor blood vessels and a large variability of results was reported for different tumors (between 5 and 70%). Despite this aspect of angiogenesis was investigated in many pathologic conditions, no data are available about the role of EPCs in the thymus-related angiogenesis. We investigated the existence of EPCs in the normal and tumoral thymus using the immunohistochemical expression of AC133, Tie2 and VEGFR2 *(unpublished)*. Their co-localization most probably reflects immature EPCs intercalated in the endothelium. We did not find AC133+/ VEGFR2+/ Tie2+ ECs in the fetal and postnatal normal thymus. This finding could indicate a limited (if any) contribution of EPCs in the development of thymic vasculature in normal conditions. AC133 positive ECs that co-express Tie2 and VEGFR2 were found in thymoma high grade either as isolated or small groups of flat cells located within the endothelial layer (Fig. **12** and Fig. **13**). This observation suggests a significant contribution of EPCs in tumor angiogenesis, and on the other hand, correlates with the proliferation rate found in the same cases *(unpublished)*.

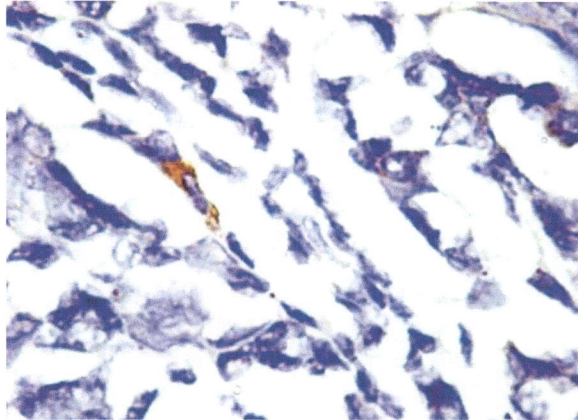

Fig. (12). Thymoma. Single AC133 positive cell, x400.

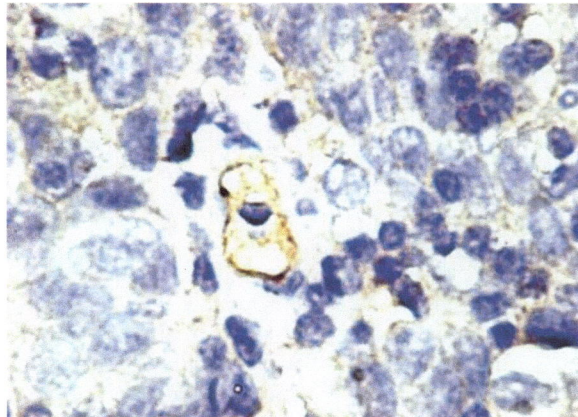

Fig. (13). Small capillary with the entire endothelium stained for AC133. x900.

3. CELL PARTNERS

Macrophages: Macrophages are usually found in the normal thymus and are preferentially located in the deep cortex and medulla. Until now, there are no evidences that could imply macrophages in normal thymus angiogenesis. Many macrophages are found in thymoma, but their number does not correlate with MVD. Based on findings on other human tumors, it is possible that macrophages secrete angiogenic factors, but this aspect remains to be clarified.

Mast cells: Mast cells were found in the thymus many years ago in the interlobular connective tissue, but their functional significance is still unknown. These

cells are involved in angiogenesis by secretion of different cytokines and mainly VEGF [27]. Based on the immunohistochemical expression of mast cell tryptase, we found mast cells in the fetal and postnatal human thymus not only interlobular but also in the medulla (Fig. **14**), but not in the cortex. Usually they are located close to the blood vessels, but in the normal thymus, a correlation was not found between blood vessels and mast cells densities. Only rare mast cells are found in the involution of the thymus, constantly arranged around perivascular spaces (PVS).

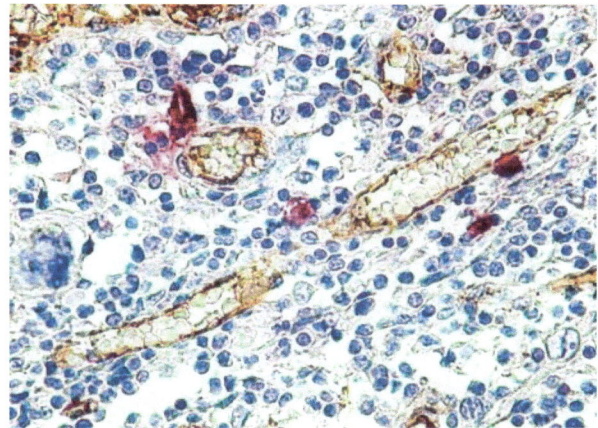

Fig. (14). Fetal human thymus, mast cells (red) and blood vessels (brown) in the medulla. CD34/mast cell tryptase double immunostaining, x400.

A significant increase in the number of intralobular but not interlobular mast cells was found in patients with myasthenia gravis (6.53 mast cells/x400 in the normal thymus versus 21.4 in myasthenia gravis), and this is associated with an increased MVD. Similar data were found in patients with myasthenia gravis with associated thymoma. It can be speculated that myasthenia gravis could stimulate mast cell progenitors that are thought to be present in the thymus [28]. On the other hand, currently there are not convincing data about the presence of mast cell progenitors in the human thymus.

In thymoma, tryptase positive mast cells are found between tumor cells, concentrated at the interface with tumor stroma and usually are rare in the stroma. The mast cell density is significantly higher in thymoma than in the normal thymus, and also their diameter is higher than in normal conditions. Based on a study on 28 cases with thymoma, we found no correlation between mast cell density and MVD on slides with double immunostaining for CD34 and mast cell tryptase. On the other hand, very few mast cells were found in thymoma type A, AB and B1, and in numerous in types B2, B3 and C (see Fig. **15** and **16**). Usually, mast cells were found in high number around and within PVS in low grade thymoma, and mainly between tumor cells in high grade cases. These data support the hypothesis that MCD correlates with histologic classification of thymoma.

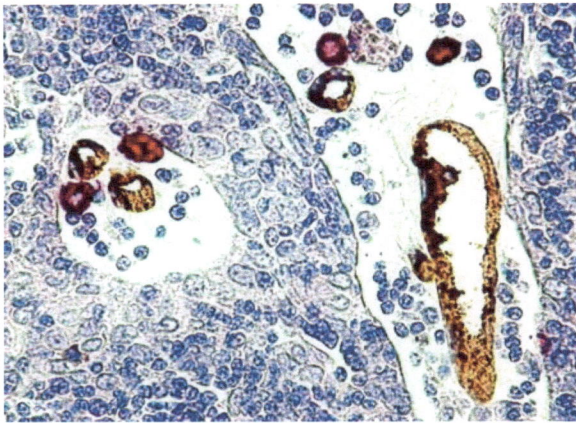

Fig. (15). Mast cells within the perivascular space in low grade thymoma. Double immunostaining CD34/mast cell tryptase, x400.

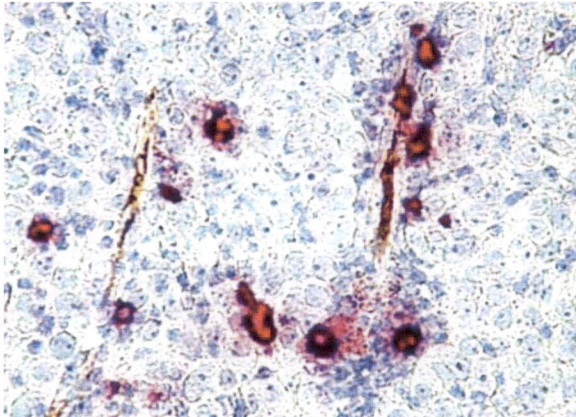

Fig. (16). Accumulation of tryptase positive mast cells in high grade thymoma, Double immunostaining CD34/ mast cell tryptase, x400.

The precise significance of mast cells in the thymus is not known, but it seems that the thymus plays a role in the development of some mast cells, as it was demonstrated many years ago in the athymic mice and interleukin-3 induction [29, 30]. Despite the role of mast cells in thymoma is not clarified, a correlation was found in grade and stage of the tumor. Whether mast cells secrete proangiogenic factors in thymoma remains to be further investigated.

4. GROWTH FACTORS AND THEIR RECEPTORS

The vascular network of the normal thymus consists of branching and anastomosing blood vessels but the molecular basis involved in the formation of the typical vasculature is unknown. In humans, the expression of angiogenesis-associated growth factors in normal and malignant thymic tissues is less investigated.

Vascular endothelial growth factor (VEGF): VEGF-A plays an important role in angiogenesis in normal conditions and its expression is upregulated in many solid tumors. It is involved in wound healing, the reproductive cycle, mechanically induced changes of the cartilage in osteoarthitris [31], and tumor angiogenesis and progression. In tumor microenvironment, an upregulation of both VEGF and its receptors occurs, leading to a high concentration of occupied receptors on tumor vascular endothelium. This growth factor is involved in the development and progression of malignant tumors and represents the only accepted target for the antiangiogenic therapy using humanized monoclonal antibody treatment [32]. VEGF is involved in the development of the normal vascular network of the human thymus. This process depends on the high concentration of VEGF in epithelial cells of the thymus. After birth, the levels of VEGF rapidly decrease in the normal human thymus. In human fetal thymuses aged between 16-22 weeks of gestation, messenger RNA encoding VEGF-A was minimally detected [33]. Stromal epithelial cells of the normal thymus expressed VEGF. Positive reaction was found as a subcapsular network of epithelial cells, isolated epithelial cells in the cortex and weak to moderate in almost all epithelial cells of the thymus medulla. All types of Hassall corpuscles expressed VEGF. For the juvenile type, the reaction was present in the entire corpuscle. The outer cells of the Hassall corpuscles were positive for VEGF with cytoplasmic, granular pattern in the periphery of mature and senescent types previously described by *Raica et al* [4]. In acute thymic involution, the positive islands of epithelial cells were grouped around dilated blood vessels with severe stasis. The positive reaction of epithelial cells for VEGF in this type of involution was correlated with lymphocytes-depleted areas. The thymic tissue from the cords of age-related thymic involution contained few positive cells with weak intensity in the periphery, near the adipose tissue between these cords.

The intensity of reaction was higher in the thymic tissue from patients with myasthenia gravis, with diffuse distribution of positive epithelial cells. This is correlated with high density of blood vessels. There were no differences of expression between thymoma-associated myasthenia gravis and myasthenia gravis without this association. Lymphoid follicles from the medulla also display positive reaction for VEGF. All types of thymomas express VEGF-A. In thymoma type A, the spindle cells are weak to moderately positive for VEGF with diffuse distribution. The same pattern was found in spindle areas from thymoma type AB (Fig. **17**). The majority of neoplastic epithelial cells from B2 thymoma show moderate expression of VEGF that was more intense around perivascular spaces. Type B3 thymoma is characterized by positive reaction in all neoplastic cells with strong, granular

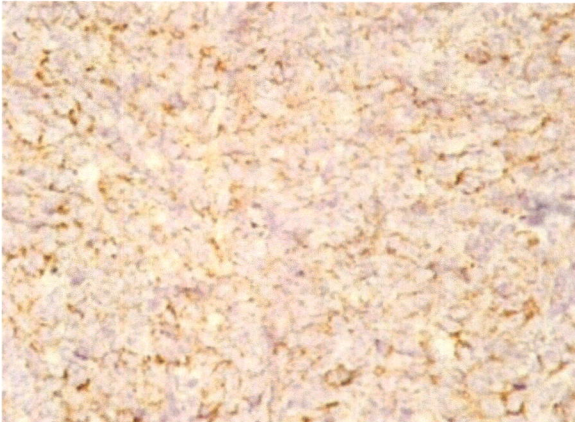

Fig. (17). VEGF expression in thymoma. Spindle positive cells of thymoma type AB, x200.

cytoplasmic pattern (Fig. **18**). It was reported that, focally, the stroma adjacent to the tumor is positive for VEGF, a feature also detected in the endothelium of large vessels around the tumor [18]. In these zones, the highest vessel density was noticed for CD105 compared with other thymomas. The remnant thymus near the type B3 thymoma expresses VEGF with weak intensity, compared with the neoplastic tissue, and has the same pattern like the normal thymus.

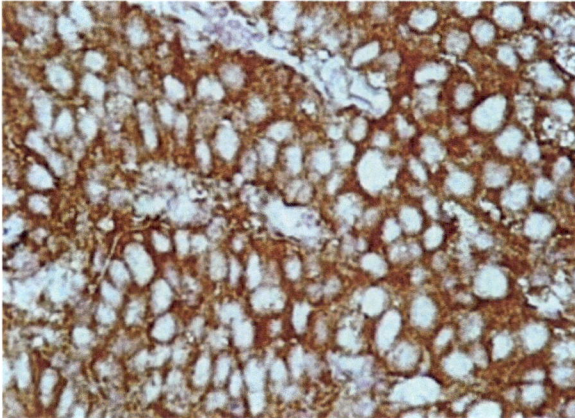

Fig. (18). Strong immunoreaction in all neoplastic cells from thymoma type B3 (x400).

It appears to be a correlation between tumor angiogenesis and the invasiveness in thymomas, with a correlation between microvascular density, VEGF expression, and Masaoka clinical stage [34]. There is a strong correlation between the expression of VEGF in thymomas and the microvascular density calculated on slides stained for CD105. *Cimpean et al* [18] reported a higher microvascular density for CD105 in type B3 thymomas, which had a strong immunoreactivity for VEGF. Expression of such a marker in thymoma could be a target for antiangiogenic therapy focusing on both tumor blood vessels and cells that produce high levels of VEGF. Increased circulating levels of VEGF are found in patients with thymic carcinoma but not

thymomas [35]. A phase II study of Erlotinib plus Bevacizumab given to patients with advanced thymomas and thymic carcinoma is going on in order to determine the objective response rate to this combination. One of the aims of this study is to correlate the expression of VEGF in tumor samples, circulating VCAM1 and urine VEGF levels pre-therapy with the tumor response to therapy. Preliminary data of this study reported at ASCO conference 2008 showed that the combination of Erlotinib and Bevacizumab has only a limited activity in thymic malignancies, but has a well tolerated side effect profile [36].

VEGF B and VEGF C *mRNA* were detected in only one case of thymoma by *Salven et al* [37]. VEGF C shared very low levels of mRNA distribution in thymomas.

VEGF receptors: Normal thymus also expresses VEGFR1 and VEGFR2. All epithelial cells of the medulla are positive for both receptors, with high intensity for VEGFR 1 and weak expression for VEGFR 2. In senescent type of Hassall corpuscles, the peripheral epithelial cells are moderately positive for VEGFR1 and for VEGFR2. Thymic nurse cells from the cortex express VEGFR1 with moderate intensity and also VEGFR2, but weak and inconstantly. Subcapsular epithelial cells were negative for both receptors. Acute thymic involution shared intense positive staining of VEGFR2 in the endothelium of dilated vessels. We also detected the presence of immunostaining in the stromal epithelial cells network of involuted thymus with moderate intensity. VEGFR1 was weakly positive with the same distribution.

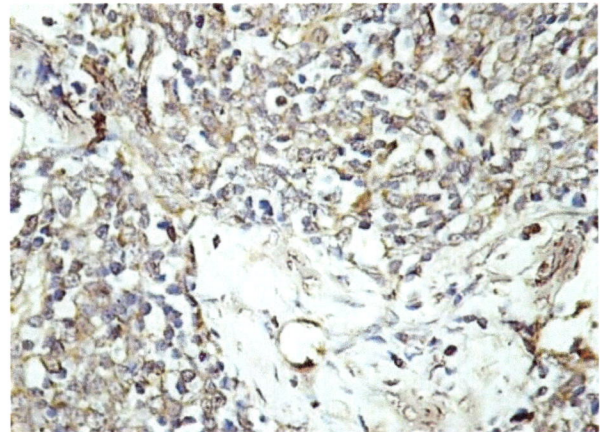

Fig. (19). Weak expression of VEGFR2 in thymoma type AB (x200).

VEGFR1 and VEGFR2 are positive in neoplastic epithelial cells and vessels of endothelium of all thymomas. There are differences in expression of receptors closely linked to the type of thymoma. In type AB thymoma we found an intense staining for VEGFR1 in spindle neoplastic cells from spindle areas, whereas lymphocytes were negative. For VEGFR2, we noticed foci with strong positive staining, which alternate with weakly positive areas (Fig. **19**). Scattered positive cells with macrophage-like morphology were observed in the connective tissue between neoplastic areas. Type B3 thymomas have a divergent expression of VEGFR1 and 2. All thymic epithelial cells are positive for VEGFR1 with the same intensity (Fig. **20**), like VEGF expression. VEGFR2 is positive in type B3 thymoma in scattered epithelial cells with weak intensity. Isolated groups of neoplastic cells showed moderate staining for VEGFR2.

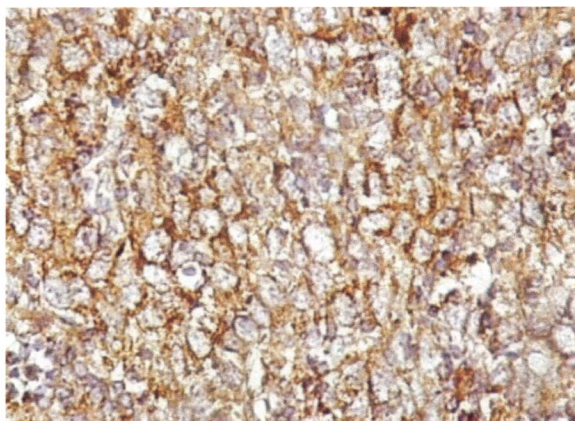

Fig. (20). Strong immunostaining for VEGFR 1 in thymoma type B3 (x400).

Thymomas in mice have been found to recruit stem cells to the vasculature during the initial phase of tumor growth. The stem cells uniformly express the receptor tyrosine kinase VEGFR2 (human homologue KDR; mouse homologue Flk1). Only 25–30% of vessels in thymomas recruit stem cells to the vasculature [38]. Inside the capsule, there are numerous invasive sites of thymoma, which share positivity for both receptors, especially for VEGFR1. Differences between thymoma type, VEGF, VEGFR 1 and 2 expression and vessels count are shown in Table 1.

The pathways through which VEGF/VEGFR1 exert autocrine activity in tumor cells is a topic of further research. In vitro, VEGFR1 activation by VEGF leads to the activation of the mitogen activated protein kinase (MAP kinase) signal transduction pathway in tumor cells [39, 40]. Activation of VEGF receptors in tumor cells leads to phenotypic changes including an increase in cell invasion and migration. Thus, we suggest that type 1 receptor for VEGF might be involved in this process by enhancement of migration and invasion potential of neoplastic thymic epithelial cells. This presumed mechanism of action of the VEGF/VEGFR1 complex could explain the paradoxical behavior of some thymomas which are of low-grade malignancy – type A and AB thymomas –

but share an extensive capsular invasion at the time of diagnosis or recurrent events after surgical treatment and chemotherapy. *Kiseleva et al.* [41] reported that VEGF not only acts as angiogenic factor, but also as an immunoregulatory factor. VEGF modulates proliferation of thymocytes and expression of VEGFR2 mRNA. *Reinders et al.* [42] described the involvement of VEGF in acute rejection of allograft. Taken together with the report of *Watanabe et al.* [3], these data support our findings concerning the positive reaction of Hassall's corpuscles cells for VEGF and its receptors. The VEGF receptors positive Hassall's corpuscles found in the normal thymus together with a strong reaction of the medulla thymic epithelial cells could be linked to the lymphocyte maturation and migration from the cortex.

Fibroblast growth factors (FGFs) and specific receptors: FGFs are a family of growth factors that can have effects on both cell proliferation and differentiation. Convincing evidences involve some members of the FGF family (FGF 7, 8, 10) in the development of the thymus stroma [43]. Initial development of the thymic bud and final positioning of the human thymus require interaction between FGF 7, 8, 10 and FGFR2IIIb [1]. In the thymus, intense FGFR1 positive reaction was seen in epithelial cells, Hassall's corpuscles, and the endothelium and smooth muscle cells of blood vessels. Expression of FGFR2, FGFR3, and FGFR4 was seen predominantly in the thymic vasculature [44]. *Tomita et al.* [16] reported cytoplasmic expression of bFGF in tumor cells from noninvasive and invasive thymoma and also from thymic carcinoma. They found positive reaction in only 8 cases from a total of 46 patients with a prevalence of FGF staining in tumor cells from invasive thymomas. Also, they found a significant correlation between bFGF expression and microvessel density assessed by FVIII related antigen. Only 3 from 8 cases of thymic carcinoma expressed bFGF [45] but with higher intensity compared with invasive thymomas. Serum VEGF and basic FGF have been noted to be elevated as compared with both normal controls and patients with thymoma, and this could be an interesting test to discriminate between thymoma and thymic carcinoma [35]. Our studies concerning immunohistochemical expression of FGFR3 in thymomas and thymic carcinomas showed an interesting distribution of membrane positive reaction, restricted only to tumor cells from type B2 and B3 thymomas (Fig. **21**). This distribution is correlated with higher microvessel density on CD105 stained slides.

PDGF AB and BB isoforms: In fetal developing human thymus aged at 28 weeks of gestation, expression of PDGF is restricted to the media of mature vessels from thymic capsule and also from connective tissue septa that impart lobulation of the organ. The vessels from thymus parenchyma are negative for this marker. In epithelial cells from thymic stroma, the expression of PDGF was observed only in the medulla of the fetal thymus. An intense staining for PDGF was also found in the peripheral epithelial cells of Hassall's corpuscles.

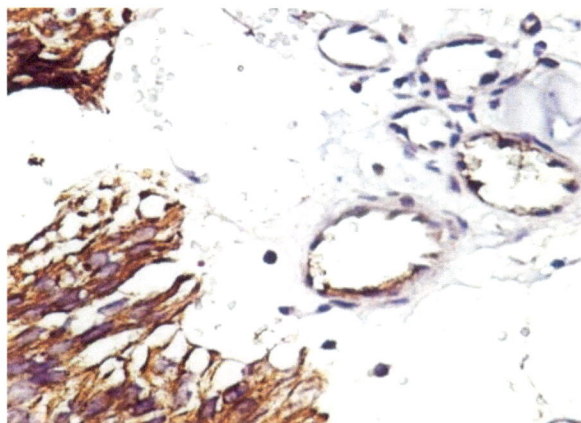

Fig. (21). All tumor cells from type B3 thymoma express FGFR3. Note that adjacent blood vessels endothelium has an intense staining for the same marker (x400).

In neoplastic lesions of the thymus, variability of positive reaction depends on thymomas type. Isolated positive vessels were observed in type AB thymomas with wide distribution. In type B1 thymoma, positive vessels tend to be grouped at the periphery of the tumor. Weak expression in tumor cells around perivascular spaces (PVS) combined with intense expression of PDGF in vessels from all PVS characterizes type B2 thymomas. Type B3 thymomas intensely express PDGF in epithelial tumor cells and also in the media of intratumoral blood vessels (Fig. **22**). Recently, *Korpisalo et al.* [46] reported in an animal model that VEGF-A and PDGF-B combination gene therapy prolongs angiogenic effects via recruitment of interstitial mononuclear cells and paracrine effects rather than improved pericyte coverage of angiogenic vessels. Type B3 thymomas express VEGF and PDGF B with high intensity and this features together with high MVD for CD105 could explain the refractory behavior and also a high incidence of recurrence for type B3 thymomas.

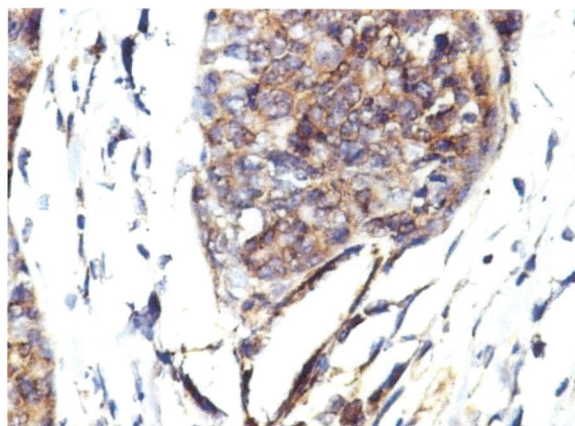

Fig. (22). Strong PDGF expression in both endothelial and tumor cells from type B3 thymoma (x400).

A Phase I pilot study of Gleevec (Imatinib) as treatment for advanced thymic carcinoma is ongoing, and this study is important to demonstrate if single agent activity is useful for patients with thymic tumors overexpressing c-kit and/or PDGF. If this current trial will be positive, it will open the door to evaluate other combinations of drugs with imatinib in thymic tumors. Table **1** summarizes the expression of mentioned growth factors together with MVD assessed for two vascular markers.

Few data are available about the involvement of growth factors in angiogenesis of thymic tumors. *Kuhn et al* [47] included VEGF and bFGF as certified molecular factors involved in a potent angiogenic activity associated with invasiveness in thymomas and thymic carcinomas. Increased levels of both serum VEGF and bFGF have been found in patients with thymic carcinomas but not thymomas.

Table 1. Comparative expression of VEGF, VEGFR1, VEGFR2, PDGF-b, and FGFR3 in thymoma and median range of microvascular density for CD34 and endoglin

Thymoma	A	AB	B2	B3
VEGF	+/++	+/++	++	+++
VEGFR1	+++	+++	+++	+++
VEGFR2	+	+	++	+/++
PDGF-B	+VM	+VM	++VM +TC	+++ vessels, TC
FGFR3	N	N	+++	+++
CD34	48	53.6	44.2	53
Cd105	20	20.8	24.2	44.8

Legend: +, weak positive; ++, moderate positive; +++, intense positive; VM= vessel media, TC= tumor cells, PVS= perivascular space, N=negative

5. LYMPHATIC VESSELS

Lymphatic vessels in the thymus have been investigated by light microscopy, electron microscopy, or a dye-injection method. New insights were given after the introduction of highly specific lymphatic endothelial cells (LECs) markers. Earlier investigators reported lymphatics in the capsule and interlobular connective tissue of the thymus [48, 49], and then in the medulla [50]. 5'-nucleotidase-positive vessels are sometimes seen in the vicinity of perivascular spaces [51, 52, 53]. The opening of the perivascular spaces into the lymphatics suggests their involvement in the transport of thymocytes and interdigitating cells in the systemic circulation.

Development of the lymphatic vessels in the thymus could be based on the VEGF-C/D and VEGFR-3 interaction. LECs produce secondary lymphoid tissue chemokine (also called Exodus-2 or CCL-21) [54, 55]. Moreover, VEGF-C binds to a nonkinase receptor neuropilin-2 [56] that is restricted to veins and lymphatics. *Yuan et al* [57] showed that neuropilin-2-defficient mouse is characterized by impeded development of lymphatic capillaries. In the mice, VEGFR-3/LYVE-1 positive vessels were found in the capsule and cortex and only rarely in the medulla, forming small plexuses or nests [53]. Some vessels were found in continuity with the capsule of the extralobular connective tissue. In an experimental model on non-obese diabetic mice, it was found that lymphatic vessels are mainly present in the corticomedullary boundary and in the proximity of the postcapillary venules [58]. These recent findings that demonstrate the presence of lymphatics in all compartments of the thymus of the mice are in contrast with previous data, which postulated the restriction of these vessels to the medulla.

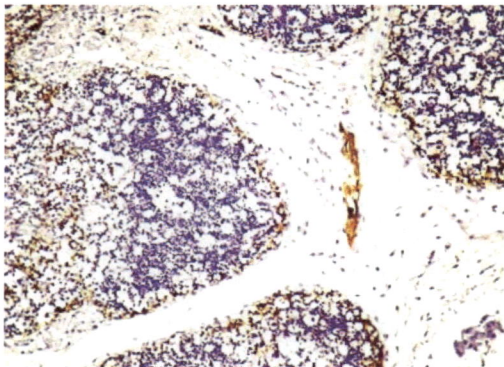

Fig. (23). Human fetal thymus, lymphatic vessel in the interlobular connective tissue, D2-40 staining, x100.

In the developing human thymus, stained with D2-40, the immunohistochemical reaction showed definite lymphatic vessels only in the medulla and interlobular connective tissue (Fig. **23**). This marker, otherwise specific for LECs, is also positive in subcapsular and a subset of medullary epithelial cells of the thymus, which renders difficult the observation of small vessels (Fig. **24**). In thymoma, lymphatic vessels are found in the fibrous connective tissue, sometimes

filled with lymphocytes and occasionally in the tumor area (Fig. 25).

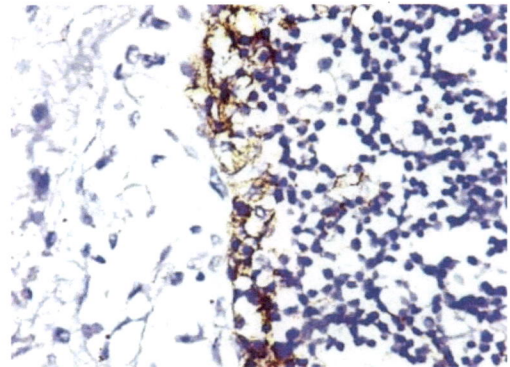

Fig. (24). Subcapsular epithelial cells positive for D2-40, x400.

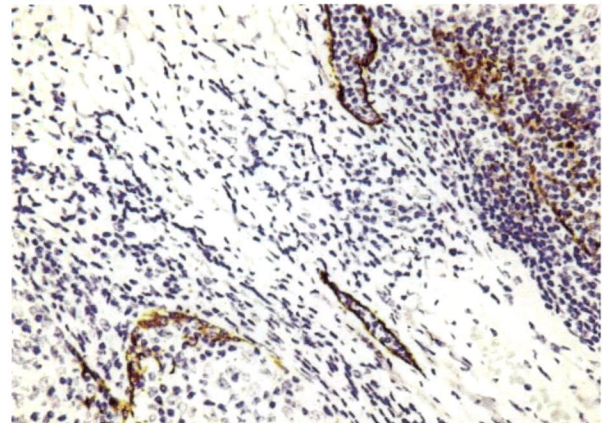

Fig. (25). Thymoma, lymphatic vessels in the stroma and tumor area, D2-40 immunostaining, x200.

VEGF-C secreted by tumor cells of the thymic carcinoma may induce LVs hyperplasia or even lymphangiomatosis, as shown in a recent case report [59]. The evaluation on lymphatic vessels may be difficult or even impossible in the tumor area of some cases, because a subset of thymoma strongly expresses podoplanin and D2-40 (Fig. **26**). On the other hand, the expression of D2-40 by both lymphatic endothelial cells and tumor cells may become an attractive target for tumor therapy [60], as an anti-human podoplanin antibody, called NZ1 was already realized [61, 62].

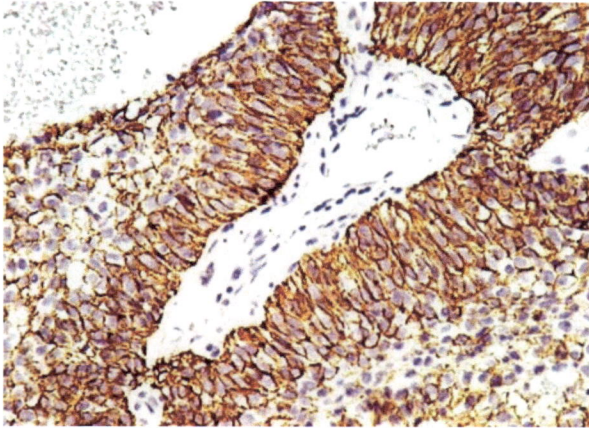

Fig. (26). Thymoma type B3, tumor cells intensely positive for D2-40, x400.

6. THYMUS AS A SOURCE OF ANGIOGENIC FACTORS

The thymus parenchyma can be regarded not only as a target but also as a source of proangiogenic factors. It was shown that epithelial cells are able to secrete growth factors directly involved in angiogenesis (VEGF, FGF or PDGF), as described before. As an example, VEGF and its receptors are expressed by epithelial cells in both infant and mature thymus, and overexpressed by some thymoma and thymic carcinoma.

An unexpected finding showed that thymic epithelial cells are able to secrete some thymic-specific substances that act like hormones. One of them, thymosin, was demonstrated to be a strong inductor of angiogenesis.

Thymosin α_1 is a highly conserved 28 amino acid peptide that has been investigated as immunomodulatory factor and affects maturation, differentiation and function of T cells [63]. In vitro and in vivo experiments showed that thymosin α_1 enhances the formation of tube-like structures by HUVECs cultured on Matrigel and acts like a chemoattractant for HUVEC migration and differentiation [64]. Based on these data, it was concluded that thymosin α_1 has potent effects on endothelial cell migration, angiogenesis and wound repair. The angiogenic effect in wound repair seems to be dose-dependent, and it was inhibited by anti-thymosin α_1 antibody [64]. The effects of thymosin α_1 in human are not known, but it can be speculated that they are the same, as the plasma concentration ranges from 400 to 1000 pg/ml. On the other hand, the tissue concentration varies with the tissue type, age and state of the immune system [65]. Actually, thymosin α_1 does not resemble any other angiogenic factor and the mechanism by which it stimulates angiogenesis needs further investigations.

Thymosin β_4 is another member of the same family of "thymic hormones" that was originally isolated from fraction 5 of the calf thymus and induces differentiation of specific subclasses of T-lymphocytes [66]. It was found extracellularly in the interstitial fluid, and intracellularly in the thymus, kidney and brain. The highest concentration of thymosin β_4 was found in the blood platelets. Thymosin β_4 seems to be involved in angiogenesis because it was found *in vivo* in growing and mature vessels in both normal and malignant tissues [67]. Moreover, thymosin β_4 is increased in the serum of patients with diseases which are associated with increased angiogenesis, like hepatitis, AIDS, or inflammatory bowel disease. In the chick chorioallantoic membrane model, thymosin β_4 was found to enhance angiogenesis [68]. Exogenous thymosin β_4 induces tube formation in Matrigel assay, stimulates endothelial cell proliferation and sprouting of coronary artery rings [67]. Studies on HUVECs showed that human endothelial cells possess a receptor or receptors for thymosin β_4, and exogenous thymosin can modify the cell cytoskeleton with increased stress fibers and F-actin [67]. Based on these data, it was suggested that thymosin β_4 plays an active role in wound healing by increasing the vessels' response to angiogenic factors and could act like a hormone on endothelial cells.

Based on these properties of thymosin β_4, a platform was developed with indications to the dermal and ophthalmic wounds, and cardiovascular diseases [69]. Thymosin β_4 was shown to be essential to the development of the prenatal heart, and it was demonstrated that it promotes myocardial and endothelial cell migration and survival [70]. The role of thymosin β_4 was found in all stages of cardiac vessel development (vasculogenesis, angiogenesis and arteriogenesis) in thymosin β_4-deficient mice [71]. Moreover, the adult epicardium was identified as a source of vascular progenitors that migrate and differentiate into smooth muscle and endothelial cells when stimulated with thymosin. These evidences support the direct involvement of thymosin in angiogenesis and its possible clinical application in chronic wound healing and cardioprotection [69, 72].

7. REFERENCES

1.　Blackburn CC, Manley NR. Developing a new paradigm for thymus organogenesis. Nat Rev Immunol 2004; 4(4): 278-289.

2.　Raica M, Cimpean AM, Encica S, Cornea R. Involution of the thymus: a possible diagnostic pitfall. Rom J Morphol Embryol 2007; 48(2):101-106

3.　Watanabe N, Wang YH, Lee HK, Ito T, Wang YH, Cao W, Liu YJ. Hassall's corpuscles instruct dendritic cells to induce CD4+CD25+ regulatory T cells in human thymus. Nature 2005; 436(7054): 1181-1185.

4.　Raica M, Encică S, Motoc A, Cîmpean AM, Scridon T, Barsan M. Structural heterogeneity and immunohistochemical profile of Hassall corpuscles in normal human thymus. Ann Anat 2006; 188(4): 345-352.

5. Manley NR, Blackburn CC. A developmental look at thymus organogenesis: where do the non-hematopoietic cells in the thymus come from? Curr Opin Immunol 2003; 15(2): 225-232.

6. Anderson M, Anderson SK, Farr AG. Thymic vasculature: organizer of the medullary epithelial compartment? Int Immunol 2000; 12(7): 1105-1110.

7. Marx A, Muller-Hermelink HK. From basic immunobiology to the upcoming WHO-classification of tumors of the thymus.The Second Conference on Biological and Clinical Aspects of Thymic Epithelial Tumors and related recent developments. Pathol Res Pract 1999; 195(8): 515-533.

8. Hale LP. Histologic and molecular assessment of human thymus. Ann Diagn Pathol 2004; 8(1): 50-60.

9. Flores KG, Li J, Sempowski GD, Haynes BF, Hale LP. Analysis of the human thymic perivascular space during aging. J Clin Invest 1999; 104(8): 1031-1039

10. Suster S, Rosai J. In: Histology for pathologists. Mills SE Ed, Lippincott Williams&Wilkins 2007; pp 507-508.

11. Ross MH, Pawlina W. Histology a text and atlas. Lippincott Williams&Wilkins, 2006.

12. Müller SM, Terszowski G, Blum C, Anquez CH, Kuschert S, Carmeliet P, Augustin HG, Rodewald H. Gene targeting of VEGF-A in thymus epithelium disrupts thymus blood vessel architecture. Proc Nat Acad Sci USA 2005; 102(30): 10587-10592.

13. Weidner N, Semple JP, Welch WR, Folkman J. N Engl J Med 1991; 324(1): 1-8.

14. Nico B, Benagiano V, Mangieri D, Maruotti N, Vacca A, Ribatti D. Evaluation of microvascular density in tumors: pro and contra. Histol Histopathol 2008; 23(5): 601-607.

15. Raica M, Cimpean AM, Encica S, Scridon T, Barsan M. Increased mast cell density and microvessel density in the thymus of patients with myasthenia gravis. Rom J Morphol Embryol 2007; 48(1): 11-16.

16. Tomita M, Matsuzaki Y, Edagawa M, Maeda M, Shimizu T, Hara M, Onitsuka T. Correlation between tumor angiogenesis and invasiveness in thymic epithelial tumors. J Thorac Cardiovasc Surg 2002; 124(3) 493-498.

17. Nabarra B, Pontoux C, Godard C, Osborne-Pellegrin M, Ezine S. Neoplastic transformation and angiogenesis in the thymus of transgenic mice expressing SV40 T and t antigen under an L-pyruvate kinase promoter (SV12 mice). Intern J Exp Pathol 2005; 86(6): 397-414.

18. Cimpean AM, Raica M, Encica S, Cornea R, Bocan V. Immunohistochemical expression of vascular endothelial growth factor A (VEGF), and its receptors (VEGFR1, 2) in normal and pathologic conditions of the human thymus. Ann Anat 2008; 190 (3): 238-245.

19. Ferrara N, Davis-Smyth T. The biology of vascular endothelial growth factor. Endocr Rev 1997; 18(1): 4-25.

20. Stalmans I, Lambrechts D, De Smet F, Jansen S, Wang J, Maity S, Kneer P, von der Ohe M, Swillen A, Maes C, Gewilling M, Molin DG, Hellings P, Boetel T, Haardt M, Compernolle V, Dewerchin M, Plaisance S, Vlietinck R, EmanuelB, Gittenberger-de Groot AC, Scambler P, Morrow B, Driscol DA, Moons L, Esguerra CV, Carmeliet G, Behn-Krapps A, Devriendt K, Collen D, Conway SJ, Carmeliet P. VEGF: a modifier of the del22q11 (DiGeorge) syndrome? Nat Med 2003; 9(2) 173-182.

21. Park HJ, Kim MN, Kim JG, Bae YH, Bae MK, Wee HJ, Kim TW, Kim BS, Kim JB, Bae SK, Yoon S. Up-regulation of VEGF expression by NGF that enhances reparative angiogenesis during thymic regeneration in adult rat. Biochim Biophys Acta 2007; 1773(9): 1462-1472.

22. Gee MG, Procopio WN, Makonnen S, Feldman MD, Yeilding NM, Lee WMF. Tumor vessel development and maturation impose limits on the effectiveness of anti-vascular therapy. Am J Pathol 2003; 162(1): 183-193.

23. Asahara T, Murohara T, Sullivan A, Silver M, van der Zee R, Li T, Witzenbichler B, Schatteman G, Isner JM. Isolation of putative progenitor endothelial cells for angiogenesis. Science 1997; 275(5302): 964-967.

24. Asahara T, Masuda H, Takahashi T.Bone marrow origin of endothelial progenitor cells responsible for postnatal vasculogenesis in physiological and pathological neovascularization. Circulation Res 1999; 85(3): 221-228.

25. Lin Y, Weisdorf DJ, Solovey A, Hebbel RP. Origins of circulating endothelial cells and endothelial outgrowth from blood. J Clin Invest 2000; 105(1): 71-77.

26. Handgretinger R, Gordon PR, Leimig T, Chen X, Buhring HJ, Niethammer D, Kuci S.Biology and plasticity of CD133+ hematopoietic stem cells. Ann N Y Acad Sci 2003; 996: 141-151.

27. Grutzkau A, Kruger-Krasagajes S, Baumeister H, Schwarz C, Kogel H, Welker P, Lippert U, Henz BM, Moller A. Synthesis, storage, and release of vascular endothelial growth factor/vascular permeability factor (VEGF/VPF) by human mast cells: implications for the biological significance of VEGF206. Mol Biol Cell 1998; 9(4): 875-884.

28. Ishizaka T Okudaira H, MauserLE, Ishizaka K. Development of rat mast cells in vitro. I. Differentiation of mast cells from thymus cells. J Immunol 1976; 116(3) 747-754.

29. Aldenborg F, Enerback L. Histamine content and mast cell numbers in tissues of normal and athymic rats. Agents Actions 1986; 17(5-6): 454-459.

30. Kawanishi H, Medicus RG, Palaszynski EW. Mast cells induced in vitro by interleukin 3 from native murine thymus cells. Scand J Immunol 1986; 24(1): 29-38.

31. Pufe T, Kurz B, Petersen W, Varoga D, Mentlein R, Kulow S, Lemke A, Tillmann B. The influence of biomechanical parameters on the expression of VEGF and endostatin in the bone and joint system. Ann Anat 2005; 187(5-6): 461-472.

32. De Gramont A, Tourniqand C, Andre T, Larsen AK, Louvet C. Targeted agents for adjuvant therapy of colon cancer. Semin Oncol 2006; 33(6 Suppl 11): S42–45.

33. Shifren JD, Doldi N, Ferrara N, Mesiano S, Jaffe RB. In the human fetus, vascular endothelial growth factor is expressed in epithelial cells and myocytes, but not vascular endothelium: implications for mode of action. J Clin Endocrinol Metab 1994; 79 (1): 316-322.

34. Papadopoulos KP, Thomas CR. Current chemotherapy options for thymic epithelial neoplasms. Expert Opin Pharmacother 2005; 6(7): 1169-1177.

35. Sasaki H, Yukiue H, Kobayashi Y, Nakashima Y, Moriyama S, Kaji M, Kiriyama M, Fukai I, Yamakawa Y, Fujii Y. Elevated serum vascular endothelial growth factor and basic fibroblast growth factor levels in patients with thymic epithelial neoplasms. Surg Today 2001; 31(11): 1038-1040.

36. Bedano PM, Perkins S, Burns M, Kessler K, Nelson R, Schneider BP, Risley L, Dropcho S, Loehrer PJ. J Clin Oncol 2008; 26 (suppl 20): A 19087.

37. Salven P, Lymboussaki A, Heikkilä P, Jääskela-Saari H, Enholm B, Aase K, von Euler G, Eriksson U, Alitalo K, Joensuu H. Vascular endothelial growth factors VEGF-B and VEGF-C are expressed in human tumors.Am J Pathol 1998; 153(1):103-108.

38. McDonald MD, Teicher BA, Stetler-Stevenson W, Ng SSW, Figg WD, Folkman J, Hanahan D, Auerbach R, O'Reilly M, Herbs R, Cheresh D, Gordon M, Eggermont A, Libutti SK. Report from the society for biological therapy and vascular biology faculty of the NCI workshop on angiogenesis monitoring. J Immunother 2004; 27(2):161-175.

39. Hicklin DJ, Ellis LM. Role of the vascular endothelial growth factor pathway in tumor growth and angiogenesis. J Clin Oncol 2005; 23(5) :1011-1015.

40. Fan F, Wey JS, McCarty MF, Belcheva A, Liu W, Bauer TW. Expression and function of vascular endothelial growth factor receptor-1 on human colorectal cancer cells. Oncogene 2005 ; 24(16) :2647-2653.

41. Kiseleva EP, Krylov AV, Lyudyno VI, Suvorov AN. Effect of VEGF on mouse thymocyte proliferation and apoptosis in vitro. Bull Exp Biol Med 2005 ; 139(5) : 576-579.

42. Reinders MEJ, Sho M, Izava A, Wang P, Mukhopadhyay D, Koss KE, Geehan C, Luster AD, Sayegh MH, Briscoe DM. Proinflammatory functions of vascular endothelial growth factor in alloimmunity. J Clin Invest 2003; 112(11): 1655-1665.

43. Holländer G, Gill J, Zuklys S, Iwanami N, Liu C, Takahama Y. Cellular and molecular events during early thymus development. Immunol. Rev 2006; 209: 28-46.

44. Hughes SE. Differential expression of the fibroblast growth factor receptor (FGFR) multigene family in normal human adult tissues. J Histochem Cytochem. 1997; 45(7): 1005-1019.

45. Tomita M, Matsuzaki Y, Edagawa M, Maeda M, Shimizu T, Hara M, Onitsuka T. Clinical and immunohistochemical study of eight cases with thymic carcinoma. BMC 2002; 23: 2-3.

46. Korpisalo P, Karvinen H, Rissanen TT, Kilpijoki J, Marjomäki V, Baluk P, McDonald DM, Cao Y, Eriksson U, Alitalo K, Ylä-Herttuala S. Vascular endothelial growth factor-A and platelet-derived growth factor-B combination gene therapy prolongs angiogenic effects via recruitment of interstitial mononuclear cells and paracrine effects rather than improved pericyte coverage of angiogenic vessels. Circ Res 2008; 103(10):1092-1099.

47. Kuhn E, Wistuba II. Molecular pathology of thymic epithelial neoplasms. Hematol Oncol Clin North Am 2008; 22(3): 443-455.

48. Hammar JA. Die normal-morphologische Thymusforschung im letzen Vierteljahrhundert, Analyse und Synthese. Barth, Leipzig, 1936.

49. Hoepke H, Peter HZ. Das Verhalten des Igelthymus nei saurer unf basischer Emachtung.Mikrosk Anat Forsch 1936; 39: 264-314.

50. Smith C. Studies on the thymus of the mammal. VIII. Intrathymic lymphatic vessels. Anat Rec 1955; 122: 173-179.

51. Ushiki T. A scanning electron-microscopic study of the rat thymus with special reference to cell types and migration of lymphocytes into the general circulation. Cell Tissue Res 1986; 244(2): 285-298.

52. Kato S. Intralobular lymphatic vessels and their relationship to blood vessels in the mouse thymus. Light- and electron-microscopic study. Cell Tissue Res 1988; 253(1): 181-187.

53. Odaka C, Morisada T, Oike Y, Suda T. Distribution of lymphatic vessels in mouse thymus: immunofluorescence analysis. Cell Tissue Res 2006; 325(1) 13-22.

54. Gunn MD, Tangermann K, Tam C, Cyster JG, Rosen SD, Williams LT. A chemokine expressed in lymphoid high endothelial venules promotes the adhesion and chemotaxis of naïve T lymphocytes. Proc. Natl. Acad. Sci. USA, 1998; 95(1): 258-263.

55. Kriehuber E, Bretender-Geleff S, Groeger M, Soleiman A, Schoppmann SF, Stingl G, Kerjanschki D, Maurer D. Isolation and characterization of dermal lymphatic and blood endothelial cells reveal stable and functionally specialized cells lineages. J. Exp. Med 2001; 194(6):797-808.

56. Karkkainen MJ, Saaristo A Jussila L, Karila KA Lawrence EC, Pajusola K, Nueler H, Eichmann A, Kauppinen R,

57. Kettunen MI, Yla-Herttuala S, Finegold DN, Ferrell RE, Alitalo K. A model for gene therapy of human hereditary lymphedema. Proc Natl Acad Sci USA 2001; 98(22) 12677-12682.

57. Yuan L, Moyon D, Pardanaud L, Breant C, Karkkainen MJ, Alitalo K, Eichmann A. Abnormal lymphatic vessel development in neuropilin-2 mutant mice. Development 2002; 129(20) 4797-4806.

58. Ji RC, Kurihara K, Kato S. Lymphatic vascular endothelial hyaluronan receptor (LYVE)-1- and CCL21-positive lymphatic compartments in the diabetic thymus. Anat Sci Intern 2006; 81(4) 201-209

59. Ikeda J, Morii E, Tomita Y, Zhang B, Tokunaga T, Inoue M, Minami M, Okumura M, Aozasa K. Mediastinal lymphangiomatosis coexisting with occult thymic carcinoma. Virchows Arch 2007; 450(2):211-214.

60. Raica M, Cimpean AM, Ribatti D. The role of podoplanin in tumor progression and metastasis. Anticancer Res 2008; 28(5B): 2997-3006.

61. Kato Y, Kaneko MK, Kuno A, Uchiyama N, Amano K, Chiba Y, Hasegawa Y, Hirabayashi J, Narimatsu H, Mishima K, Osawa M. Inhibition of tumor cell-induced platelet aggregation using a novel anti-podoplanin antibody reacting with its platelet-aggregation-stimulating domain. Biochem Biophys Res Commun 2006;349(4) :1301-1307.

62. Kato Y, Kaneko MK, Kunita A, Ito H, Kameyama A, Ogasawara S, Matsuura N, Hasegawa Y, Suzuki-Inoue K, Inoue O, Ozaki Y, Marimatsu H. Molecular analysis of the pathophysiological binding of the platelet aggregation-inducing factor podoplanin to the C-type lectin-like receptor CLEC-2.Cancer Sci 2008; 99(1): 54-61.

63. Goldstein AL. Clinical application of thymosin α_1. Cancer Invest 1994; 12(5): 545-547.

64. Malinda KM, Sidhu GS, Banaudha KK, Gaddipati JP, Majeshwari RK, Goldstein AL, Kleinman HK. Thymosin α_1 stimulates endothelial cell migration, angiogenesis, and wound healing. J Immunol 1998; 160(2): 1001-1006.

65. Naz R, Naylor PH, Goldstein AL. Thymosin α_1 levels in human seminal plasma and follicular fluid: implication in germ cell function. Int J Fertil 1987; 32(5): 375-379.

66. Low TLK, Goldstein AL. Chemical characterization of thymosin β_4. J Biol Chem 1981; 257(2): 1000-1006.

67. Grant DS, Rose W, Yaen C, Goldstein A, Martinez J, Kleinman H. Thymosin β_4 enhances endothelial cell differentiation and angiogenesis. Angiogenesis 1999; 3(2): 125-135.

68. Koutrafouri V, Leonidis L, Avgoustakis K, Livianou E, Czarnecki J, Ithakissios D, Evangelatos G. Effect of thymosin peptides on the chick chorioallantoic membrane angiogenesis model. Biochim Biophys Acta 2001; 1568 (1): 60-66.

69. Crockford D. Development of thymosin β_4 for treatment of patients with ischemic heart disease. Ann NY Acad Sci 2007; 1112: 385-395.

70. Bock-Marquette I, Saxena A, White MD, Dimaio JM, Srivastava D. Thymosin β_4 activates integrin-limked kinase and promotes cardiac cell migration, survival, and cardiac repair. Nature 2004; 432(7016): 466-472.

71. Smart N, Risebro CA, Melville AA, Moses K, Schwartz RJ, Chien KR, Rilez PR. Thymosin β_4 induces epicardial progenitor mobilization and neovascularization. Nature 2007; 445(7124): 177-182.

72. Smart N, Rossdeutsch A, Riley PR. Thymosin β_4 and angiogenesis: modes of action and therapeutic potential. Angiogenesis 2007; 10(4): 229-241.

CHAPTER 6

Zebrafish as a Tool to Study Tumor Angiogenesis

Marco Presta

Department of Biomedical Sciences and Biotechnology, University of Brescia, Italy

Correspondence to: Prof. Marco Presta, Unit of General Pathology and Immunology,Department of Biomedical Sciences and Biotechnology, University of Brescia Medical School, Viale Europa, 30, 25123 Brescia, Italy. Tel: 0039.0303717311; Fax: 0039.030303701157; Email; presta@med.unibs.it

Abstract: Zebrafish (*Danio rerio*) represents a powerful model system in cancer research. Recent observations have shown the possibility to exploit zebrafish to investigate tumor angiogenesis, a pivotal step in cancer progression and target for anti-tumor therapies. Experimental models have been established in zebrafish adults, juveniles, and embryos, each one with its own advantages and disadvantages. Novel genetic tools and high resolution *in vivo* imaging techniques are also becoming available in zebrafish. It is anticipated that zebrafish will represent an important tool for chemical discovery and gene targeting in tumor angiogenesis. This review focuses on the recently developed tumor angiogenesis models in zebrafish, with particular emphasis to tumor engrafting in zebrafish embryos.

1. INTRODUCTION

Angiogenesis plays a key role in tumor growth and metastasis [1]. Thus, the identification of anti-angiogenic drugs and of angiogenesis-related targets may have significant implications for the development of anti-neoplastic therapies, as shown by the positive outcomes in the treatment of cancer patients with the monoclonal anti-vascular endothelial growth factor-A (VEGF-A) antibody bevacizumab [2].

The teleost zebrafish (*Danio rerio*) has exceptional utility as a human disease model system and represents a promising alternative model in cancer research [3]. Zebrafish embryo allows disease-driven drug target identification and *in vivo* validation, thus representing an interesting bioassay tool for small molecule testing and dissection of biological pathways alternative to other vertebrate models [4]. Indeed, when compared to other vertebrate model systems, zebrafish offers many advantages, including ease of experimentation, drug administration, and amenability to *in vivo* manipulation. Also, zebrafish is suitable for forward genetic screens and transient or permanent gene inactivation via antisense morpholino oligonucleotide (MO) injection or "targeting-induced local lesions in genes" (TILLING), respectively [5]. Moreover, the possibility to introduce targeted heritable gene mutations into the zebrafish germ line using engineered zinc-finger nucleases has been recently reported [6]. Importantly, zebrafish is suitable for high-throughput screening of chemical compounds using robotic platforms [6, 7].

Zebrafish possesses a complex circulatory system similar to that of mammals [8]. The basic vascular plan of the developing zebrafish embryo shows strong similarity to that of other vertebrates [9]. At the 13 somite-stage, endothelial cell precursors migrating from the lateral mesoderm originate the zebrafish vasculature and a single blood circulatory loop is present at 24 hours post-fertilization (hpf). Blood vessel development continues during the subsequent days by angiogenic processes. In particular, angiogenesis occurs in the formation of the intersegmental vessels (ISVs) of the trunk that will sprout from the dorsal aorta at 20 hpf. Also, the subintestinal vein vessels (SIVs) originate from the duct of Cuvier area at 48 hpf and will form a vascular plexus across most of the dorsal-lateral aspect of the yolk ball during the next 24 hours [9].

Various animal models have been developed in rodents and in the chick embryo to investigate the angiogenesis process and for the screening of pro- and anti-angiogenic compounds, each with its own unique characteristics and disadvantages [10]. Previous studies had shown that developmental angiogenesis in the zebrafish embryo, leading to the formation of the ISVs of the trunk [11] and of the SIV plexus [12], represents a target for the screening of anti-angiogenic compounds. In these assays, low molecular weight compounds dissolved in fish water are investigated for their impact on the growth of new blood vessels driven by the complex network of endogenous, developmentally regulated signals. Recently, a novel zebrafish yolk membrane (ZFYM) assay has been proposed based on the injection of an angiogenic growth factor [e.g. recombinant fibroblast growth factor-2 (FGF2)] in the perivitelline space of zebrafish embryos in the proximity of developing SIVs. FGF2 induces a rapid and dose-dependent angiogenic response from the SIV basket, characterized by the growth of newly formed, alkaline phosphatase-positive blood vessels [13]. The ZFYM assay differs from the previous zebrafish-based angiogenesis assays since the angiogenic stimulus is represented by a well-defined, topically delivered exogenous agent that leads to the growth of ectopic blood vessels. This allows the screening of low and high molecular weight antagonists targeting a specific angiogenic growth factor and/or its receptor(s) [13].

However, the study of vascular development and on the effects of positive or negative modulators of the embryonic angiogenic process may have important limitations when translated to cancer research. Indeed, tumor-induced vessels show profound morpho-functional alterations when compared to the normal vasculature [1]. This is reflected by significant differences in gene expression profiling between normal and tumor-derived endothelium [14, 15]. Thus, the identification of therapeutic targets and the assessment of the efficacy of anti-angiogenic compounds require the development of appropriate animal models in which tumor vasculature can be investigated. To this respect, tumor models have been established in zebrafish embryos, juveniles, and adults (reviewed in [16, 17]) that may be suitable for studying the tumor angiogenesis process and its modulators. The availability of imbred, transgenic, gene knock-out/knock-in animals, of a wide array of antibodies, as well as of bioinformatic genomic, transcriptomic and proteomic information represent important tools for tumor angiogenesis studies. Several of these tools have been becoming available also for zebrafish.

This review focuses on the recently developed tumor angiogenesis models in zebrafish, with particular emphasis to tumor engrafting in zebrafish embryos.

2. TUMOR ANGIOGENESIS MODELS IN ZEBRAFISH ADULTS

Zebrafish spontaneously develops almost any type of tumor. Also, several approaches have been developed to induce cancer in zebrafish. They include treatment with chemical carcinogens, forward genetic screening, target-selected inactivation of tumor suppressor genes, and expression of mammalian oncogenes. An overview of these approaches and of their main advantages and disadvantages has been published recently [16]. Also, transplantable tumor cell lines have been generated in clonal zebrafish and maintained for several passages in syngeneic and isogeneic adults [18]. Interestingly, microarray analysis has shown that gene expression signatures are conserved in fish tumors when compared to their human counterpart [3]. Relevant to tumor angiogenesis studies in adults, a transparent *casper* zebrafish line that lacks all types of pigments has been generated, allowing the rapid identification of transplanted tumor cells [19]. Also, crossing of the *casper* mutant with transgenic lines that label vasculature or internal organs with fluorescent tags may represent an useful approach to study tumor-host interactions in zebrafish by epifluorescence

stereomicroscopy, confocal microscopy, and dual-photon confocal microscopy.

Noninvasive imaging in non-transparent zebrafish adults has been attempted. Ultrasound biomicroscopy has been used to follow the growth of liver tumors, their vascularity, and response to treatment [20]. Other imaging techniques, including microcomputerized axial tomography, micromagnetic resonance imaging, and optical projection tomography are beginning to be applied in zebrafish and will help to investigate tumor growth and vascularization in adult zebrafish [21].

3. TUMOR ANGIOGENESIS MODELS IN ZEBRAFISH JUVANILES

Human cancer cells have been successfully transplanted in the peritoneal cavity of 30 day-old zebrafish [22]. This has allowed the study of the dynamics of microtumor formation and neovascularization using high resolution imaging techniques, leading to a detailed description of the interaction among fluorescent tumor cells and the green fluorescent protein (GFP)-labeled vasculature of the host by three-dimensional reconstruction of confocal microscopy images. The results of these studies have shown that tumor cells secreting human VEGF promote fish vessel remodeling and angiogenesis and that the human metastatic gene *RhoC* drives the initial steps of the metastatic process.

Due to the fact that juvenile zebrafish has a functional immune system, dexamethasone administration is required to prevent the rejection of the tumor engraftment. Also, at variance with zebrafish embryos (see below), the MO gene targeting approach is unfeasible in zebrafish juveniles. On the other hand, the impact of the tumor graft on the mature vasculature of juvenile fishes may recapitulate more closely the events that occur during tumor angiogenesis in adult animals and cancer patients. Indeed, developing vessels of zebrafish embryos may respond differently to tumor grafts compared to the fully developed vasculature of juvenile animals [17].

4. TUMOR ANGIOGENESIS MODELS IN ZEBRAFISH EMBRYOS

The optical transparency and ability to survive for 3-4 days without functioning circulation make the zebrafish embryo amenable for vascular biology studies. Also, because of the immaturity of the immune system in zebrafish embryos, no xenograft rejection occurs at this stage [8]. Moreover, transient gene inactivation via MO injection represents a powerful tool for the identification of target genes in zebrafish embryo [5].

Recent studies have shown the feasibility of injecting human melanoma cells in zebrafish embryos to follow their fate and to study their impact on zebrafish development [23]. In these studies, tumor cells were injected at the blastula stage to explore potential bidirectional interactions between cancer cells and embryonic stem cells. The results indicate that developing zebrafish can be used as a biosensor for tumor-derived signals. However, grafting of tumor cells at this stage, well before vascular development, results in their reprogramming toward a non-tumorigenic phenotype, thus hampering any attempt to investigate tumor-driven vascularization. At variance, injection of melanoma cells into the hindbrain ventricle or yolk sac of 48 hpf embryos results in the formation of tumor masses within 4 days [24]. Immunostaining analysis of the grafts reveals the presence of blood vessels within the brain and abdominal lesions, even though the high vascularity of the invaded regions may not allow easy discrimination between developmental and tumor-induced angiogenesis [24].

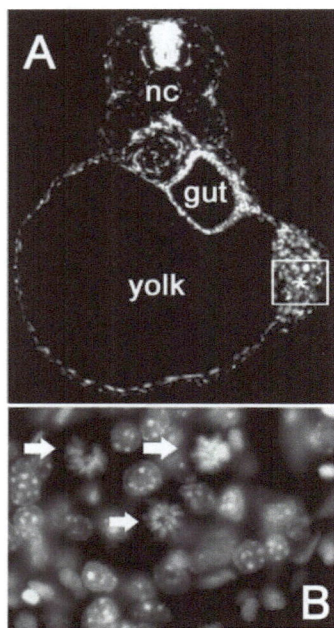

Fig. (1). Tumor cell xenograft in zebrafish embryo. Tumor cells were injected in the perivitelline space of zebrafish embryo at 48 hpf. After 24 hours, transverse sections of the embryo were stained with DAPI. In A, the graft is marked with an asterisk (nc, notochord). In B, the graft is shown at higher magnification to visualize proliferating tumor cells (arrows).

Recently, a novel zebrafish embryo/tumor xenograft angiogenesis assay has been described [25, 26]. The assay is based on the grafting of mammalian tumor cells in the proximity of the developing SIV plexus at 48 hpf (Fig. **1**). Pro-angiogenic factors released locally by the tumor graft affect the normal developmental pattern of the SIVs by stimulating the migration and growth of sprouting vessels towards the implant. One-two days after tumor cell grafting, whole mount phosphatase alkaline staining allows the macroscopic

evaluation of the angiogenic response (Fig. **2A**). The use of transgenic zebrafish embryos, in which endothelial cells express GFP under the control of endothelial-specific promoters ([27] and references therein), represents an improvement of the method, allowing the observation and time-lapse recording of newly formed blood vessels in live embryos by epifluorescence microscopy as well as by *in vivo* confocal microscopy [25, 26] (Fig. **2B**). Also, quantum dots may be used as labeling agents of the zebrafish embryo vasculature for long-lasting intravital time-lapse studies [28].

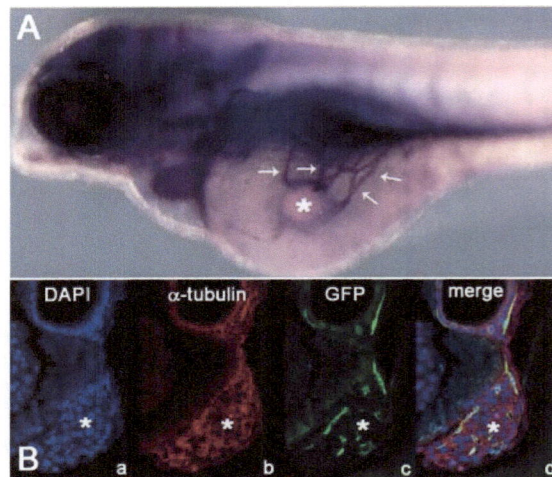

Fig. (2). Tumor angiogenesis in zebrafish embryo. Tumor cells were injected in the perivitelline space of zebrafish embryo at 48 hpf. A) After 24 hours, embryos were stained for alkaline phosphatase activity to visualize the newly formed blood vessels (arrows) converging towards the graft (asterisk). In B, cryosection of a tumor graft (asterisk) in transgenic *VEGFR2:G-RCFP* zebrafish embryo [11]. Note the GFP-tagged blood vessels within the graft (c, d). Sections were counterstained with DAPI (a) and anti-α-tubulin antibodies (b).

When compared to other *in vivo* tumor angiogenesis assays, the zebrafish embryo/tumor xenograft model presents several advantages. i) The model allows the delivery of a very limited number of cells, mimicking the initial stages of tumor angiogenesis and metastasis. ii) Labeled tumor cells (e.g. GFP-transduced or fluorescent dye-loaded cells) can be easily visualized within the embryo. Thus, analysis of the spatial/temporal relationship among tumor cells and newly formed blood vessels may represent an important feature of this model. iii) Several techniques can be applied within the constraints of paraffin or gelatin embedding, including histochemistry and immunohistochemistry. Electron microscopy can also be used in combination with light microscopy. Moreover, reverse transcriptase-polymerase chain reaction analysis with species-specific primers allows the study of gene expression by grafted tumor cells and by the host under different experimental conditions [26].

The identification of genes essential for blood vessel formation is of pivotal importance for the understanding of the angiogenesis process and for the discovery of novel therapeutic targets. In zebrafish embryos, MO injection induce a translational block in gene function [29]. Gene inactivation by this approach is easy and fast (3-4 days) when compared to the generation of knock-out mice (several months). Also, the simultaneous injection of different MOs may allow the inactivation of more than one gene at the same time. This represents a paramount advantage compared to any mammalian assay available and it can be exploited for the identification of novel gene(s) involved in tumor neovascularization. For instance, MO-induced inactivation of *VE-cadherin* [26] or *calcitonin receptor-like receptor* [30] zebrafish gene orthologs results in a significant inhibition of the angiogenic process triggered by the tumor graft in zebrafish embryos.

Because of the permeability of its embryos to small molecules, zebrafish allows disease-driven drug target identification and *in vivo* validation, thus representing an interesting bioassay tool for small molecule testing and dissection of biological pathways alternative to other vertebrate models [4]. Accordingly, systemic exposure of live zebrafish embryos to anti-angiogenic compounds dissolved in fish water results in a significant inhibition of neovascularization triggered by the tumor graft [31]. Thus, the zebrafish embryo/tumor xenograft model may represent a short-term assay suitable for the identification of novel tumor angiogenesis inhibitors. It is interesting to note the rapid response of this model to angiogenesis inhibitors (24-48 h) when compared to the chick embryo chorioallantoic membrane assay (3-4 days), the s.c. murine Matrigel plug assay (5-7 days), the murine (1 week) and rabbit (2-3 weeks) cornea assays, and the s.c. mouse syngraft and xenograft assays (several weeks) [10]. Also, a large number of zebrafish embryos can be injected and maintained in 96 well-plates, thus allowing systemic *in vivo* treatment of the animals with minimal amounts of compound. Therefore, dose-response experiments can be easily performed and numerous compounds can be tested in an effective manner. However, the metabolic fate of the drug (either in terms of its activation or inactivation) may differ in zebrafish embryo in respect to mammalian species. Also, zebrafish embryos are maintained at 28°C. This may not represent an optimal temperature for mammalian cell growth and metabolism, even though we have observed mitotic figures with no sign of apoptosis in grafted tumors throughout the whole experimental period [26] (Fig. 1B). In this respect, the possibility to raise the incubation temperature up to 35°C with no apparent gross effects on zebrafish development has been reported [24].

With its own advantages and disadvantages, the zebrafish embryo/tumor xenograft model represents a novel tool for investigating the neovascularization process exploitable for drug discovery and gene targeting in tumor angiogenesis.

5. ACKNOWLEDGEMENTS

Images shown in figures were provided by Dr. S. Nicoli. This work was supported by grants from Istituto Superiore di Sanità (Oncotechnological Program), Ministero dell'Istruzione, Università e Ricerca (Centro di Eccellenza per l'Innovazione Diagnostica e Terapeutica, Cofin projects), Associazione Italiana per la Ricerca sul Cancro, Fondazione Berlucchi, SPAFARM Project (Regione Lombardia), and NOBEL Project Cariplo.

6. REFERENCES

1. Carmeliet P, Jain RK. Angiogenesis in cancer and other diseases. Nature 2000; 407(6801): 249-257.
2. Ferrara N. Vascular endothelial growth factor: basic science and clinical progress. Endocr Rev 2004; 25(4): 581-611.
3. Lam SH, Wu YL, Vega VB, Miller LD, Spitsbergen J, Tong Y, Zhan H, Govindarajan KR, Lee S, Mathavan S, Murthy KR, Buhler DR, Liu ET, Gong Z. Conservation of gene expression signatures between zebrafish and human liver tumors and tumor progression. Nat Biotechnol 2006; 24(1): 73-75.
4. Pichler FB, Laurenson S, Williams LC, Dodd A, Copp BR, Love DR. Chemical discovery and global gene expression analysis in zebrafish. Nat Biotechnol 2003; 21(8): 879-883.
5. Thisse C, Zon LI. Organogenesis--heart and blood formation from the zebrafish point of view. Science 2002; 295(5554): 457-462.
6. Meng X, Noyes MB, Zhu LJ, Lawson ND, Wolfe SA. Targeted gene inactivation in zebrafish using engineered zinc-finger nucleases. Nat Biotechnol 2008; 26(6): 695-701.
7. Funfak A, Brosing A, Brand M, Kohler JM. Micro fluid segment technique for screening and development studies on Danio rerio embryos. Lab Chip 2007; 7(9): 1132-1138.
8. Weinstein B. Vascular cell biology in vivo: a new piscine paradigm? Trends Cell Biol 2002; 12(9): 439-445.
9. Isogai S, Horiguchi M, Weinstein BM. The vascular anatomy of the developing zebrafish: an atlas of embryonic and early larval development. Dev Biol 2001; 230(2): 278-301.
10. Hasan J, Shnyder SD, Bibby M, Double JA, Bicknel R, Jayson GC. Quantitative angiogenesis assays in vivo--a review. Angiogenesis 2004; 7(1): 1-16.
11. Cross LM, Cook MA, Lin S, Chen JN, Rubinstein AL. Rapid analysis of angiogenesis drugs in a live fluorescent zebrafish assay. Arterioscler Thromb Vasc Biol 2003; 23(5): 911-912.
12. Serbedzija GN, Flynn E, Willett CE. Zebrafish angiogenesis: a new model for drug screening. Angiogenesis 2000; 3(4): 353-359.

13.   Nicoli S, De Sena G, Presta M. Fibroblast Growth Factor 2-induced angiogenesis in zebrafish: the zebrafish yolk membrane (ZFYM) angiogenesis assay. J Cell Mol Med 2008; [Epub ahead of print].

14.   Ghilardi C, Chiorino G, Dossi R, Nagy Z, Giavazzi R, Bani M. Identification of novel vascular markers through gene expression profiling of tumor-derived endothelium. BMC Genomics 2008; 9(Apr 30): 201.

15.   St Croix B, Rago C, Velculescu V, Traverso G, Romans KE, Montgomery E, Lal A, Riggins GJ, Lengauer C, Vogelstein B, Kinzler KW. Genes expressed in human tumor endothelium. Science 2000; 289(5482): 1197-1202.

16.   Feitsma H, Cuppen E. Zebrafish as a cancer model. Mol Cancer Res 2008; 6(5): 685-694.

17.   Stoletov K, Klemke R. Catch of the day: zebrafish as a human cancer model. Oncogene 2008; 27(33): 4509-4520.

18.   Mizgireuv IV, Revskoy SY. Transplantable tumor lines generated in clonal zebrafish. Cancer Res 2006; 66(6): 3120-3125.

19.   White RM, Sessa A, Burke C, Bowman T, LeBlanc J, Ceol C, Bourque C, Dovey M, Goessling W, Burns CE, Zon LI. Transparent adult zebrafish as a tool for in vivo transplantation analysis. Cell Stem Cell 2008; 2(2): 183-189.

20.   Goessling W, North TE, Zon LI. Ultrasound biomicroscopy permits in vivo characterization of zebrafish liver tumors. Nat Methods 2007; 4(7): 551-553.

21.   Spitsbergen J. Imaging neoplasia in zebrafish. Nat Methods 2007; 4(7): 548-549.

22.   Stoletov K, Montel V, Lester RD, Gonias SL, Klemke R. High-resolution imaging of the dynamic tumor cell vascular interface in transparent zebrafish. Proc Natl Acad Sci USA 2007; 104(44): 17406-17411.

23.   Topczewska JM, Postovit LM, Margaryan NV, Sam A, Hess AR, Wheaton WW, Nickoloff BJ, Topczewski J, Hendrix MJ. Embryonic and tumorigenic pathways converge via Nodal signaling: role in melanoma aggressiveness. Nat Med 2006; 12(8): 925-932.

24.   Haldi M, Ton C, Seng WL, McGrath P. Human melanoma cells transplanted into zebrafish proliferate, migrate, produce melanin, form masses and stimulate angiogenesis in zebrafish. Angiogenesis 2006; 9(3): 139-151.

25.   Nicoli S, Presta M. The zebrafish/tumor xenograft angiogenesis assay. Nat Protoc 2007; 2(11): 2918-2923.

26.   Nicoli S, Ribatti D, Cotelli F, Presta M. Mammalian tumor xenografts induce neovascularization in zebrafish embryos. Cancer Res 2007; 67(7): 2927-2931.

27.   Baldessari D, Mione M. How to create the vascular tree? (Latest) help from the zebrafish. Pharmacol Ther 2008; 118(2): 206-230.

28.   Rieger S, Kulkarni RP, Darcy D, Fraser SE, Koster RW. Quantum dots are powerful multipurpose vital labeling agents in zebrafish embryos. Dev Dyn 2005; 234(3): 670-681.

29.   Nasevicius A, Ekker SC. Effective targeted gene 'knockdown' in zebrafish. Nat Genet 2000; 26(2): 216-220.

30.   Nicoli S, Tobia C, Gualandi L, De Sena G, Presta M. Calcitonin receptor-like receptor guides arterial differentiation in zebrafish. Blood 2008; 111(10): 4965-4972.

31.   Serbedzija GN, Flynn E, Willett CE. Zebrafish angiogenesis: a new model for drug screening. Angiogenesis 1999; 3(4): 353-359.

CHAPTER 7

The Contribution of Circulating Endothelial Cells to Tumor Angiogenesis

Francesco Bertolini[1], Patrizia Mancuso[1], Paola Braidotti[2], Yuval Shaked[3] and Robert S. Kerbel[4].

[1] *European Institute of Oncology, and [2] University of Milan, Department of Medicine, Surgery and Dentistry and San Paolo Hospital, Milan, Italy. [3] Technion- Israel Institute of Technology, Rappaport Faculty of Medicine, Department of Molecular Pharmacology, Haifa, Israel, [4] Sunnybrook Health Sciences Centre, Molecular and Cellular Biology, Department of Medical Biophysics, University of Toronto, Toronto, Ontario M4N 3M5, Canada.*

Address correspondence to: Dr Francesco Bertolini, European Institute of Oncology, via Ripamonti 435, 20141 Milan, Italy; Tel: 02-57489-535; Fax 02-574-89-537; Email: francesco.bertolini@ieo.it

Abstract: Immunohistochemistry, flow cytometry and cell culture procedures have demonstrated the presence of circulating endothelial cells (CECs) and circulating endothelial progenitors (CEPs) in the blood of vertebrates. CECs and CEPs are currently being investigated in a variety of diseases as markers of vascular turnover or damage and, also in the case of CEPs, vasculogenesis. CEPs appear to have a "catalytic" role in different steps of cancer progression and recurrence after therapy, and there are preclinical and clinical data suggesting that CEC enumeration might be useful to select and predict clinical response in patients who are candidates for anti-angiogenic treatments. In some types of cancer, CECs and CEPs might be one of the possible hidden identities of cancer stem cells. The definition of CEC and CEP phenotype and the standardization of CEC and CEP enumeration strategies are highly desirable goals in order to exploit these cells as reliable biomarkers in oncology clinical trials.

1. INTRODUCTION

By means of microscopy, cells with a possible endothelial morphology were found to circulate in the blood in the early '70s [1]. In the '90s, immunohistochemistry (IHC) studies confirmed the endothelial nature of these cells, and their enumeration by means of positive enrichment, IHC or flow cytometry (FC) indicated that levels of circulating endothelial cells (CECs) are increased in a very wide spectrum of disorders encompassing vascular, autoimmune, infectious and ischemic diseases [2-8]. Over the past ten years, increased CEC counts were observed in some cancer patients [9-21], and these cells were studied as surrogate biomarkers of angiogenesis and anti-angiogenic drug activity in preclinical models and medical oncology [22-26]. These studies also indicated that the endothelial phenotype was expressed by cells displaying a wide variety of different features [6-8]. Some CECs had a phenotype compatible with terminally differentiated endothelial cells (EC), in some cases being apoptotic or necrotic and thus most likely derived from the turnover of vessel walls. Some other cells expressed progenitor-associated antigens in addition to endothelial antigens, and were considered candidates as "circulating endothelial progenitors" (CEPs). This chapter will describe some of the most recent findings about CECs and CEPs in cancer, along with novel

(and possibly provocative) hypotheses emerging from these studies.

2. TOWARDS A MOLECULAR, ULTRA-STRUCTURAL AND PHENOTYPIC DEFINITION OF CECs AND CEPs

The two most frequently used CEC enumeration strategies, IHC and FC, have provided in many cases different CEC frequencies in health and disease [6-8]. According to IHC enumeration, CECs are large cells present in a frequency of 10-100/mL in healthy subjects [6-7]. According to FC, events with an EC phenotype show in most cases small dimensions and are counted with a frequency of 100-10,000/mL [8-11, 16-18]. Antigenic promiscuity between CECs and platelets has prompted the development and validation of new FC enumeration procedures where DNA staining reagents have allowed the count and the sorting of platelet-depleted, DNA-containing cells with an EC phenotype (CD45-,CD31+CD146+; Mancuso et al, in press). Studies which have used transmission electron microscopy (TEM), confirmed that these sorted CECs are of endothelial nature by virtue of the presence of EC-specific Weibel-Palade bodies (Fig. 1) and of RNA transcripts for the EC-specific gene VE-cadherin. Transmission electron microscopy (TEM) studies also offered an explanation of the controversies about CEC frequency in the

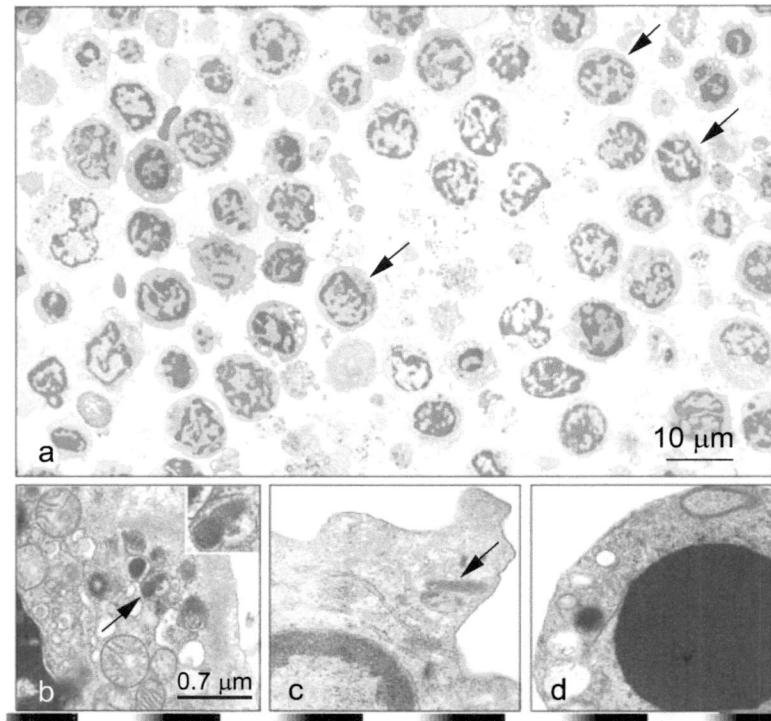

Fig. (1). Transmission electron microscopy images of sorted DNA+,CD45-CD31+CD146+ CECs (from Bertolini et al, 2009, modified).

a) Low-magnification overview of the sorted cell population, showing the presence of apoptotic/necrotic cells most likely derived from vessel wall turnover along with lymphocyte-like cells (arrows).

b) Endothelial (precursor?) cell undergoing cellular division (a centriole is present). The arrow points to a Weibel-Palade body seen more detailed in the inset.

c) A mature endothelial cell with a Weibel-Palade body (arrow).

d) An overtly apoptotic cell.

blood. The majority of sorted CECs, in fact, were found to be apoptotic or necrotic cellular fragments, most likely lost at count after the cell processing involved in IHC enumeration. Along with apoptotic CECs, however, TEM showed the presence of small, viable and lymphoid-like cells that are compatible with a progenitor cell morphology (Fig. **2**).

TEM will most likely be of help for the next crucial steps in CEC and CEP studies, namely, to dissect the functions of candidate CEC and CEP subpopulations. Both these cell families, in fact, encompass subpopulations with different roles. Multiparametric FC has shown that among DNA+,CD45-,CD31+,CD146+ CECs there are some expressing other EC-related antigens such as CD143, CD144, VEGFR1, VEGFR2, VEGFR3, along with activation antigens such as CD105 (endoglin), among others [8]. The need for a detailed phenotypic profile is particularly urgent for CEPs, because CD34 and VEGFR2 antigens, used by many investigators for CEP enumeration by FC [5, 8, 27-28], are expressed

also by mature CECs, and the use of CD133 antigen for CEP identification [29-30] has led to the sorting of cells that not all laboratories were able to differentiate in vitro and in vivo along the endothelial lineage [31-32]. Even more controversies exist for the enumeration of CEPs in mice, because the expression and function of CD34 and CD133 antigens are not well characterized in mice compared to humans. Thus a candidate phenotype for CEPs in mice is CD45-, VEGFR2(Flk)+, CD117+ [22-24], and antibodies reacting with a particular configuration of CD144 are also used [33-34].

3. CEC NUMBER AND VIABILITY IN CANCER TREATMENT

A variety of FC and IHC studies have indicated that in some types of cancer patient CEC numbers and viability are increased when compared to healthy controls [9-21]. Possible explanations for these findings involve the angiogenic switch associated with cancer growth and the robust production of angiogenic

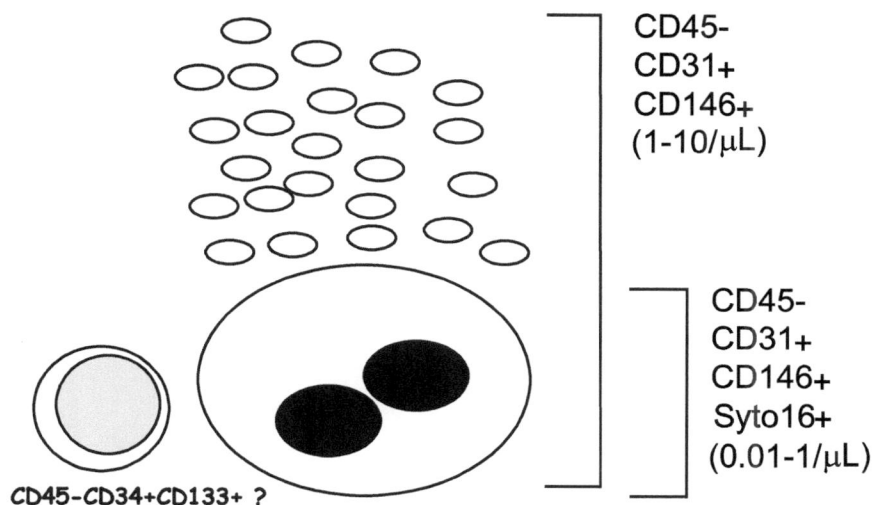

Fig. (2). Overview of cellular events with an EC phenotype enumerated by flow cytometry (from Bertolini et al, 2009, modified). The majority of CD45-,CD31+CD146+ events are apoptotic or necrotic cellular fragments (1-10/μL in the blood). The use of Syto16 allows the enumeration of DNA-containing CD45-CD31+CD146+ CECs (0.01-1/μL). Along with CECs, TEM showed the presence of some small, viable and lymphoid-like cells that are compatible with a progenitor cell morphology, lack CD45 expression and may express CD133 and/or CD34 (Mancuso et al, in press).

growth factors such as VEGF, bFGF, HGF and many others by cancer cells and/or various host cells [8]. The recent and unexpected finding of an autocrine loop in ECs [35] is of particular interest, because it might be that the increase of viable CECs in the blood of cancer patients mirrors an aberrant vascular turnover/remodeling associated with high local levels of VEGF produced by cancer cells.

Following the preclinical evidence that CEC count can be used as a surrogate biomarker for angiogenesis and anti-angiogenic drug activity by means of determining the optimal biological dosage of anti-angiogenic drugs [24-26], their numbers and viability have also been measured in different clinical trials involving cancer patients treated with various anti-angiogenic therapies [10-21]. An increase in the number of apoptotic CECs after 60 days of therapy was associated with prolonged progression-free survival and overall survival in metastatic breast cancer patients treated with a doublet low-dose metronomic (antiangiogenic) chemotherapy regimen [16]. When the humanized anti-VEGF antibody, bevacizumab, was added to the metronomic chemotherapy for the treatment of metastatic breast cancer patients who showed a clinical response in a phase II clinical trial (as well as a larger population of patients who had a clinical benefit from the treatment) had significantly greater baseline levels of viable CECs than did patients who failed to respond; furthermore, the number of apoptotic CECs before therapy initiated was associated with prolonged progression-free survival [36]. In patients with renal cancer treated with the small molecule anti-angiogenic

agent, sunitinib, changes in CECs differed between the patients with clinical benefit and those with progressive disease [18]. Taken together, these data suggest that the investigation of CEC number and viability by FC has potential for the stratification of cancer patients who are more likely to benefit from anti-angiogenic treatments [8, 25, 37]. This possibility awaits confirmation in prospective randomized clinical trials.

4. THE CATALYTIC CEP ROLE IN DEVELOPMENT OF MACROMETAS-TASES AND RESISTANCE TO CHE-MOTHERAPY, VDAS AND ANTI-ANGIOGENIC DRUGS

Asahara et al first proposed the concept of CEP-dependent new blood vessel formation in adult life in 1997 [27], a few months before a similar proposal from Shi et al in 1998 [28]. These two seminal studies identified endothelial progenitors as cells that are capable of generating mature ECs in vitro and in vivo. A study from Lyden et al [38] was the first to identify a role for CEPs in cancer growth using $Id (Id1^{+/-}Id3^{-/-})$ deficient mice. These mice have a severe CEP defect leading to impaired angiogenesis and tumor growth. More recently it was found that CEP generation depends on the ability of Id to restrain the expression of its target gene p21 [39]. Genetic ablation of p21 rescued CEP generation in Id1 deficient mice, re-establishing normal tumor growth [39]. Understanding whether all types of tumor rely, at least in part, on

CEP-dependent vessel generation has been elusive, primarily because the relative contribution of CEP-derived vessels was found to be extremely variable, and in most cases low, in different preclinical models of cancer [38-43]. Clinical studies in patients who received a gender-mismatched bone marrow transplant before cancer recurrence [44] indicated that CEP-derived vessels were indeed present, albeit at a low frequency (on average, 5% of all vessels).

Benezra's group reconciled these apparently conflicting data by demonstrating that the recruitment of CEPs into tumor vasculature depends on the tumor grade [43] and also by showing that CEPs are key contributors in the first steps of tumor vascularization in small tumors. However, following the establishment of cancer vessels, their relative contribution to neoplastic angiogenesis is quantitatively less relevant as these cells become progressively diluted with the division of differentiated endothelial cells [33].

Three previously unrecognized and crucial roles for CEPs in tumor progression have been recently suggested. Angiogenesis-mediated progression from micro- to lethal macro-metastasis is a leading cause of death in cancer patients. Using preclinical models of pulmonary metastasis, the Mittal laboratory reported that tumors induce Id1 expression in CEPs. Id1 suppression after metastatic colonization blocked CEP mobilization, caused angiogenesis inhibition, impaired pulmonary macrometastases, and increased survival of tumor-bearing animals [34]. In addition, a new perspective has recently emerged regarding what could be a critical role for CEPs in tumor angiogenesis, namely, following acute types of cytotoxic therapy. For example, Shaked et al [45] found that treatment of tumor-bearing mice with vascular disrupting agents (VDAs), i.e., drugs which target the established but abnormal tumor vasculature, causing a rapid shutdown of blood flow followed by extensive tumor hypoxia and necrosis, leads to an acute mobilization of CEPs, which subsequently home to the viable tumor rim that usually remains after such therapy, and drives 'rebound revascularization' and tumor regrowth/recovery following VDA therapy. In another study, we [46] found that certain chemotherapy drugs (taxanes in particular) administered at maximum tolerated doses (MTDs) can also induce a rapid CEP mobilization, most likely generated – at least in part - by the modulation of circulating SDF-1 levels. Prevention of the CEP spike by concurrent treatment with targeted antiangiogenic drugs, e.g. treatment with anti-VEGFR-2 or anti-VEGF monoclonal antibodies, or by genetic manipulation strategies (e.g.,undertaking treatment of tumors in Id mutant mice), or by the use of anti-SDF-1 neutralizing antibodies, resulted in enhanced antitumor activity of the administered cytotoxic chemotherapeutic drug. These findings raise the possibility that therapeutic strategies which aim to reduce CEP mobilization, might enhance the efficacy of certain cytotoxic anti-cancer therapies and – at the same time – reduce the risk of cancer metastases.

These results point to a sudden and "catalytic" function for CEPs, which may be a consequence of the aforementioned cytotoxic drugs not only being able to induce rapid mobilization of CEPs from the bone marrow, but also because the agents can damage the tumor vasculature, thereby creating the need and favorable circumstances for their physical incorporation into damaged vessels as part of a rapid host repair response. Indeed, cardiovascular researchers have for a number of years been studying the hypotheses that rapid mobilization of CEPs following damage to blood vessels caused by such pathologic events as stroke or infarcts represents such an adaptive (reactive) host repair process. Interestingly, when certain chemotherapy drugs are administered at much lower doses in a frequent repetitive fashion (i.e., "metronomic" chemotherapy), the acute CEP mobilization response seen with MTDs is not only avoided, but that such cells are actually targeted [23, 26]. This may be one of the mechanisms by which low-dose metronomic chemotherapy can cause an antiangiogenic effect [47].

5. CEC AND CEPs AS POSSIBLE BIOMARKERS OF OCCULT CANCER

A number of investigators have suggested that vessel-lining ECs in tumors might express a specific antigenic profile. The St Croix group compared gene expression patterns of ECs obtained from normal resting tissues, tumors, and regenerating liver [48]. They identified 25 transcripts overexpressed in tumor versus normal ECs, including 13 that were not found in the angiogenic endothelium of regenerating liver. Those EC tumor-specific antigens were primarily cell surface molecules of uncertain function. Should the tumor–specific expression of these antigens be confirmed in CECs, it would be possible – following the intuition of the late Judah Folkman [49] - to monitor tumor-specific CECs in subjects at high risk for cancer development or recurrence after therapy, in order to treat them with low-toxic anti-angiogenic (or other) targeted drugs before overt cancer symptoms or recurrence. In other words, it might be possible to monitor a nascent cancer before it becomes malignant, and try to keep it dormant and avoid development of metastases. Anti-angiogenic drugs, given in this way, may play a role similar to that of statins for the prevention of vascular diseases.

6. GENETICALLY ABERRANT CEC/CEPs

At variance with genetically unstable cancer cells, tumor-lining ECs have long been considered for many

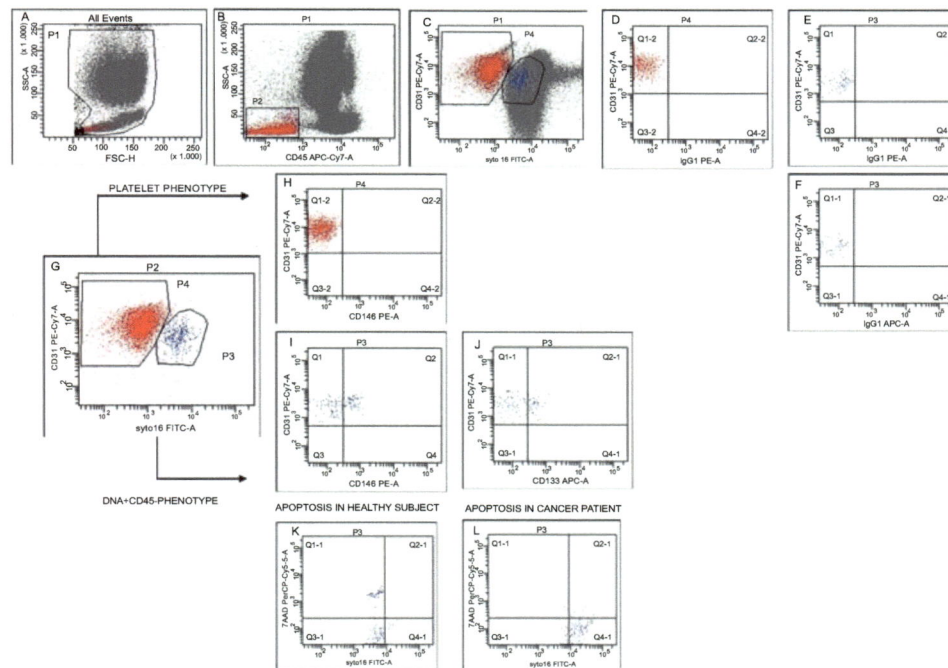

Fig. (3). Representative CEC/CEP count by flow cytometry (from Mancuso et al, 2009, modified). Panels A and B show the gate used to exclude necrotic/dead cell fragments and debris (panel A), and the gate made to depict CD45-negative (ie non-hematopoietic) cells (panel B). Panel C shows CD31 expression and Syto16 staining. Red and blue dots are from the CD45- events gate in Panel B. Panels D-F show the negative controls (Panel D for Panel H; Panel E for Panel I; Panel F for Panel J). Panel G shows the gates made on CD31bright/Syto16dim platelets (P4, red dots) and on CD31+Syto16+ CEC/CEPs (P3, blue dots) for further phenotypic investigation and enumeration. Panel H from the platelet gate (P4) shows the lack of CD146 expression in platelets. Panels I-J from the CEC/CEP gate show CECs (DNA/Syto16+,CD31+,CD146+, panel I) and CEP (DNA/Syto16+,CD31+,CD133+, panel J) counts. Panels K and L from the CEC gate show the frequency of viable, apoptotic and necrotic CECs in representative healthy subjects (panel K) and cancer patients at diagnosis (panel L). Quadrants to identify necrotic, apoptotic and viable cells are determined according to van der Pol et al [15]. The combination of syto 16 and 7AAD is used to identify necrotic cells (syto16low/7AAD+), apoptotic cells (syto16low/7AAD-) and viable cells (syto16bright/7AAD-). In Panel K, 7AAD+ cells are used as a reference to set the quadrants, which are copied in panel L.

years a genetically stable host cell drug target [50]. Preclinical and clinical evidence has recently challenged this view, and in hematological malignancies such as non-Hodgkin's lymphoma, myeloma, chronic and acute leukemias and myelodysplastic syndromes there is evidence that ECs might share the same genetic abnormalities found in cancer cells [51-55]. Although it is still not clear whether these unexpected findings were due to a common cancer/EC progenitor, to cancer-to-EC trans-differentiation, or to fusion between cancer and ECs [8], there are at least two related questions that deserve investigation.

First, are oncogene-bearing CEC/CEPs potentially able to cause cancer recurrence, and if so, should they be investigated as a new 'site' for minimal residual disease after therapy?

The second question stems from the recent findings of Shen et al [56]. These authors have found that in some

preclinical tumor models, most blood vessels were derived from precancerous cancer stem cells (pCSCs). These pCSCs expressed VEGFR-2, and were much more potent in tumor vasculogenesis than the differentiated tumor monocytic cells from the same tumor. They also observed tumor-cell related vasculogenesis in human cervical cancer and breast cancers. These findings suggest that oncogene-bearing CEC/CEPs might be one of the possible hidden identities of cancer stem cells, and suggest a possible mechanism for resistance to anti-angiogenic drug therapy of cancer, currently a subject of considerable interest and importance [57].

7. CONCLUSION: WHAT IS AND WILL BE THE ROLE OF CEC AND CEP IN CLINICAL ONCOLOGY

Under the light of the results summarized above, one can foresee two separate fields of clinical investigation for CEPs and CECs. Some CEPs (along with other hematopoietic cells) appear to have a transient "catalytic" but critical role [58] in promoting angiogenesis during tumor growth, in stimulating growth of micro- to macro-metastases, and in 'rebound' revascularization after certain therapies are stopped [30, 33-34, 38-39, 45, 58-59]. These cells are potentially promising targets for anti-cancer therapies and for adjuvant therapeutic strategies in patients at risk for cancer relapse. Also, one can try to exploit the tumor tropism of these cells for delivering anti-cancer drugs specifically at tumor site (reviewed in [8]). On the other side of the coin, these catalytic functions are in most cases associated with a pulsating presence of these cells in the blood and in the tissues, and thus it might be difficult to exploit measurement of these cells as biomarkers for selection and stratification of patients.

CECs in most cases are apoptotic or necrotic cells, being released into the circulation as a consequence of vascular turnover, and thus they would not represent a "druggable" target for anticancer therapies. On the other hand, CEC presence in the blood seems less pulsating (i.e., more stable) than CEPs and there is increasing evidence of their potential as surrogate biomarkers of cancer angiogenesis and of anti-angiogenic drug activity [8-21].

8. ACKNOWLEDGMENTS

We apologize to the numerous investigators whose papers could not be cited because of space limitations.

Supported in part by AIRC (Associazione Italiana per la Ricerca sul Cancro), ISS (Istituto Superiore di Sanità), Ministero della Salute grant RF-IMI-2006-411189 and the the sixth EU Framework Programme (Integrated Project 'Angiotargeting; contract no 504743) in the area of 'Life sciences, genomics and biotechnology for health". FB is a scholar of the US National Blood Foundation. RSK is a recipient of a Tier I Canada Research Chair and is supported by grants from the National Institutes of Health, USA (CA-41233), the Ontario Institute for Cancer Research (OICR), and the National Cancer Institute of Canada (NCIC).

9. REFERENCES

1.   Hladovec J, Rossmann P., Circulating endothelial cells isolated together with platelets and the experimental modification of their counts in rats, Thromb Res 1973; 3: 665-674.
2.   Moldovan NI, Moldovan L, Simionescu N. Binding of vascular anticoagulant alpha (annexin V) to the aortic intima of the hypercholesterolemic rabbit. An autoradiographic study, Blood Coagul Fibrinolysis 1994; 5(6): 921-928.
3.   Dignat-George F, Sampol J Circulating endothelial cells in vascular disorders: new insights into an old concept, Eur J Haematol 2000; 65(4): 215–220.
4.   Lin Y, Weisdorf DJ Solovey A, Hebbel RP. Origins of circulating endothelial cells and endothelial outgrowth from blood, J. Clin. Invest 2000; 105(1): 71-77.
5.   Rosenzweig A. Circulating Endothelial Progenitors – Cells as biomarkers. N Engl J Med 2005; 353(10): 1055-1057.
6.   Blann AD, Woywodt A, Bertolini F, Bull TM, Buyon JP, Clancy RM, Haubitz M, Hebbel RP, Lip GY, Mancuso P, Sampol J, Solovey A, Dignat-GeorgeF. Circulating endothelial cells. Biomarker of vascular disease, Thromb Haemost 2005; 93(2): 228-235.
7.   Woywodt A,. Blann AD, Kirsch T, Erdbruegger U, Banzet N, Haubitz M, Dignat-George F. Isolation and enumeration of circulating endothelial cells by immunomagnetic isolation: proposal of a definition and a consensus protocol. J Thromb Haemost 2006; 4(3): 671-677.
8.   Bertolini F, Shaked Y, Mancuso P, Kerbel RS. The multifaceted circulating endothelial cell in cancer: towards marker and target identification, Nat Rev Cancer 2006; 6(11): 835-845.
9.   Mancuso P, Burlini A, Pruneri G, Goldhirsch A, Martinelli G, Bertolini F. Resting and activated endothelial cells are increased in the peripheral blood of cancer patients, Blood 2001; 97(11): 3658-3661.
10.   Rabascio C, Muratori E, Mancuso P, Calleri A, Raia V, Foutz T, Cinieri S, Veronesi G, Pruneri G, Lampertico P, Iavarone M, Martinelli G, Goldhirsch A, Bertolini F. Assessing tumor angiogenesis: increased circulating VE-cadherin RNA in patients with cancer indicates viability of circulating endothelial cells, Cancer Res 2004; 15(12): 4373-4377
11.   Willett CG, Boucher Y, di Tomaso E, Duda DG, Munn LL, Tong RT, Chung DC, Sahani DV, Kalva SP, Kozin SV, Mino M, Cohen KS, Scadden DT, Hartford AC, Fischman AJ, Clark JW, Ryan DP, Zhu AX, Blaszkowsky LS, Chen HX, Shellito PC, Lauwers GY, Jain RK. Direct evidence that the VEGF-specific antibody bevacizumab has antivascular effects in human rectal cancer, Nat Med 2004; 10(2): 145-147.
12.   Beaudry P, Force J, Naumov GN, Wang A, Baker CH, Ryan A, Soker S, Johnson BE, Folkman J, Heymach JV. Differential effects of vascular endothelial growth factor receptor-2 inhibitor ZD6474 on circulating endothelial progenitors and mature circulating endothelial cells: implications for use as a surrogate marker of antiangiogenic activity, Clin Cancer Res 2005; 11(9): 3514-3522
13.   Zhang H, Vaki V, Braunstein M, Smith EL, Maroney J, Chen L, Dai K, Berenson JR, Hussain MM, Klueppelberg U, Norin AJ, Akman HO, Özcelik T, Batuman OA. Circulating endothelial progenitor cells in multiple myeloma: implications and significance, Blood 2005; 105(8): 3286-3294.
14.   Goon PK, Lip GY, Boos CJ, Stonelake PS, Blann AD. Circulating endothelial cells, endothelial

progenitor cells, and endothelial microparticles in cancer, Neoplasia 2006; 8(2): 79-88.

15. Duda DG, Cohen KS, di Tomaso E, Au P, Klein RJ, Scadden DT, Willett CG, Jain RK. Differential CD146 expression on circulating versus tissue endothelial cells in rectal cancer patients: implications for circulating endothelial and progenitor cells as biomarkers for antiangiogenic therapy, J Clin Oncol 2006; 24(9): 1449-1453.

16. Mancuso P, Colleoni M, Calleri A, Orlando L, Maisonneuve P, Pruneri G, Agliano A , Goldhirsch A, Shaked Y, Kerbel RS, Bertolini F. Circulating endothelial cell kinetics and viability predict survival in breast cancer patients receiving metronomic chemotherapy, Blood 2006; 108(2): 452-459.

17. Fürstenberger G, von Moos R, Lucas R, Thürlimann B, Senn HJ, Hamacher J, Boneberg EM. Circulating endothelial cells and angiogenic serum factors during neoadjuvant chemotherapy of primary breast cancer, Br J Cancer 2006; 94(4): 524-531.

18. Norden-Zfoni A, Desai J, Manola J, Beaudry P, Force J, Maki R, Folkman J, Bello C, Baum C, DePrimo SE, Shalinsky DR, Demetri GD, Heymach JV. Blood-based biomarkers of SU11248 activity and clinical outcome in patients with metastatic imatinib-resistant gastrointestinal stromal tumor, Clin Cancer Res 2007; 13(9): 2643-2650.

19. Beerepoot LV, Radema SA, Witteveen EO, Thomas T, Wheeler C, Kempin S, Voest EE. Phase I clinical evaluation of weekly administration of the novel vascular-targeting agent, ZD6126, in patients with solid tumors, J Clin Oncol 2006; 24(10): 1491-1498.

20. Rademaker-Lakhai JM, Beerepoot LV, Mehra N, Radema SA, van Maanen R. Phase I pharmacokinetic and pharmacodynamic study of the oral protein kinase C beta-inhibitor enzastaurin in combination with gemcitabine and cisplatin in patients with advanced cancer, Clin Cancer Res 2007; 13(15Pt1): 4474-4481.

21. Farace F, Massard C, Borghi E, Bidart JM, Soria JC. Vascular disrupting therapy-induced mobilization of circulating endothelial progenitor cells, Ann Oncol 2007; 18(8): 1421-1422.

22. Monestiroli S, Mancuso P, Burlini A, Pruneri G, Dell'Agnola C, Gobbi A, Martinelli G, Bertolini F. Kinetics and viability of circulating endothelial cells as surrogate angiogenesis marker in an animal model of human lymphoma, Cancer Res 2001; 61(11): 4341-4344.

23. Bertolini F, Paul S, Mancuso P, Monestiroli S, Gobbi A, Shaked Y, Kerbel RS. Maximum tolerable dose and low-dose metronomic chemotherapy have opposite effects on the mobilization and viability of circulating endothelial progenitor cells. Cancer Res 2003; 63(15): 4342-4346.

24. Shaked Y , Bertolini F, Man S, Rogers MS, Cervi D, Foutz T, Rawn K, Voskas D, Dumont DJ, Ben-David Y, Lawler J, Henkin J, Huber J, Hicklin DJ, D'Amato RJ, Kerbel RS. Genetic heterogeneity of the vasculogenic phenotype parallels angiogenesis; Implications for cellular surrogate marker analysis of antiangiogenesis, Cancer Cell 2005; 7(1): 101-111.

25. Schneider M, Tjwa M, Carmeliet P. A surrogate marker to monitor angiogenesis at last, Cancer Cell 2005; 7(1): 3-4.

26. Shaked Y, Emmenegge U, Man S, Cervi D, Bertolini F, Ben-David Y, Kerbel RS. Optimal biologic dose of metronomic chemotherapy regimens is associated with maximum antiangiogenic activity, Blood 2005; 106(9): 3058-3061.

27. Asahara T, Murohara T, Sullivan A, Silver M, van der Zee R, Li T, Witzenbichler B, Schatteman G, Isner JM. Isolation of putative progenitor endothelial cells for angiogenesis, Science 1997; 275(5302): 964-967.

28. Shi Q, Rafii S, Wu MH, Wijelath ES, Yu C, Ishida A, Fujita Y, Kothari S, Mohle R, Sauvage LR, Moore MA, Storb RF, Hammond WP. Evidence for circulating bone marrow-derived endothelial cells. Blood 1998; 92(2): 362–367.

29. Peichev M, Naiyer AJ, Pereira D, Zhu Z, Lane WJ, Williams M, Oz MC, Hicklin DJ, Witte L, Moore MA, Rafii S. Expression of VEGFR-2 and AC133 by circulating human CD34(+) cells identifies a population of functional endothelial precursors, Blood 2000; 95(3): 952-958.

30. Rafii S, Lyden D,Benezra R, Hattori K, Heissig B. Vascular and haematopoietic stem cells: novel targets for anti-angiogenesis therapy?, Nat Rev Cancer 2002; 2(11): 826-835.

31. Yoder MC, Mead LE, Prater D, Krier TR, Mroueh KN, Li F, Krasich R, Temm CJ, Prchal JT, Ingram DA. Redefining endothelial progenitor cells via clonal analysis and hematopoietic stem/progenitor cell principals, Blood 2007; 109(5): 1801-1809.

32. Case J, Mead LE, Bessler WK, Prater D, White HA, .Saadatzadeh MR, Bhavsar JR, Yoder MC, Haneline LS, Ingram DA. Human CD34+AC133+VEGFR-2+ cells are not endothelial progenitor cells but distinct, primitive hematopoietic progenitors, Exp Hematol 2007; 35(7): 1109-1118.

33. Nolan DJ, Ciarrocchi A, Mellick AS , Jaggi JS, Bambino K, Gupta S, Heikamp E, McDevitt MR, Scheinberg DA, Benezra R,.Mittal V. Bone marrow-derived endothelial progenitor cells are a major determinant of nascent tumor neovascularization. Genes Dev 2007; 21(12): 1546-1558.

34. Gao D, Nolan DJ, Mellick AS, Bambino K, McDonnell K, Mittal V. Endothelial progenitor cells control the angiogenic switch in mouse lung metastasis, Science 2008; 319(5860): 195-1998.

35. Lee S, Chen TT, Barber CL, Jordan MC, Murdock J, Desai S, Ferrara N, Nagy A, Roos KP , Iruela-Arispe ML. Autocrine VEGF signaling is required for vascular homeostasis, Cell 2007; 130(4): 691-703.

36. Dellapasqua S, Bertolini F, Bagnardi V, Campagnoli E, Scarano E, Torrisi R, Shaked Y, Mancuso P, Goldhirsch A, Rocca A, Pietri E, Colleoni M. Metronomic cyclophosphamide and capecitabine combined with bevacizumab in advanced breast cancer, J Clin Oncol 2008; 26(30): 4899-4905.

37. Kerbel RS, Folkman J. Clinical translation of angiogenesis inhibitors. Nat Rev Cancer 2002; 2(10): 727-739.

38. Lyden D, Hattori K, Dias S, Costa C, Blaikie P, Butros L, Chadburn A, Heissig B, Marks W, Witte

L, Wu Y, Hicklin D, Zhu Z, Hackett NR, Crystal RG, Moore MA, Hajjar KA, Manova K, Benezra R, Rafii S. Impaired recruitment of bone-marrow-derived endothelial and hematopoietic precursor cells blocks tumor angiogenesis and growth, Nat Med 2001; 7(11): 1194-1201.

39. Ciarrocchi A, Jankovic V, Shaked Y, Nolan DJ, Mittal V, Kerbel RS, Nimer SD, Benezra R. Id1 Restrains p21 Expression to Control Endothelial Progenitor Cell Formation, PLoS ONE 2007; 2(12): 1338.

40. De Palma M, Venneri MA, Roca C, Naldini L. Targeting exogenous genes to tumor angiogenesis by transplantation of genetically modified hematopoietic stem cells. Nat Med 2003; 9(6): 789-795.

41. Göthert JR, Gustin SE, van Eekelen JA, Schmidt U, Hall MA, Jane SM, Green AR, Göttgens B, Izon DJ, Begley CG. Genetically tagging endothelial cells in vivo: bone marrow-derived cells do not contribute to tumor endothelium, Blood 2004; 104(6): 1769-1777.

42. Spring H, Schüler T, Arnold B, Hämmerling GJ, Ganss R. Chemokines direct endothelial progenitors into tumor neovessels, Proc. Natl Acad. Sci. USA 2005; 102(50): 18111-18116.

43. Ruzinova MB, Schoer RA, Gerald W, Egan JE, Pandolfi PP, Rafii S, Manova K, Mittal V, Benezra R. Effect of angiogenesis inhibition by Id loss and the contribution of bone-marrow-derived endothelial cells in spontaneous murine tumors, Cancer Cell 2003; 4(4): 277-289.

44. Peters BA, Diaz LA, Polyak K, Meszler L, Romans K, Guinan EC, Antin JH, Myerson D, Hamilton SR, Vogelstein B, Kinzler KW, Lengauer C. Contribution of bone marrow-derived endothelial cells to human tumor vasculature, Nat Med 2005; 11(3): 261-262.

45. Shaked Y, Ciarrocchi A, Franco M, Lee CR, Man S, Cheung AM, Hicklin DJ, Chaplin D, Foster FS, Benezra R, Kerbel RS. Therapy-induced acute recruitment of circulating endothelial progenitor cells to tumors, Science 2006; 22(5794): 1785-1787.

46. Shaked Y, Henke E, Roodhart JM, Mancuso P, Langenberg MH, Colleoni M, Daenen LG, Man S, Xu P, Emmenegger U, Tang T, Zhu Z, Witte L, Strieter RM, Bertolini F, Voest EE, Benezra R, Kerbel RS. Rapid chemotherapy-induced acute endothelial progenitor cell mobilization: implications for antiangiogenic drugs as chemosensitizing agents, Cancer Cell 2008; 14(3): 263-273.

47. Kerbel RS, Kamen BA. The anti-angiogenic basis of metronomic chemotherapy, Nat Rev Cancer 2004; 4(6): 423-436.

48. Seaman S, Stevens J, Yang MY, Logsdon D, Graff-Cherry C, St.Croix B. Genes that distinguish physiological and pathological angiogenesis, Cancer Cell 2007; 11(6): 539-554.

49. Folkman J, Kalluri R. Cancer without disease, Nature 2004; 427(6977): 787.

50. Kerbel RS. Inhibition of tumor angiogenesis as a strategy to circumvent acquired resistance to anti-cancer therapeutic agents, Bioassays 1991; 13(1): 31-36.

51. Gunsilius E. Evidence from a leukaemia model for maintenance of vascular endothelium by bone-marrow-derived endothelial cells, Adv Exp Med Biol 2003; 522: 17-24

52. Hida K, Hida Y, Amin DN, Flint AF, Panigrahy D, Moton CC, Klgasbrun M. Tumor-associated endothelial cells with cytogenetic abnormalities, Cancer Res 2004; 64(22): 8249–8255.

53. Streubel B, Chott A, Huber D, Exner M, Jäger U, Wagner O, Schwarzinger I. Lymphoma-specific genetic aberrations in microvascular endothelial cells in B-cell lymphomas, N Engl J Med 2004; 351(3): 250-259.

54. Rigolin GM, Fraulini C, Ciccone M, Mauro E, Bugli AM, De Angeli C, Negrini M, Cuneo A, Castaldi G. Neoplastic circulating endothelial cells in multiple myeloma with 13q14 deletion, Blood 2006; 107(6): 2531-2535.

55. Della Porta MG, Malcovati L, Rigolin GM, Rosti V, Bonetti E, Travaglino E, Boveri E, Galli A, Boggi S, Ciccone M, Pramparo T, Mazzini G, Invernizzi R, Lazzarino M, Cazzola M. Immunophenotypic, cytogenetic and functional characterization of circulating endothelial cells in myelodysplastic syndromes., Leukemia 2008; 22(3): 530-537.

56. Shen R, Ye Y, Chen L, Yan Q, Barsky SH, Gao JX. Precancerous stem cells can serve as tumor vasculogenic progenitors, PLoS ONE 2008; 3(2): e-1652

57. Bergers G, Hanahan D. Models of resistance of anti-angiogenic therapy, Nat Rev Cancer 2008; 8(8): 592-603.

58. Seande M, Butler J, Lyden D, Rafii S. A catalytic role for proangiogenic marrow-derived cells in tumor neovascularization, Cancer Cell 2008; 13(3): 181-183.

59. Kaplan RN, Riba RD, Zacharoulis S, Bramley AH, Vincent L, Costa C, MacDonald DD, Jin DK, Shido K, Kerns SA, Zhu Z, Hicklin D, Wu Y, Port JL, Altorki N, Port ER, Ruggero D, Shmelkov SV, Jensen KK, Rafii S, Lyden D. VEGFR1-positive haematopoietic bone marrow progenitors initiate the pre-metastatic niche, Nature 2005; 8(7069): 820-827.

CHAPTER 8

Role of Thymidine Phosphorylase/Platelet-Derived Endothelial Cell Growth Factor in Tumor Progression

Sandra Liekens

Department of Microbiology and Immunology, Rega Institute for Medical Research, B-3000 Leuven, Belgium

Address correspondence to: Dr. Sandra Liekens, Rega Institute for Medical Research, Minderbroedersstraat 10, B-3000 Leuven, Belgium; Tel: +32-16-337355; Fax: +32-16-337340; Email: sandra.liekens@rega.kuleuven.be

Abstract: Thymidine phosphorylase/platelet-derived endothelial cell growth factor (TP/PD-ECGF) has diverse functions within cells, including the regulation of thymidine levels, the mediation of angiogenesis and apoptosis and the activation of prodrugs of the cancer chemotherapeutic agent 5-fluorouracil (5FU). The purpose of this review is to provide an overview of the pro-tumor effects of TP, including the molecular mechanisms of angiogenesis stimulation and apoptosis inhibition by TP.

1. INTRODUCTION

Thymidine phosphorylase (TP) is an important enzyme of the nucleoside salvage pathway [1]. The enzyme was first described and isolated from mammalian tissues more than 50 years ago [2]. TP catalyses the (reversible) phosphorolysis of thymidine and 2'-deoxyuridine to their respective base and α-2'-deoxy-*D*-ribose-1-phosphate (2dR-1P) (Fig. **1**). The latter is rapidly converted to 2-deoxy-*D*-ribose (2dR) [3].

In 1987, a novel "endothelial cell growth factor" was purified from human platelets. This protein did not bind heparin, was found to stimulate the incorporation of [³H]thymidine in endothelial cells,

but not in fibroblasts, and was therefore named platelet-derived endothelial cell growth factor (PD-ECGF) [4]. In 1992, recombinant human PD-ECGF was shown to possess TP activity [5]. Finally, amino acid sequence analysis and gel chromatography revealed that PD-ECGF is identical to TP [6,7]. Thus, the increased uptake of [³H]thymidine in endothelial cells treated with PD-ECGF was not related to any growth-promoting activity, i.e. due to its TP activity, PD-ECGF reduces cellular thymidine pools, resulting in the rapid uptake of a pulse of radiolabeled thymidine [7,8].

PD-ECGF/TP was also found to be identical to gliostatin, a protein isolated from neurofibroma [9]. Gliostatin inhibits the growth of glial tumor cell lines and astrocytes but promotes the survival of cortical

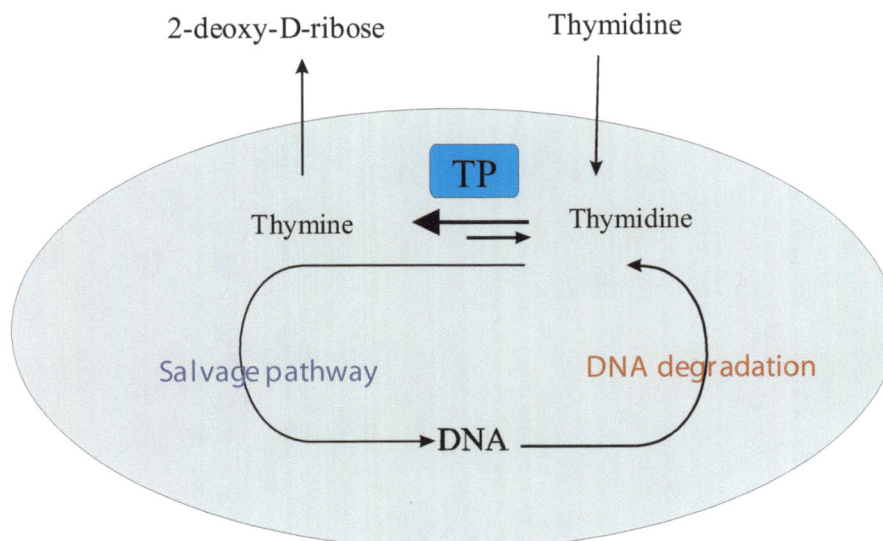

Fig. (1). TP catalyzes the conversion of thymidine to thymine and 2-deoxy-D-ribose-1-phosphate. The latter is rapidly dephosphorylated after which it can diffuse out of the cell. Thus, TP removes thymidine from the cytoplasm driving the nucleoside salvage pathway.

Domenico Ribatti (Ed.)

neurons [10]. Although the 3 names refer to the same protein, "PD-ECGF" and "TP" are used throughout the literature, whereas the use of "gliostatin" is mainly confined to arthritis and neurological research.

2. ANGIOGENIC ACTIVITY OF TP (Fig. 2)

TP has been shown to stimulate (i) chemotaxis of endothelial cells (ECs), (ii) tube formation of ECs in a collagen gel, (iii) outgrowth of vessels from rings of rat aorta and (iv) angiogenesis in several *in vivo* models, including the CAM assay, gelatin sponges and matrigel plugs implanted in mice and a freeze-injured skin graft model [11-16].

Overexpression of TP in various tumor cell lines did not confer a growth advantage to the cells *in vitro* [11,13,16,17]. However, transfection of RT112 bladder carcinoma cells with a retroviral vector containing TP cDNA resulted in enhanced regeneration of a wounded monolayer and increased invasion *in vitro*. [16,18]. Also MKN-45 and YCC-3 gastric cancer cell lines overexpressing TP showed increased adhesion, migration and invasion *in vitro* [19]. The *in vivo* effects of TP transfection were found to vary depending on the cell type used. Upon subcutaneous inoculation of Ha-ras-transformed 3T3 cells transfected with TP cDNA, tumors were formed that contained significantly more blood vessels than tumors from mock-transfected cells, but tumor

growth itself was not affected by TP [11]. Also, TP overexpression in a rat carcinoma cell line (PROb) had a relatively minor effect on tumor growth and this effect concerned only the initial stages of tumour expansion. However, the number of endothelial cells was consistently higher in TP-expressing tumors than in controls [20]. In contrast, overexpression of TP in MCF-7 breast carcinoma cells markedly increased both the vascular density and the tumor growth rate *in vivo* [14]. Also TP-overexpressing RT112 cells were characterized by a significantly greater xenograft growth rate than mock-transfected RT112 cells [18]. Nude mice inoculated with TP-overexpressing KB (human epidermoid carcinoma) cells had shorter survival times than those injected with control KB cells, and KB/TP tumors were more invasive than control tumors. [21]. TP also induced invasiveness and metastasis in lung adenocarcinoma [17]. Finally, lung colonization and spontaneous metastasis of A-07 melanoma cells were inhibited by treatment with a neutralizing antibody against TP, indicating that TP might promote lung metastasis of melanomas [22].

Thus, although the effect of TP on tumor growth rate *in vivo* is cell-type dependent, these studies clearly demonstrate the malignant potential of TP and its capacity to increase tumor vascularization and invasion.

The angiogenic activity of TP was inhibited by the TP inhibitor 6-amino-5-chlorouracil and by neutralizing antibodies to TP [11-13]. Moreover, lysates of COS-7

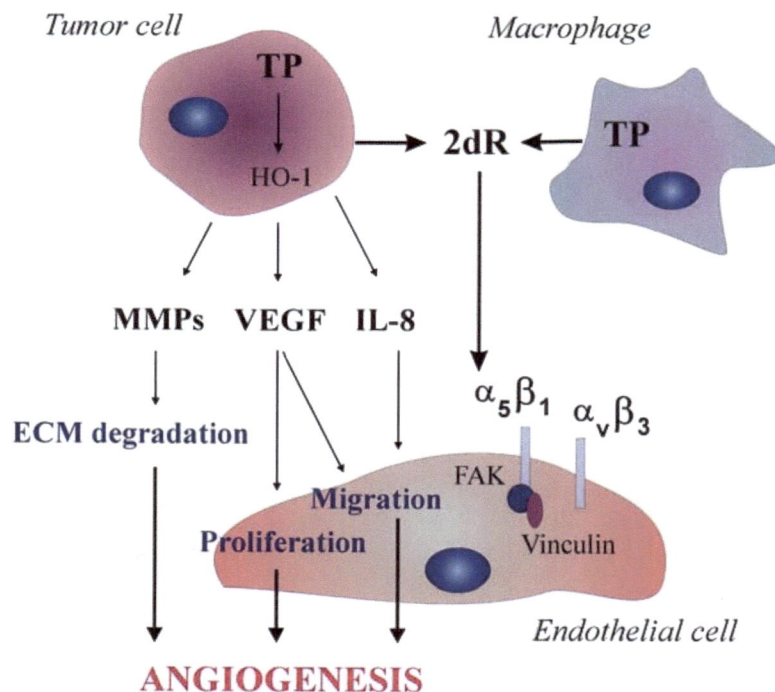

Fig. (2). Various conditions of cellular stress, such as low pH, hypoxia, inflammatory cytokines, radio- and chemotherapy may induce the expression of TP. Degradation of thymidine by TP results in the formation of 2dR-1P, which causes oxidative stress, resulting in the increased expression and secretion of several oxidative stress-response angiogenic factors. 2dR can also leave the cell and induce integrin expression and activation in endothelial cells.

cells transfected with three enzymatically inactive TP mutants, K115E, L148R and R202S did not possess angiogenic activity in contrast to wild-type transfectants [13].

Also the role of TP substrate (thymidine) and enzymatic products were extensively studied. TP, its catalytic product 2dR-1P, and the subsequent metabolite 2dR promoted endothelial tubulogenesis *in vitro*, and the regeneration of a wounded monolayer of ECs without exerting any mitogenic effect. *In vivo*, 2dR promoted blood vessel formation in an avascular sponge and in the CAM assay [12,16].

TP, 2dR-1P and 2dR were also found to induce chemotaxis of human umbilical vein endothelial cells (HUVEC). Migration induced by 2dR-1P was blocked by an alkaline phosphatase inhibitor, suggesting that the chemotactic activity of 2dR-1P first requires its conversion to 2dR. In a co-culture assay, U937 and THP1 human monocyte cells, which constitutively express high levels of TP, and TP-overexpressing carcinoma cells strongly induced HUVEC migration. Cell-stimulated HUVEC migration was inhibited by the TP inhibitor 5-chloro-6(1-imidazolylmethyl)uracil but not by a neutralizing antibody to TP, although the latter completely blocked migration induced by purified TP [23]. Together, these experimental data indicate that the angiogenesis-stimulating properties of TP (i) require its enzymatic activity and (ii) are mediated by the degradation product 2dR. So, although a receptor for TP has never been identified and TP is mainly retained intracellularly, the protein can elicit its angiogenic activity *via* the intracellular metabolism of thymidine and subsequent extracellular release of 2dR, which forms a chemotactic gradient. Interestingly, several of the biological effects induced by 2dR were found to be inhibited by its stereoisomer 2-deoxy-*L*-ribose [24-26].

Only recently, molecular mediators of TP and signaling pathways associated with TP-induced angiogenesis have been identified. Both TP and 2dR were found to stimulate the formation of focal adhesions and the phosphorylation of focal adhesion kinase (FAK) at tyrosine 397 in HUVEC and this effect was blocked by antibodies to either integrin α5β1 or αvβ3. TP and 2dR also increased the cell surface expression of integrin α5β1 and the association of FAK and vinculin with α5β1 [27].

A complementary DNA microarray was used to identify genes that are induced during *in vitro* migration of TP-overexpressing DLD-1 colon cancer cells. Rho-associated coiled-coil domain kinase (ROCK1) was found to be significantly overexpressed in TP transfectants compared with

mock-transfected cells. TP transfectants also showed higher cell motility than control cells. Also addition of recombinant TP increased cell migration of wild-type DLD-1 cells, and motility was blocked by a neutralizing antibody to TP and by Y-27632, a specific inhibitor of ROCK1. Moreover, actin fiber polymerization, which is a marker of activation of ROCK1, was higher in TP transfectants than in control cells [28].

Addition of TP to AGS and MKN-45 gastric carcinoma cell lines resulted in increased cancer cell invasion through matrigel, which was accompanied by actin filament remodeling and increased activation of the phosphatidylinosital-3-kinase (PI3K) pathway. In addition, TP-overexpressing MKN-45 cells showed increased activity of mammalian target of rapamycin (mTOR) and p70 ribosomal S6 kinase (p70^{S6K}) compared with control cells, suggesting the involvement of the PI3K/mTOR/ p70^{S6K} pathway in TP-induced migration and invasion of gastric carcinoma cells [19].

Transfection of RT112 human bladder carcinoma cells with TP resulted in the secretion of vascular endothelial growth factor (VEGF), interleukin (IL)-8, and matrix metalloproteinase (MMP)-1 [29]. Secretion of these angiogenic factors was only evident after supplementing the culture medium with thymidine, which recapitulates the tumor microenvironment in which thymidine concentrations are raised due to the hydrolysis of DNA from necrotic cells in hypoxic areas. Thymidine was shown to increase cellular levels of heme-oxygenase (HO-1), a marker for oxidative stress, in RT112/TP cells. This effect was abrogated by thymine, which may reverse thymidine catabolism by capturing 2dR-1P. These data suggest that 2dR-1P is responsible for the TP-induced oxidative stress, possibly by generating oxygen radical species during the early stages of protein glycation [29]. A time-dependent increase in HO-1 expression was also observed during monolayer regeneration of RT112/TP cells [16].

Increased mRNA expression and activity of MMP-9 were observed in KB/TP cell cultures and tumors compared with their mock-transfected counterparts and this was suggested to reflect the increased invasive potential of KB/TP cells/tumors [26]. KK47 bladder cancer cells that overexpress TP had higher levels of MMP-7 and MMP-9 than control cells, whereas overexpression of TP in prostate cancer cells resulted in increased expression of MMP-1 and MMP-7. Moreover, in bladder cancers from 72 randomly selected patients, the expression level of TP was found to correlate with that of urokinase-type plasminogen activator (uPA), MMP-1, MMP-9, plasminogen activator inhibtor (PAI)-1 and VEGF. Taken together, these data indicate that the TP-induced production and secretion of VEGF and various MMPs may contribute its angiogenic and invasive properties [30].

TP gene transfer was found to induce angiogenesis and decrease ischemia in a rabbit hindlimb model by promoting arteriogenesis [31]. TP was also evaluated for it ability to ameliorate chronic myocardial ischemia in dogs. Direct injection of a plasmid vector encoding TP cDNA into the ischemic area decreased the size of the infarct and reduced the number of apoptotic myocardial cells and the expression of the pro-apoptotic proteins active caspase-3 and Bax in the TP-treated group compared with the control group. Moreover, double immunohistochemical staining for von Willebrand factor and alpha-actin smooth muscle cells demonstrated an increase in angiogenesis and arteriogenesis after TP treatment, which was paralleled by increased myocardial blood flow and myocardial function [32,33]. TP gene transfer did not induce neoplasms in remote organs, suggesting that this gene may be a promising therapeutic strategy for peripheral vascular disease and myocardial ischemia.

In an *in vitro* angiogenesis assay TP was shown to increase VEGF-induced tube formation. Thus, to improve angiogenic gene therapy, a combination plasmid, encoding the VEGF gene and the TP gene was constructed. Upon transfection in COS-7 cells both gene products were expressed and functional as shown by Western blots, ELISAs and bioassays. However, the therapeutic potential of the phVEGF165-TP.MB plasmid has not yet been evaluated *in vivo* [34].

3. PHYSIOLOGICAL ROLE OF TP

Mice deficient in TP don't show any vascular defects, indicating that TP does not play an important role during vasculogenesis and/or developmental angiogenesis [35]. However, a recent study aimed at identifying factors secreted by endothelial progenitor cells (EPCs) demonstrated a key role for TP in the survival and angiogenic potential of EPCs. Inhibition of TP by 6-amino-5-bromouracil or gene silencing caused a significant increase in basal and oxidative stress-induced apoptosis. Moreover, 2dDR-1P produced by EPC cultures stimulated the migration of ECs in a paracrine manner, as demonstrated in transmigration and wound repair assays. Finally, the effect of conditioned medium from EPC cultures on endothelial migration was attenuated by RGD peptides and inhibitory antibodies to integrin $\alpha v \beta 3$ [36].

The highest TP activity has been detected in blood platelets suggesting a role for this protein in wound healing [37]. High levels of TP have also been observed in the placenta, where TP was shown to be present throughout pregnancy [38]. TP is also produced in the human endometrium where its expression was found to be inversely correlated with oestradiol concentrations during the menstrual cycle [39,40]. Furthermore, the expression of TP was increased in human endometrial stromal cells by the addition of progesterone, which induces differentiation of the stromal cells into decidualized cells [41]. Thus TP may play a physiological role in the process of decidualization of human endometrium. Taken together, TP does not seem to contribute to developmental angiogenesis, but its presence in the endometrium and placenta point to a potentially important role in the remodeling of the pre-existing vasculature.

4. ROLE OF TP IN ANGIOGENIC DISEASES

Several studies have implicated TP in angiogenic/inflammatory diseases. High expression of TP was detected in lesional psoriatic skin, wheras non-lesional skin showed minimal TP mRNA production and weak epidermal immunostaining [42]. TP immunoreactivity was also correlated with lesional microvessel density in coronary atherosclerotic plaques [43].

Furthermore, high concentrations of TP have been detected in the serum and synovial fluid of rheumatoid arthritis (RA) patients, compared with osteoarthritis patients [44]. Conversely, purified recombinant human TP administered to rabbit knee joints resulted in the development of diffuse synovitis resembling RA. Surprisingly, intra-articular injection of an enzymatically inactive mutant of TP induced the same effect, indicating that human TP can cause RA-like synovitis in rabbit knee joints via a mechanism other than its TP enzymatic activity [45]. In fibroblast-like synoviocytes (FLSs) obtained from patients with RA, the expression of TP mRNA was significantly increased by stimulation with IL-1β. TP mRNA levels in IL-1β-stimulated FLSs were reduced by treatment with aurothioglucose and dexamethasone, suggesting that the anti-rheumatic activity of these compounds may be mediated by the suppression of TP production [46]. TP was also found to induce the expression and secretion of VEGF, MMP-1 and MMP-3 in FLSs. Thus, VEGF and MMPs may mediate TP-induced angiogenesis and joint destruction in RA [47,48].

5. TP AND CANCER

Over the past years, an increasing number of studies have demonstrated a clinical role for TP in the progression of a variety of tumors and their metastases. Elevated levels of TP were found in the tumors compared with the non-neoplastic tissue of the corresponding organ and in the serum of tumor-bearing patients. Serum TP is likely to result from cellular turnover in the tumor and may also be released from trapped blood platelets. However, also tumor-infiltrating macrophages were found to express high levels of TP. Moreover, TP was proposed to be a marker of pro-tumor monocytes in breast cancer [49]. In addition, elevated TP levels were associated with increased vascular density in colorectal, gastric, esophageal, pancreatic, renal, endometrial, breast, ovarian, cervical, prostate, non-small cell lung cancer and glioblastoma, pointing to a role for TP in tumor angiogenesis [50-62]. Moreover, TP expression correlated well with tumor grade, metastasis and shorter patient survival in colorectal, pancreatic, renal, ovarian, cervical, bladder and non-small cell lung cancer [50,51, 54,55,58,59,61,63-68].

Although these studies have linked TP expression in the tumor to angiogenesis and/or malignancy, a number of reports did not find TP to be correlated with tumor progression. Several reasons may account for these discrepancies. In some cases where tumor TP levels are not predictive for survival, the concentration of TP in the serum of cancer patients may have prognostic value. Indeed, high serum TP levels in patients with esophageal squamous cell carcinoma were found to be associated with depth of tumor invasion, poor response to treatment and poor survival [69]. In addition, TP is not always produced by tumor cells but often by the infiltrating stromal cells. For example, in invasive breast cancer, the TP expression in stromal cells was found to predict overall survival as well as nodal status and tumor size [70].

In most cell lines *in vitro* TP mRNA levels are very low. However, several inflammatory mediators, including interferons (IFN)-α, -β, and -γ, IL-1α and tumor necrosis factor (TNF)-α, were found to upregulate TP expression by both transcriptional and posttranscriptional mechanisms. IFN-α and IFN-β induced an increase in TP mRNA levels and enzyme activity in HT29 human colon carcinoma cells due to the induction of nuclear factors that bind to a putative IFN response element in the TP promoter. TP mRNA was also shown to contain a pyrimidine-rich sequence at its 3' end that has been reported to mediate increased mRNA stability in other genes [71]. IFN-γ was found to be the most effective inducer of TP expression in human monocytic U937 cells by increasing signal transducers and activators of transcription 1 (STAT1) binding to the gamma-activated sequence-like element in the TP promoter [72]. A role for the Janus kinase (JAK)-STAT pathway in IFN-induced TP expression was also shown in human T98G cells [73]. However,

Fukushima *et al.* [74] demonstrated that IFN only affects human cancer cells with low TP activity. Tumor cells that already have high TP activity are no longer susceptible to induction by IFN due to the high level of STAT1 in these cells.

TP expression was also found to be upregulated by TNFα. In human colon carcinoma cells, the Sp1 transcription factor was found to contribute to the TNFα-induced expression of TP [75]. In the human monocyte cell line THP-1 both TP mRNA and enzyme activity were found to be up-regulated by TNFα and this regulation involved TNFα-receptor R2 and nuclear factor (NF)κB [76]. Conversely, prolonged exposure of THP-1 cells to sulfasalazine, an anti-inflammatory drug and inhibitor of NFκB, resulted in down-regulation of TP (mRNA, protein and activity) along with elimination of TP induction by TNFα [77].

TP expression may also be upregulated by environmental factors, such as low pH (6.3-6.7) and hypoxia, which may explain why TP expression is highest close to areas of necrosis, and is increased by occlusion of the tumor vasculature [78].

Finally, X-ray irradiation and various chemotherapeutic agents have been shown to induce TP expression, some of which by increasing TNF-α levels [79,80]. These findings have lead to the hypothesis that a combination of TP-inducible chemotherapy and capecitabine, a prodrug of 5FU that requires TP for its activation, might enhance the effectiveness of anti-cancer therapy [79-83]. So far, capecitabine showed promising synergistic anti-tumor activity with IFN-α, cisplatin, docetaxel, mitomycin C and radiotherapy in several phase II studies [reviewed in 84]. In addition, a phase III trial enrolling metastatic breast cancer patients has shown that addition of capecitabine to standard TP-inducible chemotherapy like paclitaxel, cisplatin, cyclophosphamide or irradiation results in increased response rate, time to progression and survival of patients compared with standard treatment alone [85]. Capecitabine is currently approved by the FDA for use as first-line therapy in patients with metastatic colorectal cancer. The drug is also approved in metastatic breast cancer patients in combination with docetaxel after failure of anthracycline-based chemotherapy [reviewed in 84].

VEGF and TP are frequently co-expressed in highly vascularized tissues and tumors [38,62,86,87]. Co-expression of TP and VEGF may be explained by the presence of SP1 transcription factor binding sites in the TP and VEGF promoters suggesting similar transcriptional activation of both genes [88,89]. However, TP may also directly induce VEGF production and secretion *via* an autocrine manner in tumor cells [29].

Besides being co-expressed, VEGF and TP have also been shown to co-operate in stimulating neovascularization. Hotchkiss *et al.* [27] showed that the combined effects of TP and VEGF on migration of HUVEC are additive up to the maximum of each individual agent, suggesting that both proteins may use similar signal transduction pathways. However, TP-induced endothelial cell migration was mediated by integrins $\alpha_5\beta_1$ and $\alpha_v\beta_3$, whereas VEGF-induced migration only involved $\alpha_v\beta_3$ [27].

In vivo studies suggest a synergistic function of VEGF and TP, based on the finding that VEGF and TP are often expressed by different cell types. In particular VEGF may be expressed exclusively in cancer cells, whereas TP expression is often particularly evident in stromal cells [60,90]. In endometrial carcinoma, the most potent angiogenic phenotype was observed when VEGF (in the tumor cells) and TP (in fibroblasts and macrophages) were co-expressed [60]. Moreover, patients with stage I lung adenocarcinoma that showed expression of TP in the stromal cells and VEGF in the tumor cells had a significantly worse prognosis than patients in the TP-negative or VEGF-negative group [90].

6. TP PROTECTS TUMOR CELLS AGAINST APOPTOSIS

TP may also stimulate tumor growth independent of its pro-angiogenic activity. KB cells transfected with TP cDNA were found to be resistant to hypoxia-induced apoptosis. Also 2dR and thymine partially prevented hypoxia-induced apoptosis, suggesting that the enzymatic activity of TP is required for the anti-apoptotic effect [91]. In human leukemia HL-60 cells, 2dR was found to inhibit several events related to hypoxia-induced apoptosis, such as the upregulation of hypoxia-inducible factor (HIF)-1α, loss of mitochondrial transmembrane potential and subsequent cytochrome c release, downregulation of Bcl-2 and Bcl-x(L), increase of Bax and caspase 3 activation. Moreover, 2dR was found to inhibit hypoxia-induced phosphorylation of p38 mitogen-activated protein kinase (MAPK) in HL-60 cells [92,93]. In Jurkat cells, hypoxia-induced apoptosis was prevented at least in part by TP or 2dR-induced suppression of BNIP3 (Bcl2/adenovirus E1B 19kDa interacting protein) expression [94].

Overexpression of TP was also found to protect KB tumor cells against Fas-induced apoptosis (i.e. caspase-8 cleavage, loss of mitochondrial membrane potential, release of cytochrome c, activation of caspase-3) [95]. Treatment with the TP inhibitor TPI did not affect survival of KB/TP cells, indicating that the enzymatic activity of TP is not required for suppression of Fas-induced apoptosis [96]. Also

protection of Jurkat/TP and U937 cells against apoptosis induced by various DNA damaging agents, such as cisplatin, doxorubicin, paclitaxel and vincristine, was unrelated to TP enzymatic activity [97-99]. The protective effect of TP in U937 cells was mediated by increased activation of the PI3K/Akt survival pathway [99].

The anti-apoptotic effect of TP may explain why in some clinical studies TP was shown to be a prognostic factor although no correlation could be established between TP and intratumoral vascular density. In these tumors, where other angiogenic factors are likely to be more important for tumor neovascularization, TP may contribute to tumor malignancy by preventing apoptosis in the presence of low oxygen tension and/or chemotherapeutic agents.

7. TP INHIBITORS

For more than 30 years, the reference compounds for TP inhibition were 6-aminothymine (6AT) and 6-amino-5-bromouracil (6A5BU) with 50% inhibitory concentrations (IC_{50}) around 30 μM [100]. As the stimulatory role of TP in angiogenesis and cancer became evident, interest was raised in the synthesis of novel TP inhibitors with improved solubility, specificity and inhibitory activity against TP. Most of these compounds are pyrimidine analogues, which compete with thymidine for binding to TP and inhibit the enzyme with IC_{50} values in the micromolar range [for an extensive review see 101].

The most potent and specific TP inhibitor that has been developed till now is 5-chloro-6-[1-(2-iminopyrroli-dinyl)methyl]uracil hydrochloride (TPI) with anti-TP activity in the nanomolar range, i.e. 1000-fold more active than the reference compounds [102]. TPI was found to inhibit the migration and invasion of TP-overexpressing KB cells *in vitro*, and angiogenesis in a mouse dorsal air sac assay [103]. In addition, TPI decreased the growth rate and increased the apoptotic index of KB/TP cells, xenografted into nude mice, and suppressed experimental liver metastases of these cells [103,104]. Analysis of the crystal structure of human TP bound to TPI indicates that the inhibitor mimics the substrate transition state of the enzyme, which may explain its potency [105].

Based on its potent activity and oral bioavailability, TPI was considered for combination therapy with trifluorothymidine (TFT), an anti-tumor agent which, based on its homology with thymidine, is rapidly degraded by TP [102,106]. TFT is being used clinically as an antiviral agent for use against herpes simplex virus-induced keratoconjunctivitis. Clinical studies to determine its anti-tumor potential were discontinued because of a poor pharmacokinetic profile [107]. TAS-102 (Fig. **3**), an orally administrable combination of

TFT (1M) and TPI (0.5M) was found to suppress TP-induced angiogenesis, enhance the antitumor efficacy of TFT in nude mice xenografted with human gastrointestinal cancer cell lines, and decrease TFT toxicity [108]. TAS-102 is currently being evaluated in Phase I studies enrolling patients with various solid tumors [107,109].

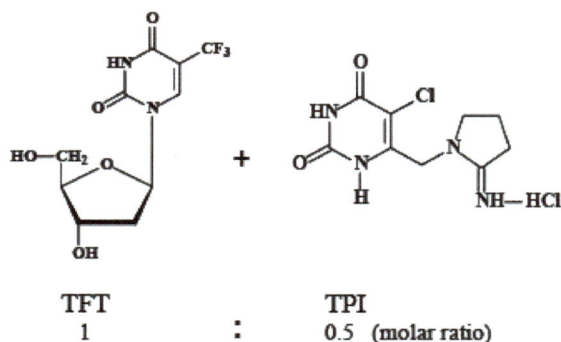

TFT
1

:

TPI
0.5   (molar ratio)

Fig. (3). Chemical structure of TAS-102.

TP is a dimer, consisting of two identical subunits (with a molecular mass ranging from 45 kD in *E. coli* to 55 kD in mammals) that are non-covalently associated. The nucleic acid sequence of TP is highly conserved, i.e. human TP shares 39% sequence identity with *E. coli* TP. Also the crystal structures of *E. coli* and human TP show a similar overall folding, each subunit being composed of a small α-helical domain containing the thymidine-binding site and, separated by a cleft, a large α/β domain containing the phosphate-binding site [105,110,111]. In its inactive conformation, the substrate-binding sites of TP are too far apart for the two substrates to directly interact. Movement of the α domains was suggested to be critical for enzymatic activity by closing the active site cleft, leading to the exclusion of water [112].

The reference TP inhibitors 6AT and 6A5BU were modeled into the active site of *E. coli* TP, based on the position of thymine as proposed by Walter *et al.* [110]. In order to create extra stabilizing interactions, a second ring was added onto the pyrimidine base. This resulted in 7-deazaxanthine (7DX), the first purine derivative with anti-TP activity similar to the reference compounds [113]. 7DX was also found to inhibit angiogenesis in the CAM assay.

As domain movement is thought to be critical for TP activity, immobilization of TP in its inactive conformation was considered as a new strategy to inhibit TP enzymatic activity. In its open, inactive conformation, the distance between the thymidine- and phosphate-binding sites of *E. coli* TP is approximately 8-10 Å. Thus, compounds were designed that contain a base, interacting at the thymidine-binding site and, connected by a linker, a phosphonate moiety, interacting at the phosphate-binding site [114]. Replacement of the thymine base by 7DX resulted in TP65, the first multi-substrate analogue inhibitor of TP [114]. Enzyme kinetic studies showed that TP65 acts as a competitive inhibitor with regard to thymidine and phosphate, indicating that the compound interacts with both substrate-binding sites of the TP enzyme, as originally designed [115]. However, TP65 did not prove to be a more potent inhibitor of TP than 7DX with IC_{50} values of 20 to 60 μM against *E. coli* and human TP [116].

We recently described the inhibitory activity of KIN59 (5'-O-tritylinosine) and analogues against TP enzymatic activity (IC_{50} value of 30 μM) and TP-induced angiogenesis in the CAM assay [117,118]. KIN59 is a very unusual TP inhibitor; i.e. it is a purine nucleoside with an intact ribose moiety. Moreover, in contrast to previously described TP inhibitors, KIN59 does not compete with the nucleoside- or phosphate-binding site of the enzyme. In the CAM assay, KIN59 was shown to completely inhibit TP-induced angiogenesis. The compound also caused the degradation of pre-existing immature vessels, without eliciting systemic toxicity [117] (Fig. **4**). These data suggest that the enzymatic and angiogenic activities of TP are not solely directed through its substrate-binding sites, but that a yet unidentified allosteric site in TP contributes to its biological properties. Efforts are undergoing to identify the amino acid residues in TP that interact with KIN59, as they might offer new insights into the mechanism of action of TP.

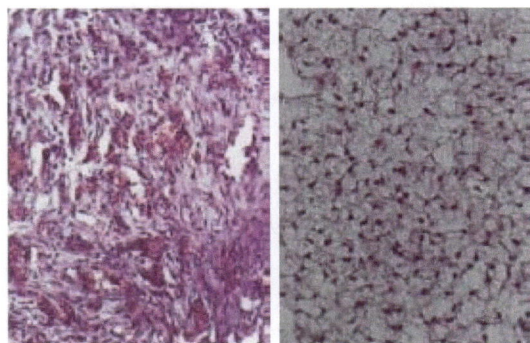

Fig. (4). Inhibition of TP-induced angiogenesis (left) by KIN59 (right) in the CAM assay.

7. CONCLUSIONS

TP is a unique enzyme, which may fulfill diverse roles within cells. Stimulation of angiogenesis by TP requires its enzymatic activity, resulting in integrin activation, the induction of oxidative stress and the upregulation and release of angiogenic mediators, such as VEGF, IL-8 and MMPs. However, the mechanism by which TP inhibits apoptosis depends upon the apoptotic stimulus, and may be independent of its enzymatic activity. Increased TP expression in tumors is correlated with increased angiogenesis, tumor progression, metastasis and low prognosis, implying the need for TP inhibitors in cancer treatment.

In contrast, as TP expression is highly upregulated in the tumor microenvironment, TP is being used for the tumor-specific activation of 5FU prodrugs, such as capecitabine. Identification of the angiogenic mediators and nucleoside metabolizing enzymes in individual tumors should aid in determining the right treatment strategy (TP inhibition *versus* TP stimulation combined with 5FU treatment).

8. ACKNOWLEDGMENTS

SL is a postdoctoral research fellow of the "Fonds voor Wetenschappelijk Onderzoek (FWO)". This work was funded by grants from the Centers of Excellence of the K.U. Leuven (Krediet nr EF-05/15), the FWO (Krediet nr G. 0486.08) and "Geconcerteerde Onderzoeksactie-Vlaanderen" (GOA-2005/19).

9. REFERENCES

1. Iltzsch MH, El Kouni MH, Cha S. Kinetic studies of thymidine phosphorylase from mouse liver. Biochemistry 1985; 24(24): 6799-6807.

2. Friedkin M, Roberts D. The enzymatic synthesis of nucleosides. I. Thymidine phosphorylase in mammalian tissue. J Biol Chem 1954; 207(1): 245-256.

3. de Bruin M, van Capel T, Van der Born K, Kruyt FA, Fukushima M, Hoekman K, Pinedo HM, Peters GJ. Role of platelet-derived endothelial cell growth factor/thymidine phosphorylase in fluoropyrimidine sensitivity. Br J Cancer 2003; 88(6): 957-964.

4. Miyazono K, Okabe T, Urabe A, Takaku F, Heldin CH. Purification and properties of an endothelial cell growth factor from human platelets. J Biol Chem 1987; 262(9): 4098-4103.

5. Barton GJ, Ponting CP, Spraggon G, Finnis C, Sleep D. Human platelet-derived endothelial cell growth factor is homologous to Escherichia coli thymidine phosphorylase. Protein Sci 1992; 1(5): 688-690.

6. Moghaddam A, Bicknell R. Expression of platelet-derived endothelial cell growth factor in Escherichia coli and confirmation of its thymidine phosphorylase activity. Biochemistry 1992; 31(48): 12141-12146.

7. Usuki K, Saras J, Waltenberger J, Miyazono K, Pierce G, Thomason A, Heldin CH. Platelet-derived endothelial cell growth factor has thymidine phosphorylase activity. Biochem Biophys Res Commun 1992; 184(3): 1311-1316.

8. Finnis C, Dodsworth N, Pollitt CE, Carr G, Sleep D. Thymidine phosphorylase activity of platelet-derived endothelial cell growth factor is responsible for endothelial cell mitogenicity. Eur J Biochem 1993; 212(1): 201-210.

9. Asai K, Hirano T, Kaneko S, Moriyama A, Nakanishi K, Isobe I, Eksioglu YZ, Kato T. A novel glial growth inhibitory factor, gliostatin, derived from neurofibroma. J Neurochem 1992; 59(1): 307-317.

10. Asai K, Nakanishi K, Isobe I, Eksioglu YZ, Hirano A, Hama K, Miyamoto T, Kato T. Neurotrophic action of gliostatin on cortical neurons. Identity of gliostatin and platelet-derived endothelial cell growth factor. J Biol Chem 1992; 267(28): 20311-20316.

11. Ishikawa F, Miyazono K, Hellman U, Drexler H, Wernstedt C, Hagiwara K, Usuki K, Takaku F, Risau W, Heldin CH. Identification of angiogenic activity and the cloning and expression of platelet-derived endothelial cell growth factor. Nature 1989; 338(6216): 557-562.

12. Haraguchi M, Miyadera K, Uemura K, Sumizawa T, Furukawa T, Yamada K, Akiyama S, Yamada Y. Angiogenic activity of enzymes. Nature 1994; 368(6468): 198.

13. Miyadera K, Sumizawa T, Haraguchi M, Yoshida H, Konstanty W, Yamada Y, Akiyama S. Role of thymidine phosphorylase activity in the angiogenic effect of platelet derived endothelial cell growth factor/thymidine phosphorylase. Cancer Res 1995; 55(8): 1687-1690.

14. Moghaddam A, Zhang HT, Fan TP, Hu DE, Lees VC, Turley H, Fox SB, Gatter KC, Harris AL, Bicknell R. Thymidine phosphorylase is angiogenic and promotes tumor growth. Proc Natl Acad Sci USA 1995; 92(4): 998-1002.

15. Stevenson DP, Milligan SR, Collins WP. Effects of platelet-derived endothelial cell growth factor/thymidine phosphorylase, substrate, and products in a three-dimensional model of angiogenesis. Am J Pathol 1998; 152(6): 1641-1646.

16. Sengupta S, Sellers LA, Matheson HB, Fan TP. Thymidine phosphorylase induces angiogenesis in vivo and in vitro: an evaluation of possible mechanisms. Br J Pharmacol. 2003; 139(2): 219-231.

17. Sato J, Sata M, Nakamura H, Inoue S, Wada T, Takabatake N, Otake K, Tomoike H, Kubota I. Role of thymidine phosphorylase on invasiveness and metastasis in lung adenocarcinoma. Int J Cancer 2003; 106(6): 863-70.

18. Jones A, Fujiyama C, Turner K, Cranston D, Williams K, Stratford I, Bicknell R, Harris AL. Role of thymidine phosphorylase in an in vitro model of human bladder cancer invasion. J Urol 2002; 167(3): 1482-1486.

19. Yu EJ, Lee Y, Rha SY, Kim TS, Chung HC, Oh BK, Yang WI, Noh SH, Jeung HC. Angiogenic factor thymidine phosphorylase increases cancer cell invasion activity in patients with gastric adenocarcinoma. Mol Cancer Res 2008; 6(10): 1554-1566.

20. Marchetti S, Chazal M, Dubreuil A, Fischel JL, Etienne MC, Milano G. Impact of thymidine phosphorylase surexpression on fluoropyrimidine activity and on tumour angiogenesis. Br J Cancer 2001; 85(3): 439-445.

21. Nakajima Y, Haraguchi M, Furukawa T, Yamamoto M, Nakanishi H, Tatematsu M, Akiyama S. 2-Deoxy-L-ribose inhibits the invasion of thymidine phosphorylase-overexpressing tumors by suppressing

matrix metalloproteinase-9. Int J Cancer. 2006; 119(7): 1710-1716.

22.   Rofstad EK, Halsor EF. Vascular endothelial growth factor, interleukin 8, platelet-derived endothelial cell growth factor, and basic fibroblast growth factor promote angiogenesis and metastasis in human melanoma xenografts. Cancer Res 2000; 60(17): 4932-4938.

23.   Hotchkiss KA, Ashton AW, Klein RS, Lenzi ML, Zhu GH, Schwartz EL. Mechanisms by which tumor cells and monocytes expressing the angiogenic factor thymidine phosphorylase mediate human endothelial cell migration. Cancer Res 2003; 63(2): 527-533.

24.   Uchimiya H, Furukawa T, Okamoto M, Nakajima Y, Matsushita S, Ikeda R, Gotanda T, Haraguchi M, Sumizawa T, Ono M, Kuwano M, Kanzaki T, Akiyama S. Suppression of thymidine phosphorylase-mediated angiogenesis and tumor growth by 2-deoxy-L-ribose. Cancer Res 2002; 62(10): 2834-2839.

25.   Nakajima Y, Gotanda T, Uchimiya H, Furukawa T, Haraguchi M, Ikeda R, Sumizawa T, Yoshida H, Akiyama S. Inhibition of metastasis of tumor cells overexpressing thymidine phosphorylase by 2-deoxy-L-ribose. Cancer Res 2004(5); 64: 1794-1801.

26.   Nakajima Y, Haraguchi M, Furukawa T, Yamamoto M, Nakanishi H, Tatematsu M, Akiyama S. 2-Deoxy-L-ribose inhibits the invasion of thymidine phosphorylase-overexpressing tumors by suppressing matrix metalloproteinase-9. Int J Cancer 2006; 119(7): 1710-1716.

27.   Hotchkiss KA, Ashton AW, Schwartz EL. Thymidine phosphorylase and 2-deoxyribose stimulate human endothelial cell migration by specific activation of the integrins alpha 5 beta 1 and alpha V beta 3. J Biol Chem 2003; 278(21): 19272-19279.

28.   Yoshinaga K, Inoue H, Tanaka F, Mimori K, Utsunomiya T, Mori M. Platelet-derived endothelial cell growth factor mediates Rho-associated coiled-coil domain kinase messenger RNA expression and promotes cell motility. Ann Surg Oncol 2003; 10(5): 582-587.

29.   Brown NS, Jones A, Fujiyama C, Harris AL, Bicknell R. Thymidine phosphorylase induces carcinoma cell oxidative stress and promotes secretion of angiogenic factors. Cancer Res 2000(22); 60: 6298-6302.

30.   Gotanda T, Haraguchi M, Tachiwada T, Shinkura R, Koriyama C, Akiba S, Kawahara M, Nishiyama K, Sumizawa T, Furukawa T, Mimata H, Nomura Y, Akiyama S, Nakagawa M. Molecular basis for the involvement of thymidine phosphorylase in cancer invasion. Int J Mol Med 2006; 17(6): 1085-1091.

31.   Yamada N, Li W, Ihaya A, Kimura T, Morioka K, Uesaka T, Takamori A, Handa M, Tanabe S, Tanaka K. Platelet-derived endothelial cell growth factor gene therapy for limb ischemia. J Vasc Surg 2006; 44(6): 1322-1328.

32.   Li W, Tanaka K, Ihaya A, Fujibayashi Y, Takamatsu S, Morioka K, Sasaki M, Uesaka T,

Kimura T, Yamada N, Tsuda T, Chiba Y. Gene therapy for chronic myocardial ischemia using platelet-derived endothelial cell growth factor in dogs. Am J Physiol Heart Circ Physiol 2005; 288(1): H408-415.

33.   Li W, Tanaka K, Morioka K, Takamori A, Handa M, Yamada N, Ihaya A. Long-term effect of gene therapy for chronic ischemic myocardium using platelet-derived endothelial cell growth factor in dogs. J Gene Med 2008; 10(4): 412-420.

34.   Bouis D, Boelens MC, Peters E, Koolwijk P, Stob G, Kema IP, Klinkenberg M, Mulder NH, Hospers GA. combination of vascular endothelial growth factor (VEGF) and thymidine phosphorylase (TP) to improve angiogenic gene therapy. Angiogenesis 2003; 6(3): 185-192.

35.   Haraguchi M, Tsujimoto H, Fukushima M, Higuchi I, Kuribayashi H, Utsumi H, Nakayama A, Hashizume Y, Hirato J, Yoshida H, Hara H, Hamano S, Kawaguchi H, Furukawa T, Miyazono K, Ishikawa F, Toyoshima H, Kaname T, Komatsu M, Chen ZS, Gotanda T, Tachiwada T, Sumizawa T, Miyadera K, Osame M, Yoshida H, Noda T, Yamada Y, Akiyama S. Targeted deletion of both thymidine phosphorylase and uridine phosphorylase and consequent disorders in mice. Mol Cell Biol 2002; 22(14): 5212-5221.

36.   Pula G, Mayr U, Evans C, Prokopi M, Vara DS, Yin X, Astroulakis Z, Xiao Q, Hill J, Xu Q, Mayr M. Proteomics Identifies Thymidine Phosphorylase As a Key Regulator of the Angiogenic Potential of Colony-Forming Units and Endothelial Progenitor Cell Cultures. Circ Res 2009; 104(1): 32-40.

37.   Shaw T, Smillie RH, MacPhee DG. The role of blood platelets in nucleoside metabolism: assay, cellular location and significance of thymidine phosphorylase in human blood. Mutat Res 1988; 200(1-2): 99-116.

38.   Jackson MR, Carney EW, Lye SJ, Ritchie JW. Localization of two angiogenic growth factors (PDECGF and VEGF) in human placentae throughout gestation. Placenta 1994; 15(4): 341-353.

39.   Fujimoto J, Ichigo S, Sakaguchi H, Hirose R, Tamaya T. Expression of platelet-derived endothelial cell growth factor and its mRNA in uterine endometrium during the menstrual cycle. Mol Hum Reprod 1998; 4(5): 509-513.

40.   Zhang L, Mackenzie IZ, Rees MC, Bicknell R. Regulation of the expression of the angiogenic enzyme platelet-derived endothelial cell growth factor/thymidine phosphorylase in endometrial isolates by ovarian steroids and cytokines. Endocrinology 1997; 138(11): 4921-4930.

41.   Osuga Y, Toyoshima H, Mitsuhashi N, Taketani Y. The presence of platelet-derived endothelial cell growth factor in human endometrium and its characteristic expression during the menstrual cycle and early gestational period. Hum Reprod 1995; 10(4): 989-993.

42.   Creamer D, Jaggar R, Allen M, Bicknell R, Barker J. Overexpression of the angiogenic factor platelet-derived endothelial cell growth factor/thymidine phosphorylase in psoriatic epidermis. Br J Dermatol 1997; 137(6): 851-855.

43.   Ignatescu MC, Gharehbaghi-Schnell E, Hassan A, Rezaie-Majd S, Korschineck I, Schleef RR, Glogar

HD, Lang IM. Expression of the angiogenic protein, platelet-derived endothelial cell growth factor, in coronary atherosclerotic plaques: In vivo correlation of lesional microvessel density and constrictive vascular remodeling. Arterioscler Thromb Vasc Biol 1999; 19(10): 2340-2347.

44.   Takeuchi M, Otsuka T, Matsui N, Asai K, Hirano T, Moriyama A, Isobe I, Eksioglu YZ, Matsukawa K, Kato T. Aberrant production of gliostatin/platelet-derived endothelial cell growth factor in rheumatoid synovium. Arthritis Rheum 1994; 37(5): 662-672.

45.   Waguri-Nagaya Y, Otsuka T, Sugimura I, Matsui N, Asai K, Nakajima K, Tada T, Akiyama S, Kato T. Synovial inflammation and hyperplasia induced by gliostatin/platelet-derived endothelial cell growth factor in rabbit knees. Rheumatol Int 2000; 20(1): 13-19.

46.   Kusabe T, Waguri-Nagaya Y, Tanikawa T, Aoyama M, Fukuoka M, Kobayashi M, Otsuka T, Asai K. The inhibitory effect of disease-modifying anti-rheumatic drugs and steroids on gliostatin/platelet-derived endothelial cell growth factor production in human fibroblast-like synoviocytes. Rheumatol Int 2005; 25(8): 625-630.

47.   Muro H, Waguri-Nagaya Y, Mukofujiwara Y, Iwahashi T, Otsuka T, Matsui N, Moriyama A, Asai K, Kato T. Autocrine induction of gliostatin/platelet-derived endothelial cell growth factor (GLS/PD-ECGF) and GLS-induced expression of matrix metalloproteinases in rheumatoid arthritis synoviocytes. Rheumatology (Oxford) 1999; 38(12): 1195-1202.

48.   Tanikawa T, Waguri-Nagaya Y, Kusabe T, Aoyama M, Asai K, Otsuka T. Gliostatin/thymidine phosphorylase-regulated vascular endothelial growth-factor production in human fibroblast-like synoviocytes. Rheumatol Int 2007; 27(6): 553-559.

49.   Toi M, Ueno T, Matsumoto H, Saji H, Funata N, Koike M, Tominaga T. Significance of thymidine phosphorylase as a marker of protumor monocytes in breast cancer. Clin Cancer Res 1999; 5(5): 1131-1137.

50.   Takebayashi Y, Akiyama S, Akiba S, Yamada K, Miyadera K, Sumizawa T, Yamada Y, Murata F, Aikou T. Clinicopathologic and prognostic significance of an angiogenic factor, thymidine phosphorylase, in human colorectal carcinoma. J Natl Cancer Inst 1996; 88(16): 1110-1117.

51.   Matsuura T, Kuratate I, Teramachi K, Osaki M, Fukuda Y, Ito H. Thymidine phosphorylase expression is associated with both increase of intratumoral microvessels and decrease of apoptosis in human colorectal carcinomas. Cancer Res 1999; 59(19): 5037-5040.

52.   Maeda K, Chung YS, Ogawa Y, Takatsuka S, Kang SM, Ogawa M, Sawada T, Onoda N, Kato Y, Sowa M. Thymidine phosphorylase/platelet-derived endothelial cell growth factor expression associated with hepatic metastasis in gastric carcinoma. Br J Cancer 1996; 73(8): 884-888.

53.   Igarashi M, Dhar DK, Kubota H, Yamamoto A, El-Assal O, Nagasue N. The prognostic significance of microvessel density and thymidine phosphorylase

expression in squamous cell carcinoma of the esophagus. Cancer 1998; 82(7): 1225-1232.

54.   Takao S, Takebayashi Y, Che X, Shinchi H, Natsugoe S, Miyadera K, Yamada Y, Akiyama S, Aikou T. Expression of thymidine phosphorylase is associated with a poor prognosis in patients with ductal adenocarcinoma of the pancreas. Clin Cancer Res 1998; 4(7): 1619-1624.

55.   Imazano Y, Takebayashi Y, Nishiyama K, Akiba S, Miyadera K, Yamada Y, Akiyama S, Ohi Y. Correlation between thymidine phosphorylase expression and prognosis in human renal cell carcinoma. J Clin Oncol 1997; 15(7): 2570-2578.

56.   Mazurek A, Kuc P, Terlikowski S, Laudanski T. Evaluation of tumor angiogenesis and thymidine phosphorylase tissue expression in patients with endometrial cancer. Neoplasma 2006; 53(3): 242-246.

57.   Relf M, LeJeune S, Scott PA, Fox S, Smith K, Leek R, Moghaddam A, Whitehouse R, Bicknell R, Harris AL. Expression of the angiogenic factors vascular endothelial cell growth factor, acidic and basic fibroblast growth factor, tumor growth factor beta-1, platelet-derived endothelial cell growth factor, placenta growth factor, and pleiotrophin in human primary breast cancer and its relation to angiogenesis. Cancer Res 1997; 57(5): 963-969.

58.   Reynolds K, Farzaneh F, Collins WP, Campbell S, Bourne TH, Lawton F, Moghaddam A, Harris AL, Bicknell R. Association of ovarian malignancy with expression of platelet-derived endothelial cell growth factor. J Natl Cancer Inst 1994; 86(16): 1234-1238.

59.   Fujimoto J, Sakaguchi H, Hirose R, Ichigo S, Tamaya T. Expression of platelet-derived endothelial cell growth factor (PD-ECGF) and its mRNA in uterine cervical cancers. Br J Cancer 1999; 79(7-8): 1249-1254.

60.   Sivridis E, Giatromanolaki A, Papadopoulos I, Gatter KC, Harris AL, Koukourakis MI. Thymidine phosphorylase expression in normal, hyperplastic and neoplastic prostates: correlation with tumour associated macrophages, infiltrating lymphocytes, and angiogenesis. Br J Cancer 2002; 86(9): 1465-1471.

61.   Koukourakis MI, Giatromanolaki A, O'Byrne KJ, Comley M, Whitehouse RM, Talbot DC, Gatter KC, Harris AL. Platelet-derived endothelial cell growth factor expression correlates with tumour angiogenesis and prognosis in non-small-cell lung cancer. Br J Cancer 1997; 75(4): 477-481.

62.   Yao Y, Kubota T, Sato K, Kitai R. Macrophage infiltration-associated thymidine phosphorylase expression correlates with increased microvessel density and poor prognosis in astrocytic tumors. Clin Cancer Res 2001; 7(12): 4021-4026.

63.   Fujioka S, Yoshida K, Yanagisawa S, Kawakami M, Aoki T, Yamazaki Y. Angiogenesis in pancreatic carcinoma: thymidine phosphorylase expression in stromal cells and intratumoral microvessel density as independent predictors of overall and relapse-free survival. Cancer 2001; 92(7): 1788-1797.

64.   Mizutani Y, Wada H, Yoshida O, Fukushima M, Kawauchi A, Nakao M, Miki T. The significance of thymidine phosphorylase/platelet-derived endothelial cell growth factor activity in renal cell carcinoma. Cancer 2003; 98(4): 730-736.

65. Hata K, Kamikawa T, Arao S, Tashiro H, Katabuchi H, Okamura H, Fujiwaki R, Miyazaki K, Fukumoto M. Expression of the thymidine phosphorylase gene in epithelial ovarian cancer. Br J Cancer 1999; 79(11-12): 1848-1854.

66. Fujimoto J, Sakaguchi H, Hirose R, Wen H, Tamaya T. Clinical implication of expression of platelet-derived endothelial cell growth factor (PD-ECGF) in metastatic lesions of uterine cervical cancers. Cancer Res 1999; 59(13): 3041-3044.

67. Arima J, Imazono Y, Takebayashi Y, Nishiyama K, Shirahama T, Akiba S, Furukawa T, Akiyama S, Ohi Y. Expression of thymidine phosphorylase as an indicator of poor prognosis for patients with transitional cell carcinoma of the bladder. Cancer 2000; 88(5): 1131-1138.

68. O'Byrne KJ, Koukourakis MI, Giatromanolaki A, Cox G, Turley H, Steward WP, Gatter K, Harris AL. Vascular endothelial growth factor, platelet-derived endothelial cell growth factor and angiogenesis in non-small-cell lung cancer. Br J Cancer 2000; 82(8): 1427-1432.

69. Shimada H, Takeda A, Shiratori T, Nabeya Y, Okazumi S, Matsubara H, Funami Y, Hayashi H, Gunji Y, Kobayashi S, Suzuki T, Ochiai T. Prognostic significance of serum thymidine phosphorylase concentration in esophageal squamous cell carcinoma. Cancer 2002; 94(7): 1947-1954.

70. Nagaoka H, Iino Y, Takei H, Morishita Y. Platelet-derived endothelial cell growth factor/thymidine phosphorylase expression in macrophages correlates with tumor angiogenesis and prognosis in invasive breast cancer. Int J Oncol 1998; 13(3): 449-454.

71. Schwartz EL, Wan E, Wang FS, Baptiste N. Regulation of expression of thymidine phosphorylase/platelet-derived endothelial cell growth factor in human colon carcinoma cells. Cancer Res 1998; 58(7): 1551-1557.

72. Goto H, Kohno K, Sone S, Akiyama S, Kuwano M, Ono M. Interferon gamma-dependent induction of thymidine phosphorylase/platelet-derived endothelial growth factor through gamma-activated sequence-like element in human macrophages. Cancer Res 2001; 61(2): 469-473.

73. Yao Y, Kubota T, Sato K, Takeuchi H, Kitai R, Matsukawa S. Interferons upregulate thymidine phosphorylase expression via JAK-STAT-dependent transcriptional activation and mRNA stabilization in human glioblastoma cells. J Neurooncol 2005; 72(3): 217-223.

74. Fukushima M, Okabe H, Takechi T, Ichikawa W, Hirayama R. Induction of thymidine phosphorylase by interferon and taxanes occurs only in human cancer cells with low thymidine phosphorylase activity. Cancer Lett 2002; 187(1-2): 103-110.

75. Zhu GH, Lenzi M, Schwartz EL. The Sp1 transcription factor contributes to the tumor necrosis factor-induced expression of the angiogenic factor thymidine phosphorylase in human colon carcinoma cells. Oncogene 2002; 21(55): 8477-8485.

76. Zhu, GH, Schwartz EL. Expression of the angiogenic factor thymidine phosphorylase in THP-1 monocytes: induction by autocrine tumor necrosis factor-alpha and inhibition by aspirin. Mol Pharmacol 2003; 64(5): 1251-1258.

77. de Bruin M, Peters GJ, Oerlemans R, Assaraf YG, Masterson AJ, Adema AD, Dijkmans BA, Pinedo HM, Jansen G. Sulfasalazine down-regulates the expression of the angiogenic factors platelet-derived endothelial cell growth factor/thymidine phosphorylase and interleukin-8 in human monocytic-macrophage THP1 and U937 cells. Mol Pharmacol 2004; 66(4): 1054-1060.

78. Griffiths L, Dachs GU, Bicknell R, Harris AL, Stratford IJ. The influence of oxygen tension and pH on the expression of platelet-derived endothelial cell growth factor/thymidine phosphorylase in human breast tumor cells grown in vitro and in vivo. Cancer Res 1997; 57(4): 570-572.

79. Sawada N, Ishikawa T, Fukase Y, Nishida M, Yoshikubo T, Ishitsuka H. Induction of thymidine phosphorylase activity and enhancement of capecitabine efficacy by taxol/taxotere in human cancer xenografts. Clin Cancer Res 1998; 4(4): 1013-1019.

80. Sawada N, Ishikawa T, Sekiguchi F, Tanaka Y, Ishitsuka H. X-ray irradiation induces thymidine phosphorylase and enhances the efficacy of capecitabine (Xeloda) in human cancer xenografts. Clin Cancer Res 1999; 5(10): 2948-2953.

81. Endo M, Shinbori N, Fukase Y, Sawada N, Ishikawa T, Ishitsuka H, Tanaka Y. Induction of thymidine phosphorylase expression and enhancement of efficacy of capecitabine or 5'-deoxy-5-fluorouridine by cyclophosphamide in mammary tumor models. Int J Cancer 1999; 83(1): 127-134.

82. Kikuno N, Moriyama-Gonda N, Yoshino T, Yoneda T, Urakami S, Terashima M, Yoshida M, Kishi H, Shigeno K, Shiina H, Igawa M. Blockade of paclitaxel-induced thymidine phosphorylase expression can accelerate apoptosis in human prostate cancer cells. Cancer Res 2004; 64(20): 7526-7532.

83. Fujimoto-Ouchi K, Tanaka Y, Tominaga T. Schedule dependency of antitumor activity in combination therapy with capecitabine/5'-deoxy-5-fluorouridine and docetaxel in breast cancer models. Clin Cancer Res 2001; 7(4): 1079-1086.

84. Walko CM, Lindley C. Capecitabine: a review. Clin Ther 2005; 27(1): 23-44.

85. O'Shaughnessy J, Miles D, Vukelja S, Moiseyenko V, Ayoub JP, Cervantes G, Fumoleau P, Jones S, Lui WY, Mauriac L, Twelves C, Van Hazel G, Verma S, Leonard R. Superior survival with capecitabine plus docetaxel combination therapy in anthracycline-pretreated patients with advanced breast cancer: phase III trial results. J Clin Oncol 2002; 20(12): 2812-2823.

86. Toi M, Inada K, Hoshina S, Suzuki H, Kondo S, Tominaga T. Vascular endothelial growth factor and platelet-derived endothelial cell growth factor are frequently coexpressed in highly vascularized human breast cancer. Clin Cancer Res 1995; 1(9): 961-964.

87. Amaya H, Tanigawa N, Lu C, Matsumura M, Shimomatsuya T, Horiuchi T, Muraoka R. Association of vascular endothelial growth factor

expression with tumor angiogenesis, survival and thymidine phosphorylase/platelet-derived endothelial cell growth factor expression in human colorectal cancer. Cancer Lett 1997; 119(2): 227-235.

88.   Hagiwara K, Stenman G, Honda H, Sahlin P, Andersson A, Miyazono K, Heldin CH, Ishikawa F, Takaku F. Organization and chromosomal localization of the human platelet-derived endothelial cell growth factor gene. Mol Cell Biol 1991; 11(4): 2125-2132.

89.   Ryuto M, Ono M, Izumi H, Yoshida S, Weich HA, Kohno K, Kuwano M. Induction of vascular endothelial growth factor by tumor necrosis factor alpha in human glioma cells. Possible roles of SP-1. J Biol Chem 1996; 271(45): 28220-28228.

90.   Kojima H, Shijubo N, Abe S. Thymidine phosphorylase and vascular endothelial growth factor in patients with Stage I lung adenocarcinoma. Cancer 2002; 94(4): 1083-1093.

91.   Kitazono M, Takebayashi Y, Ishitsuka K, Takao S, Tani A, Furukawa T, Miyadera K, Yamada Y, Aikou T, Akiyama S. Prevention of hypoxia-induced apoptosis by the angiogenic factor thymidine phosphorylase. Biochem Biophys Res Commun 1998; 253(3): 797-803.

92.   Ikeda R, Furukawa T, Kitazono M, Ishitsuka K, Okumura H, Tani A, Sumizawa T, Haraguchi M, Komatsu M, Uchimiya H, Ren XQ, Motoya T, Yamada K, Akiyama S. Molecular basis for the inhibition of hypoxia-induced apoptosis by 2-deoxy-D-ribose. Biochem Biophys Res Commun 2002; 291(4): 806-812.

93.   Ikeda R, Che XF, Ushiyama M, Yamaguchi T, Okumura H, Nakajima Y, Takeda Y, Shibayama Y, Furukawa T, Yamamoto M, Haraguchi M, Sumizawa T, Yamada K, Akiyama S. 2-Deoxy-D-ribose inhibits hypoxia-induced apoptosis by suppressing the phosphorylation of p38 MAPK. Biochem Biophys Res Commun 2006; 342(1): 280-285.

94.   Ikeda R, Tajitsu Y, Iwashita K, Che XF, Yoshida K, Ushiyama M, Furukawa T, Komatsu M, Yamaguchi T, Shibayama Y, Yamamoto M, Zhao HY, Arima J, Takeda Y, Akiyama S, Yamada K. Thymidine phosphorylase inhibits the expression of proapoptotic protein BNIP3. Biochem Biophys Res Commun 2008; 370(2): 220-224.

95.   Mori S, Takao S, Ikeda R, Noma H, Mataki Y, Wang X, Akiyama S, Aiko T. Role of thymidine phosphorylase in Fas-induced apoptosis. Hum Cell 2001; 14(4): 323-330.

96.   Mori S, Takao S, Ikeda R, Noma H, Mataki Y, Wang X, Akiyama S, Aikou T. Thymidine phosphorylase suppresses Fas-induced apoptotic signal transduction independent of its enzymatic activity. Biochem Biophys Res Commun 2002; 295(2): 300-305.

97.   Ikeda R, Furukawa T, Mitsuo R, Noguchi T, Kitazono M, Okumura H, Sumizawa T, Haraguchi M, Che XF, Uchimiya H, Nakajima Y, Ren XQ, Oiso S, Inoue I, Yamada K, Akiyama S. Thymidine phosphorylase inhibits apoptosis induced by

98.   cisplatin. Biochem Biophys Res Commun 2003; 301(2): 358-363.

98.   Jeung HC, Che XF, Haraguchi M, Furukawa T, Zheng CL, Sumizawa T, Rha SY, Roh JK, Akiyama S. Thymidine phosphorylase suppresses apoptosis induced by microtubule-interfering agents. Biochem Pharmacol 2005; 70(1): 13-21.

99.   Jeung HC, Che XF, Haraguchi M, Zhao HY, Furukawa T, Gotanda T, Zheng CL, Tsuneyoshi K, Sumizawa T, Roh JK, Akiyama S. Protection against DNA damage-induced apoptosis by the angiogenic factor thymidine phosphorylase. FEBS Lett 2006; 580(5): 1294-1302.

100.   Langen P, Etzold G, Barwolff D, Preussel B. Inhibition of thymidine phosphorylase by 6-aminothymine and derivatives of 6-aminouracil. Biochem Pharmacol 1967; 16(9): 1833-1837.

101.   Pérez-Pérez MJ, Priego EM, Hernández AI, Camarasa MJ, Balzarini J, Liekens S. Thymidine phosphorylase inhibitors: recent developments and potential therapeutic applications. Mini Rev Med Chem 2005; 5(12): 1113-1123.

102.   Fukushima M, Suzuki N, Emura T, Yano S, Kazuno H, Tada Y, Yamada Y, Asao T. Structure and activity of specific inhibitors of thymidine phosphorylase to potentiate the function of antitumor 2'-deoxyribonucleosides. Biochem Pharmacol 2000; 59(10): 1227-1236.

103.   Takao S, Akiyama SI, Nakajo A, Yoh H, Kitazono M, Natsugoe S, Miyadera K, Fukushima M, Yamada Y, Aikou T. Suppression of metastasis by thymidine phosphorylase inhibitor. Cancer Res 2000; 60(19): 5345-5348.

104.   Matsushita S, Nitanda T, Furukawa T, Sumizawa T, Tani A, Nishimoto K, Akiba S, Miyadera K, Fukushima M, Yamada Y, Yoshida H, Kanzaki T, Akiyama S. The effect of a thymidine phosphorylase inhibitor on angiogenesis and apoptosis in tumors. Cancer Res 1999; 59(8): 1911-1916.

105.   Norman RA, Barry ST, Bate M, Breed J, Colls JG, Ernill RJ, Luke RW, Minshull CA, McAlister MS, McCall EJ, McMiken HH, Paterson DS, Timms D, Tucker JA, Pauptit RA. Crystal structure of human thymidine phosphorylase in complex with a small molecule inhibitor. Structure 2004; 12(1): 75-84.

106.   Nakayama C, Wataya Y, Meyer RB Jr, Santi DV, Saneyoshi M, Ueda T. Thymidine phosphorylase. Substrate specificity for 5-substituted 2'-deoxyuridines. J Med Chem 1980; 23(8): 962-964.

107.   Temmink OH, Emura T, de Bruin M, Fukushima M, Peters GJ. Therapeutic potential of the dual-targeted TAS-102 formulation in the treatment of gastrointestinal malignancies. Cancer Sci 2007; 98(6): 779-789.

108.   Emura T, Suzuki N, Fujioka A, Ohshimo H, Fukushima M. Potentiation of the antitumor activity of alpha, alpha, alpha-trifluorothymidine by the co-administration of an inhibitor of thymidine phosphorylase at a suitable molar ratio in vivo. Int J Oncol 2005; 27(2): 449-455.

109.   Hong DS, Abbruzzese JL, Bogaard K, Lassere Y, Fukushima M, Mita A, Kuwata K, Hoff PM. Phase I study to determine the safety and pharmacokinetics of

oral administration of TAS-102 in patients with solid tumors. Cancer 2006; 107(6): 1383-1390.

110. Walter MR, Cook WJ, Cole LB, Short SA, Koszalka GW, Krenitsky TA, Ealick SE. Three-dimensional structure of thymidine phosphorylase from Escherichia coli at 2.8 A resolution. J Biol Chem 1990; 265(23): 14016-14022.

111. El Omari K, Bronckaers A, Liekens S, Pérez-Pérez MJ, Balzarini J, Stammers DK. Structural basis for non-competitive product inhibition in human thymidine phosphorylase: implications for drug design.Biochem J 2006; 399(2): 199-204.

112. Pugmire MJ, Ealick SE. The crystal structure of pyrimidine nucleoside phosphorylase in a closed conformation. Structure. 1998; 6(11): 1467-1479.

113. Balzarini J, Gamboa AE, Esnouf R, Liekens S, Neyts J, De Clercq E, Camarasa MJ, Pérez-Pérez MJ. 7-Deazaxanthine, a novel prototype inhibitor of thymidine phosphorylase. FEBS Lett 1998; 438(1-2): 91-95.

114. Esteban-Gamboa A, Balzarini J, Esnouf R, De Clercq E, Camarasa MJ, Pérez-Pérez MJ. Design, synthesis, and enzymatic evaluation of multisubstrate analogue inhibitors of Escherichia

coli thymidine phosphorylase. J Med Chem 2000; 43(5): 971-983.

115. Balzarini J, Degrève B, Esteban-Gamboa A, Esnouf R, De Clercq E, Engelborghs Y, Camarasa MJ, Pérez-Pérez MJ. Kinetic analysis of novel multisubstrate analogue inhibitors of thymidine phosphorylase. FEBS Lett. 2000; 483(2-3): 181-185.

116. Liekens S, Bilsen F, De Clercq E, Priego EM, Camarasa MJ, Pérez-Pérez MJ, Balzarini J. Anti-angiogenic activity of a novel multi-substrate analogue inhibitor of thymidine phosphorylase. FEBS Lett 2002; 510(1-2): 83-88.

117. Liekens S, Hernández AI, Ribatti D, De Clercq E, Camarasa MJ, Pérez-Pérez MJ, Balzarini J. The nucleoside derivative 5'-O-trityl-inosine (KIN59) suppresses thymidine phosphorylase-triggered angiogenesis via a noncompetitive mechanism of action. J Biol Chem 2004; 279(28): 29598-29605.

118. Liekens S, Bronckaers A, Hernández AI, Priego EM, Casanova E, Camarasa MJ, Balzarini J. 5'-O-tritylated nucleoside derivatives: inhibition of thymidine phosphorylase and angiogenesis. Mol Pharmacol 2006; 70(2): 501-509.

CHAPTER 9

Role of Stromal Cells in Neovascularization of Multiple Myeloma

Maria Fico[1], Giuseppe Mangialardi[1], Roberto Ria[1], Michele Moschetta[1], Domenico Ribatti[2] and Angelo Vacca[1]

[1]*Department of Biomedical Sciences and Human Oncology, University of Bari Medical School, I-70124 Bari, Italy*

[2]*Department of Human Anatomy and Histology, University of Bari Medical School, I-70124 Bari, Italy*

Address correspondence to: Dr. Angelo Vacca, Department of Internal Medicine and Clinical Oncology, Unit of Allergology and Clinical Immunology, Policlinico – Piazza Giulio Cesare, 11, 70124 Bari, Italy; Tel: +39-080-559.34.44; Fax: +39-080-559.21.89; Email: a.vacca@dimo.uniba.it

Abstract: Angiogenesis plays a pivotal role in progression of both solid and hematologic tumors. We have focused on multiple myeloma (MM) and its bone marrow stromal cells which are not only a support for tumor cell survival, but also active inducers of angiogenesis by releasing a broad number of angiogenic cytokines. Also, stromal cells such as macrophages and mast cells can participate in blood vessels formation in MM through other processes, such as a vasculogenic mimicry. Finally, it has been discovered that hematopoietic stem and progenitor cells (HSPCs) are involved in the vasculogenesis of MM.

1. INTRODUCTION

Multiple myeloma (MM) is a disease caused by the accumulation of malignant plasma cells that usually, but not in every case, actively produces antibodies [1]. During cell maturation, after the switch into the lymph nodes, B cells express a large number of adhesion molecules that facilitate their homing in the bone marrow where they afterwards differentiate. Once in the bone marrow, the adhesion molecules mediate the homotropic interactions between plasma cells and B cells, and the heterotropic interactions between plasma cells and both extracellular matrix and bone marrow stromal cells [2]. In MM, the expression of these molecules changes in the disease course, especially when plasma cells pass from the bone marrow into the peripheral blood [3]. Therefore, MM progression is characterized by three separate events: loss of the capacity to enhance apoptosis, expansion of transformed plasma cells into the bone marrow, and dissemination of malignant cells along the body. The last two steps need angiogenesis to develop.

2. ANGIOGENESIS IN ACTIVE MULTIPLE MYELOMA

The angiogenesis in MM allows the formation of new vessels that provide nutrients for transformed cells, thus supporting their high level of replication, and simultaneously facilitate the egress of MM cells into the blood circulation. These newly-formed vessels have not an ordered architecture, and show a discontinuous endothelial surface [4]. Transformed plasma cells participate to the angiogenic process by producing a large number of cytokines that act directly on endothelial cells (ECs) and stromal cells which, in turn, release enzymes and other cytokines that amplify angiogenesis. Adhesion of MM cells to the bone marrow stroma is mediated by different types of surface receptors. MM plasma cells express very late-activating antigen-4 and -5 (VLA-4 and VLA-5), and β2-integrin lymphocyte function-associated antigen-1 (LFA-1) that allow the aggregation of homotropic cells ad the link to heterotropic cells [5]. These cell-cell interactions induce the release of interleukin-6 (IL-6) and transforming growth factor-β (TGF-β) by bone marrow stromal cells [6,7], and of IL-1β, tumor necrosis factor-α (TNF-α), IL-6 and vascular endothelial growth factor (VEGF) by tumor cells [8-11]. These growth factors stimulate clonal expansion of plasma cells and contribute to bone destruction [12]. In particular, IL-6 hides the pro-apoptotic signals of FAS antigen [13].

Moreover, IL-6 synthesized not only by tumor cells but also by bone marrow stromal cells exerts an angiogenic activity both directly and indirectly, through the release of VEGF [14]. In turn, the production of IL-6 by stromal cells is due to the activity of fibroblast growth factor-2 (FGF-2) released by the plasma cells. (Fig. **1**) summarizes the interplay between various cells present in the bone marrow microenvironment and various growth factors promoting angiogenesis in MM.

3. ROLE OF MACROPHAGES AND THEIR VASCULOGENIC MIMICRY IN MULTIPLE MYELOMA

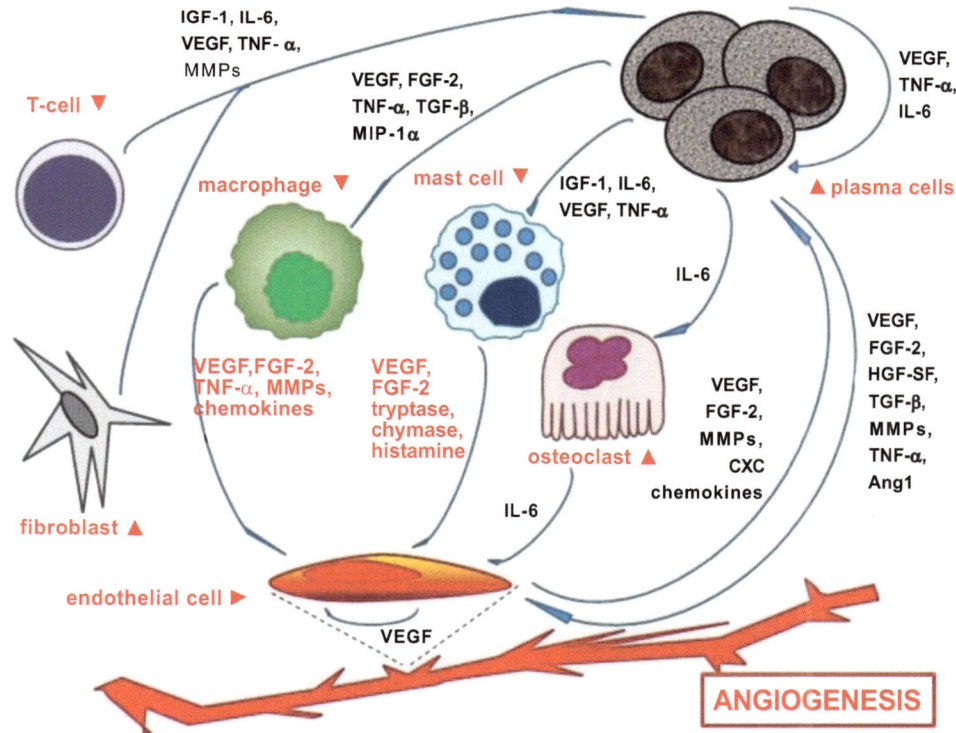

Fig. (1). Interplay between various microenvironment cells and factors promoting angiogenesis in multiple myeloma.

Tumor macrophages are a source of pro-angiogenic cytokines, such as VEGF, FGF-2, IL-8, TNF-α, and TGF-β. In addition, tumor macrophages synthesize a broad spectrum of matrix metalloproteinases (MMPs), such MMP-2, MMP-7, MMP-9 and MMP-12 [15]. All these factors contribute to the angiogenic phase in MM.

Recently, Scavelli et al. [16] have demonstrated that bone marrow macrophages of active MM patients (i.e., patients at diagnosis, relapse, or leukemic phase) are involved in the formation of new vessels through vasculogenic mimicry. In fact, when these macrophages were exposed to VEGF and FGF-2 (i.e., cytokines secreted by MM plasma cells into the microenvironment), they transformed into cells functionally and phenotypically similar to paired ECs (or MMECs), and generated capillary-like networks mimicking those of MMECs. Authors also found the macrophages (positive for their lineage marker, CD68) inside the neovessel wall which cooperated with classical MMECs (positive for Factor VIII-related antigen - FVIII-RA) in building the new vessel wall. Also, macrophages from patients with non-active MM (i.e., with complete/objective response or plateau-phase), and those from patients with monoclonal gammopathy of undetermined significance (MGUS) diplayed similar, albeit weaker features. At ultrastructural level, macrophages from active MM patients appeared as long-shaped cells with thin cytoplasmic protrusions, short microvilli, fillipodes and pseudopodes. Also, their cytoplasmic protrusions formed tubular structures anastomosed with each other and those of nearby macrophages, reminiscent of vascular structures.

4. ROLE OF MAST CELLS IN VAS-CULOGENIC MIMICRY IN MULTI-PLE MYELOMA

Mast cells are usually involved in type I hypersensitivity reactions. However, their granules contain a large number of cytokines, including angiogenic factors, such as VEGF, FGF-2, TNF-α and IL-8 [17-19], proteases, such as tryptase and chymase responsible for both basement membrane matrix degradation and activation of preformed growth factors [20, 21] .

Moreover, heparin and histamin, contained in mast cell secretory granules, exert an angiogenic activity [22]. Mast cells are involved in tumor angiogenesis [23], through the release of angiogenic factors stored in their secretory granules in a typical piecemeal degranulation mode [24]. Ribatti et al. [25] have demonstrated that in MM bone marrow, angiogenesis and mast cell counts are highly correlated, and increase in parallel in patients with active and non-active disease, as compared to those with MGUS.

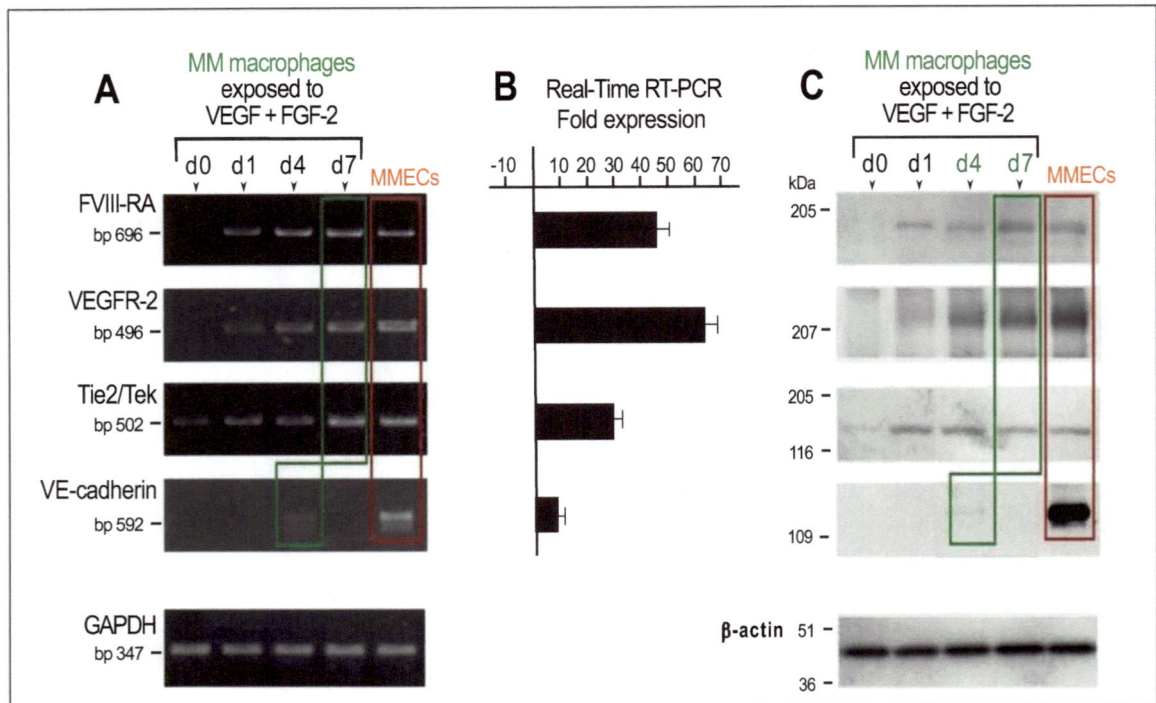

Fig. (2). Bone marrow macrophages of myeloma patients overlap phenotypically paired endothelial cells (MMECs) upon exposure to VEGF and FGF-2 for 7 days. (A) RT–PCR analysis showing the acquisition or enhancement of endothelial markers at similar levels of paired MMECs. (B) Real-Time RT-PCR fold expression of FVIII-RA, VEGFR-2, Tie2/Tek and VE-cadherin in MM macrophages exposed to VEGF and FGF-2. (C) Western blot analysis of cell lysates showing the endothelial proteins on VEGF-/FGF-2-stimulated MM macrophages at similar levels of MMECs (kDa, molecular weight in kilodaltons; GAPDH, glyceraldehyde-3-phosphate dehydrogenase; β-actin, control protein).

More recently, Nico et al. [26] have shown that mast cells are also involved in the formation of new vessels in MM through vasculogenic mimicry, similarly to macrophages. At ultrastructural level, they clearly showed that vessels in MM are lined by mast cells with characteristic electron dense granules in their cytoplasm, and these data were confirmed by confocal laser microscopy showing vessels simultaneously marked by an antibody to tryptase (a mast cell marker) and an antibody to FVIII-RA (the MMEC marker) [26].

5.   ENDOTHELIAL DIFFERENTIA-TION OF HEMATOPOIETIC STEM AND PROGENITOR CELLS IN MULTIPLE MYELOMA

Several data suggest the existence of endothelial progenitor cells (ECPs), their derivation from bone marrow, and their contribution to the formation of blood vessels in postnatal and adult life [27]. EPCs are closed associated with hematopoietic stem and progenitor cells (HSPCs) with a typical phenotype including the CD133, CD34 and VEGFR-2 molecules [28, 29].

In patients with active MM, plasma cells and stromal cells in the bone marrow microenvironment recruit HSPCs, and induce their transformation into mature MMECs [30]. In fact, when HSPCs of MM patients are incubated with VEGF, FGF-2 and insulin-like growth factor (IGF) (i.e., typical cytokines secreted by both plasma cells and stromal cells into the miroenvironment) cells differentiate into ECs-like cells expressing typical endothelial markers, such as FVIII-RA, VEGFR-2 and VE-cadherin, and form capillary-like networks *in vitro* [31]. Bone marrow biopsies revealed HPSCs inside the neovessel wall in patients with MM, but not in those with MGUS, suggesting that in the former HSPCs contribute to the new vessel building together with MMECs [32]. Therefore, besides angiogenesis, HSPC-linked vasculogenesis contributes to neovascularization in MM patients.

6. CONCLUSIONS

Overall, these data indicate that in active MM patients, macrophages, mast cells and HSPCs contribute to neovascularization through a vasculogenic pathway, and that in non-active MM and MGUS they are prone to behave accordingly, marching in step with progression, hence with the vascular switch.

7. ACKNOWLEDGMENTS

This work was supported in part by Fondazione Cassa di Risparmio di Puglia, Bari, the Associazione Italiana per la Ricerca sul Cancro (AIRC), Milan, and Ministry of Health, Progetto Oncologia 2006, Humanitas Mirasole S.P.A., Rome, Italy.

8. REFERENCES

1. Dalton WS. The tumor microenvironment: focus on myeloma. Cancer Treatment Reviews 2003; 29(1): 11-9.
2. Anderson KC, Bast Jr RC, Kufe DW, Pollack RE, Weichselbaum RR, Holland JR, Frei E, Gansler TS (eds.). Plasma cell tumors, 5th ed. Cancer Medicine. BC Decker; Hamilton, Ont 2001. p 2066–2085.
3. Shain KH, Landowski TH, Dalton WS. The tumor microenvironment as a determinant of cancer cell survival; a possible mechanism for de novo drug resistance. Curr Opin Oncol 2000; 12(6): 557-63.
4. Ribatti D, Nico B, Crivellato E, Vacca A. The structure of the vascular network of tumors. Cancer Lett 2007; 248(1): 18-23.
5. Kawano MM, Huang N, Tanaka H, Ishikawa H, Sakai A, Tanabe O, Nobuyoshi M, Kuramoto A. Homotypic cell aggregations of human myeloma cells with ICAM-1 and LFA- 1 molecules. Br J Haematol 1991; 79(4): 583-8.
6. Uchiyama H, Barut BA, Mohrbacher AF, Chauhan D, Anderson KC. Adhesion of human myeloma-derived cell lines to bone marrow stromal cells stimulates interleukin-6 secretion. Blood 1993; 82(12): 3712-20.
7. Gimble JM, Pietrangeli C, Henley A, Dorheim MA, Silver J, Namen A, Takeichi M, Goridis C, Kincade PW. Characterization of murine bone marrow and spleen-derived stromal cells; analysis of leukocyte marker and growth factor mRNA transcript levels. Blood 1989; 74(1): 303-11.
8. Hideshima T, Chauhan D, Schlossman R, Richardson P, Anderson KC. The role of tumor necrosis factor alpha in the pathophysiology of human multiple myeloma; therapeutic applications. Oncogene 2001; 20(33): 4519-27.
9. Dankbar B, Padro T, Leo R, Feldmann B, Kropff M, Mesters RM, Serve H, Berdel WE, Kienast J. Vascular endothelial growth factor and interleukin-6 in paracrine tumor–stromal cell interactions in multiple myeloma. Blood 2000; 95(8): 2630-6.
10. Urashima M, Chauhan D, Uchiyama H, Freeman GJ, Anderson KC. CD40 ligand triggered interleukin-6 secretion in multiple myeloma. Blood 1995; 85(7): 1903-12.
11. Lacy MQ, Donovan KA, Heimbach JK, Ahmann GJ, Lust JA. Comparison of interleukin-1 beta expression by in situ hybridization in monoclonal gammopathy of undetermined significance and multiple myeloma. Blood 1999; 93(1): 300-5.
12. Tricot G. New insights into role of microenvironment in multiple myeloma. Lancet 2000; 355(9200): 248-50.
13. Chauhan D, Kharbanda S, Ogata A, Urashima M, Teoh G, Robertson M, Kufe DW, Anderson KC. Interleukin-6 inhibits Fas-induced apoptosis and stress-activated protein kinase activation in multiple myeloma cells. Blood 1997; 89(1): 227-34.
14. Ribatti D, Nico B, Vacca A. Importance of the bone marrow microenvironment in inducing the angiogenic response in multiple myeloma. Oncogene 2006; 25(31): 4257-66.
15. Vacca A, Ribatti D, Presta M, Minischetti M, Iurlaro M, Ria R, Albini A, Bussolino F, Dammacco F. Bone marrow neovascularization, plasma cell angiogenic potential and matrix metalloproteinase- 2 secretion parallel progression of human multiple myeloma. Blood 1999; 93(9): 3064-73.
16. Scavelli C, Nico B, Cirulli T, Ria R, Di Pietro G, Mangieri D, Bacigalupo A, Mangialardi G, Coluccia AML, Caravita T, Molica S, Ribatti D, Dammacco F, Vacca A. Vasculogenic mimicry by bone marrow macrophages in patients with multiple myeloma. Oncogene 2008; 27(5): 663-74.
17. Moller A, Lippert U, Lessmann D, Kolde G, Hanrann K, Welker P, Schadendorf D, Rosenbach T, Luger T, Czarnetzki BM. Human mast cells produce IL-8. Journal of Immunology 1993; 151(6): 3261-6.
18. Grutzkau A, Kruger-Krasagakes S, Baumeister H, Schwarz C, Kogel H, Welker P, Lippert U, Henz BM, Moller A. Synthesis, storage and release of vascular endothelial growth factor (VEGF/VPF) by human mast cells; implications for the biological significance of VEGF206. Mol Biol Cell 1998; 9(4): 875-84.
19. Sayama S, Iozzo RV, Lazarus GS, Schechter NM. Human skin chymotrypsin like proteinase chymase. Subcellular localization to mast cell granules and interaction with heparin and other glycosaminoglycans. J Biol Chem 1987; 262(14): 6808-15.
20. Taipale J, Lohi J, Saarinen J, Kovanen PT, Keshi-Oja J. Human mast cell chymase and leukocyte elastase release latent transforming growth factor beta-1 from the extracellular matrix of cultured human epithelial and endothelial cells. J Biol Chem 1995; 270(9): 4689-96.
21. Ribatti D, Roncali L, Nico B, Bertossi M. Effects of exogenous heparin on the vasculogenesis of the chorioallantoic membrane. Acta Anat 1987; 130(3): 257-63.
22. Ribatti D, Crivellato E, Roccaro AM, Ria R, Vacca A. Mast cell contribution to angiogenesis related to tumor progression. Clin Exp Allergy 2004; 34(11): 1660-4.
23. Dvorak AM, Kissell S. Granule changes of human skin mast cells characteristic of piecemeal degranulation and associated with recovery during wound healing in situ. J Leuk Biol 1991; 49(2): 197-210.

24.   Ribatti D, Vacca A, Nico B, Crivellato E, Roncali L, Dammacco F. The role of mast cells in tumour angiogenesis. Brit J Haematol 2001; 115(3): 514-21.

25.   Ribatti D, Vacca A, Nico B, Quondamatteo F, Ria R, Minischetti M, Marzullo A, Herken R, Roncali L, Dammacco F. Bone marrow angiogenesis and mast cell density increase simultaneously with progression of human multiple myeloma. Br J Cancer 1999; 79(3-4): 451-5.

26.   Nico B, Mangieri D, Crivellato E, Vacca A, Ribatti D. Mast cells contribute to vasculogenic mimicry in multiple myeloma. Stem Cells Dev 2008; 17(1): 19-22.

27.   Ribatti D. The discovery of endothelial progenitor cells. An historical review. Leuk Res 2007; 31(4): 439-44.

28.   Yin AH, Miraglia S, Zanjani ED, Almeida-Porada G, Ogawa M, Leary AG, Olweus J, Kearney J, Buck DW. AC133, a novel marker for human hematopoietic stem and progenitor cells. Blood 1997; 90(12): 5002-12.

29.   Peichev M, Naiyer AJ, Pereira D, Zhu Z, Lane WJ, Williams M, Oz MC, Hicklin DJ, Witte L, Moore MA, Rafii S. Expression of VEGFR-2 and AC133 by circulating human CD34(+) cells identifies a population of functional endothelial precursors. Blood 2000; 95(3): 952-8.

30.   Ria R, Piccoli C, Cirulli T, Falzetti F, Mangialardi G, Guidolin D, Tabilio A, Di Renzo N, Guarini A, Ribatti D, Dammacco F, Vacca A. Endothelial differentiation of hematopoietic stem and progenitor cells from patients with multiple myeloma. Clin Cancer Res 2008; 14(6): 1678-85.

31.   Melero-Martin JM, Khan ZA, Picard A, Wu X, Paruchuri S, Bischoff J. In vivo vasculogenic potential of human blood-derived endothelial progenitor cells. Blood 2007; 109(11): 4761-8.

32.   Bruno S, Bussolati B, Grange C, Collino F, Graziano ME, Ferrando U, Camussi G. CD133+ renal progenitor cells contribute to tumor angiogenesis. Am J Pathol 2006; 169(6): 2223-35.

CHAPTER 10

Recent Advances in Angiogenesis and Antiangiogenesis: The Neuroblastoma Model

Fabio Pastorino and Mirco Ponzoni

Experimental Therapies Unit, Laboratory of Oncology, G. Gaslini Children's Hospital, Genoa, Italy.

Address correspondence to: Dr. Fabio Pastorino and Dr. Mirco Ponzon., Experimental Therapy Unit, Laboratory of Oncology, G. Gaslini Children's Hospital, Largo G. Gaslini 5, 16148 Genoa, Italy; Tel.: +39-010-5636342; Fax: +39-010-3779820; Email: fabiopastorino@ospedale-gaslini.ge.it; mircoponzoni@ospedale-gaslini.ge.it

Abstract: Promising novel antiangiogenic strategies are emerging for the treatment of cancer and the inhibition of angiogenesis might represent a powerful tool as adjuvant therapy of malignant tumors. Over the last fifteen years several reports have been published concerning the relationship between tumor progression and angiogenesis in neuroblastoma in experimental models *in vitro* and *in vivo*. Moreover, a high vascular index in neuroblastoma correlates with poor prognosis, suggesting dependence of aggressive tumor growth on active angiogenesis. Here, we present an overview of the most recent advances in antiangiogenesis in neuroblastoma, and describe tumor vascular-targeted preclinical results, as well as future perspectives.

1. ROLE OF ANGIOGENESIS IN NEUROBLASTOMA GROWTH

Angiogenesis is the formation of new blood vessels from pre-existing ones and takes place in various physiological and pathological conditions, such as embryonic development, wound healing, the menstrual cycle, chronic inflammation and tumors [1, 2]. It is generally accepted that tumor growth is angiogenesis-dependent and that every increment of tumor growth requires an increment of vascular growth [3]. Tumor angiogenesis is an uncontrolled and unlimited process essential for tumor growth, invasion and metastasis, regulated by the balanced interactions of numerous mediators and cytokines with pro-angiogenic and anti-angiogenic activity. Tumors lacking angiogenesis remain dormant indefinitely. An expanding endothelial surface also gives tumor cells more opportunities to enter the circulation and metastasize.

New vessels promote growth by conveying oxygen and nutrients and removing catabolites, whereas endothelial cells secrete growth factors for tumor cells and a variety of matrix-degrading proteinases that facilitate invasion. An expanding endothelial surface also gives tumor cells more opportunities to enter the circulation and metastasize, while release of anti-angiogenic factors by the endothelial cells explains the control exerted by primary tumors over metastasis. These observations suggest that tumor angiogenesis is linked to a switch in the equilibrium between positive and negative regulators. In normal tissues, vascular quiescence is maintained by the dominant influence of endogenous angiogenesis inhibitors over angiogenic stimuli. Tumor angiogenesis, on the other hand, is induced by increased secretion of angiogenic factors and/or downregulation of angiogenesis inhibitors.

Growth of solid and hematological tumors consists of an avascular and a subsequent vascular phase. Assuming that the latter process is dependent on angiogenesis and depends on the release of angiogenic factors, acquisition of angiogenic capability can be seen as an expression of progression from neoplastic transformation to tumor growth and metastasis.

Angiogenic factors can be produced by a number of cells such as embryonic cells, adult resident and inflammatory cells (*i.e.* fibroblasts, macrophages, T cells, plasma cells, neutrophils, and eosinophils) and neoplastic cells. Several angiogenic factors have been identified, including vascular endothelial growth factor/vascular permeability factor (VEGF/VPF), placenta growth factor (PlGF), basic fibroblast growth factor/fibroblast growth factor-2 (bFGF/FGF-2), transforming growth factor beta (TGF-β), hepatocyte growth factor (HGF), tumor necrosis factor alpha (TNF-α), interleukin-8 (IL-8), and angiopoietin-1 and –2.

Except for cancers of hematologic origin and of the central nervous system (CNS), pediatric cancers frequently originate from mesenchymal structures, such as bone or muscle. Childhood malignancies tend to have short latency periods and are frequently rapidly growing and aggressively invasive. Unlike adult cancers, most pediatric malignancies have either spread locally or have metastasized at the time of presentation and are not amenable to curative surgical excision.

Among pediatric solid tumors, neuroblastoma (NB), most commonly occurring in the adrenal gland, is predominantly a tumor of infancy with 16% of children diagnosed within the first month of life and 41% diagnosed within the first 3 months of life.

Several recent studies implicate angiogenesis in the regulation of NB growth and inhibition of angiogenesis is a promising approach in the treatment of NB because of the high degree of vascularity of these tumors. In 1994 Kleinman and co-workers published a paper in which they showed that human NB cells induce angiogenesis in nude mouse during tumorigenesis [4]. Meitar et al. (1996) evaluated the vascularity of primary untreated NB from 50 patients. They found that the vascularity of NB from patients with widely metastatic disease is significantly higher than in tumors from patients with local or regional disease [5]. Ribatti et al. (1998) investigated the angiogenic potential of two human NB cell lines demonstrating their capacity to induce *in vitro* human microvascular endothelial cells to proliferate and *in vivo* angiogenesis in the chick embryo chorioallantoic membrane assay [6].

Canete et al. (2000) in a retrospective study showed that tumor vascularity was not predictive of survival of NB patients and that neither disseminated nor local relapses were influenced by the angiogenic characteristics of the tumors [7]. Eggert et al. (2000) performed a systematic analysis of expression of angiogenic factors in 22 NB cell lines and in 37 tumor samples. They found that high expression levels of seven angiogenic factors correlated strongly with the advanced stage of NB and this suggests that several angiogenic peptides set in concert in the regulation of neovascularization [8].

Ara et al. (1998) found that increased expression of MMP-2, but not of MMP-9, in stromal tissues of NB had significant association with advanced clinical stages [9]. Sarakibara et al. (1999) have demonstrated that the higher gelatinases activation ratio resulting from high espression of a novel membrane-type matrix metalloproteinase-1 (MT-MMP-1) on NB specimens is associated significantly with advanced stage and unfavorable outcome [10]. Ribatti et al. (2001) showed that the extent of angiogenesis and the expression of the MMP-2 and MMP-9 were upregulated in advanced stages of NB [11].

MYC-N may regulate the growth of NB vessels, because its amplification or overexpression is associated with angiogenesis in experimental [12] and clinical settings [5]. Amplification of MYC-N is a frequent event in advanced stages of human NB. MYC-N amplification correlates with poor prognosis and enhanced vascularization of human NB, sugges-

ting that the MYC-N oncogene could stimulate tumor angiogenesis and thereby allow NB progression [13].

Erdreich-Epstein et al. (2000) demostrated by immunohistochemical analysis that $\alpha_v\beta_3$ integrin was expressed by 61% of microvessels in high-risk NB, but only by 18 % of microvessels in low-risk tumors [14].

It has been reported a very low tumor vascularity in Schwannian stroma-rich/stroma-dominant NB tumors and that Schwann cells produce angiogenesis inhibitors, such as tissue inhibitor of metalloproteinase-2 (TIMP-2) and pigment epithelium-derived factor (PEDF), that are capable of inducing endothelial cell apoptosis [15, 16]. Chlenski et al. (2002) isolated an angiogenic inhibitor in Schwann cell conditioned medium, identified as SPARC, which expression is inversely correlated with the degree of malignant progression in NB tumors. Furthermore, SPARC inhibited angiogenesis *in vivo* and impaired NB tumor growth [17].

Leali et al. (2003) demonstrated that FGF-2 causes osteopontin (OPN)-upregulation in endothelial cells, *in vitro* and *in vivo*, resulting in the recruitment of proangiogenic monocytes [18]. Takahashi et al. (2002) demonstrated that OPN-transfected murine NB cells significantly increased neovascularization in mice [19]. Enforced expression of OPN in NB cells significantly stimulated endothelial cells migration and induced angiogenesis in mice, as evaluated by dorsal air sac assay.

2. ANGIOGENESIS AS THERAPEUTIC TARGET

It is exhaustively reported in the literature that a functional blood supply is essential to meet the oxygen and nutrient demands of growing solid tumors [20]. Moreover, since the neovasculature that arises from the normal host vessels by the process of angiogenesis also is the principal vehicle for metastatic spread [21], we can conclude that tumor neo-vasculature is a potential therapeutic target [22] for all solid tumors, including neuroblastoma.

There are two major approaches in controlling tumor vasculature. One strategy is to prevent the development of tumor blood vessels by inhibiting the angiogenesis process (AIAs, angiogenesis inhibiting agents); the other strategy acts by compromising the function of established tumor blood vessels (VTAs/VDAs, vascular targeting/vascular disrupting agents). The latter strategy has been shown to disrupt established tumor vasculature causing rapid and sustained inhibition of tumor blood flow. By depriving tumors of the nutrients necessary to growth and survive, VTAs/VDAs induce necrosis, particularly within the core of the tumor.

Recently, the use of VTAs, such as ligand-targeted liposomes and drug conjugates, has started to fulfill its promise [23]. This strategy builds on the clinical success of nanomedicines such as Caelyx®, which are used to improved therapeutic outcome and/or minimized damage to normal tissues such as heart or bone marrow, thereby increasing the selective toxicity of chemotherapeutics in cancer [24]. Further increases in therapeutic activity can be achieved by using ligand-targeted nanomedicines that have surface-conjugated, tumor-selective antibodies or peptides [25], particularly when targeting is by internalizing ligands that facilitate the delivery of the therapeutic contents to intracellular sites of activity via the endosome/lysosome pathway [25, 26]. Indeed, compared to normal blood vessels, tumor blood vessels have an abnormal wall structure, being highly disorganized and heterogeneous, with complex branching patterns and lack of hierarchy [27]. Moreover, endothelial cells in angiogenic vessels express several proteins that are absent or barely detectable in established blood vessels, including α_v integrins [28], receptors for angiogenic growth factors [29], and other types of membrane-spanning molecules, such as the aminopeptidases N (CD13) and A (APA) [30, 31]. *In vivo* panning of phage libraries in tumor-bearing mice have proven useful for selecting peptides that bind to receptors that are either over-expressed or are selectively expressed on tumor-associated vessels and that home to neoplastic tissues [32]. Thus, it may be possible to develop ligand-targeted chemotherapy strategies, based on peptides that are selective for tumor vasculature. Among the various tumor-targeting ligands identified to date, peptides containing the asparagine-glycine-arginine (NGR) motif, which binds to CD13, have proven useful for delivering various anti-tumor compounds to tumor vasculature [33, 34]. Although there are several subpopulations of CD13 [35], relatively widely distributed in the body, only one isoform is believed to be the receptor for the NGR-containing peptides. This isoform has been shown to be expressed exclusively in angiogenic vessels, such as the neovasculature found in tumor tissues [36]. Consequently, since this CD13 isoform, recognized by NGR-containing peptides, is expressed on endothelial cells within most, if not all, solid tumors, an alternative strategy that has been pursued to increase the delivery of anti-cancer/anti-angiogenic compounds (such as doxorubicin-DXR) to tumors was based on the use of vascular targeted liposomes.

3. TUMOR VASCULAR TARGETING TECHNOLOGY

This strategy has been developed that might overcome problems of tumor cell heterogeneity by using vascular targeted liposomes to exploit the obvious advantages of anti-angiogenic therapies. Indeed, it has been shown that pronounced tumor regressions can be achieved in mice by systemic delivery of a liposomal anti-angiogenic chemotherapeutic drug that is targeted to the tumor vasculature [33]. There are several advantages of targeting chemotherapeutic agents to proliferating endothelial cells in the tumor vasculature rather than directly to tumour cells. First, acquired drug resistance, resulting from genetic and epigenetic mechanisms reduces the effectiveness of available drugs [37]. Anti-angiogenic therapy has the potential to overcome these problems or reduce their impact. This therapy targets the tumor vasculature, derived from local and circulating endothelial cells that are considered, although controversial, genetically stable. Second, the fact that a large number of cancer cells depend upon a small number of endothelial cells for their growth and survival might also amplify the therapeutic effect [38]. Third, anti-angiogenic therapies may also circumvent what may be a major mechanism of intrinsic drug resistance, namely insufficient drug penetration into the interior of a tumor mass due to high interstitial pressure gradients within tumors [39]. A strategy that targets both the tumor vasculature and the tumor cells themselves may be more effective than strategies that target only tumor vasculature, since this strategy can leave a cuff of unaffected tumor cells at the tumor periphery that can subsequently re-grow and kill the animals [40]. Fourth, oxygen consumption by neoplastic and endothelial cells, along with poor oxygen delivery, creates hypoxia within tumors. These characteristics of solid tumors compromise the delivery and effectiveness of conventional cytotoxic therapies as well as molecularly targeted therapies [38, 39]. Finally, the therapeutic target is partially independent of the type of solid tumor; killing of proliferating endothelial cells in the tumor microenvironment can be effective against a variety of malignancies.

In order to better mimic physiological and pathological features of the tumor microenvironment observed in patients suffering with cancer and, consequently, to build novel and more specific tumor- and vasculature-targeted therapies, the importance of choosing the correct animal models to be used, became mandatory. Most preclinical studies on tumor angiogenesis and anti-angiogenic therapy usually employ rapidly growing transplantable mouse tumors, or human tumor xenografts, which are grown as solid, localized tumors in the subcutaneous space. For several reasons this approach almost certainly exaggerates the anti-tumor responses. Principally, in such experimental situations, unlike in the clinic, distant metastases are usually not the focus of the treatment, but it is precisely such secondary tumors which are ultimately responsible for cancer's lethality.

For these reasons and to elucidate possible influences of the host microenvironment, angiogenesis-specific studies of tumors have been carried out in an orthotopic location. Heterotopic and orthotopic xenograft models in rodents, as a follow up to cell culture studies, have been the most widely used models to date for studies of drug efficacy. However, the use of orthotopically transplanted NB tumors may be preferable for these studies, not only to induce or enhance the incidence of metastases but also because the response of a tumor mass growing ectopically may be abnormal compared with the same tumor growing in a physiologically relevant site [41-43]. Thus, the optimal xenograft model of NB would be in an orthotopic site at an appropriate development stage to mimic the environment of endogenous neuroblastoma. [44, 45].

In the past we have shown neuroblastoma tumor regression, pronounced destruction of tumor vasculature and increased life span in orthotopic neuroblastoma-bearing mice treated with doxorubicin-loaded liposomes and coupled at the external surface with a NGR-containing peptide, able to specifically recognize the angiogenic endothelial cell marker aminopeptidase N [33, 45]. Moreover, pharmacokinetic studies indicated that systemically administered liposomes coupled to NGR peptide had long-circulating profiles in blood. They are removed only slightly more rapidly than the non-targeted formulation, with approximately 30 % of both drug and carrier remaining in the blood 24 h after liposome inoculation. Their uptake into NB tumors was at least 3 times higher than that of non-targeted liposomes after 24 hours, with doxorubicin spreading outside the blood vessels into the tumors. Five % of both the liposomes and the drug had localized to tumor by 24 h post-injection and this had increased to about 13% by 48 h post-injection. No uptake was observed with liposomes coupled with a control peptide [33].

More recently, we validated the potential of this "vascular targeting/vascular disrupting agents" strategy, by evaluating NGR-targeted liposomal doxorubicin (TVT-DOX) in several murine xenografts of doxorubicin-resistant human cancer, including lung, ovarian and, again, neuroblastoma [46]. Contrary to our previous experiments [33, 45], the TVT-DOX used in this study was manufactured as large-scale Good Manufacturing Practice (GMP) preparation [47], suited to human clinical trials. Specifically, the anti-tumor potential of several concentrations of TVT-DOX have been validated, using different treatment schedules, designed to act specifically against more or less mature neovasculature within the tumor mass.

Compared to an untargeted formulation of DOX (Caelyx®), in clinical use for the treatment of ovarian

cancer and other solid tumors [48, 49], the GMP preparation of TVT-DOX was able to more effectively kill angiogenic tumor blood vessels and, indirectly, the tumor cells that these vessels support. Moreover, the anti-tumor activity of TVT-DOX was higher than that of Caelyx®, in all three solid tumor murine models, particularly when administered at the higher dose treatment, suggesting that TVT-DOX should be evaluated as a novel VTA/VDA strategy for adjuvant therapy of solid tumors.

In order to assess the effect of TVT-DOX on controlling minimal residual disease (MRD) and helping to prevent tumor relapse, a new neuroblastoma model was set up. Briefly, mice were orthotopically injected with luciferase-transfected NB cells on day 0 and half of the mice had their tumors surgically resected on day 20, as previously reported [26]. The resected NB animal model, referred to in future as "NB-resected", was used to visualize, by bioluminescence imaging (BLI) and magnetic resonance imaging (MRI) evaluation, the response of minimal residual disease (MRD) to therapy, after surgical removal of the primary mass, as well as to monitor orthotopic expansion over time and organ-specific homing of tumor cells [46]. Interestingly, the comparison between two different imaging devises became very important in controlling primary tumor growth, relapse and minimal residual disease.

Cancer therapeutics have achieved success in the treatment of a variety of malignancies, however, relapse of disease from small numbers of persistent tumor cells remains a major obstacle. Advancement of treatment regimens that effectively control minimal residual disease (MRD) and prevent relapse would be greatly accelerated if sensitive and non invasive assays were used to quantitatively assess tumor burden in animal models of MRD that are predictive of the human response. Over the last five years there has also been a proliferation of high-resolution devices for *in vivo* imaging in animal models of human diseases [50-52]. *In vivo* bioluminescence imaging (BLI) is an assay for the detection of small numbers of cells non invasively and enables the quantification of tumor growth within internal organs [53-55]. *In vivo* BLI has enabled the study of tumor cell growth and offers sensitivity as well as a broad dynamic range of quantification. In the presence of oxygen, magnesium, and ATP the reporter gene luciferase produces visible light from a small molecule substrate, luciferin. Since visible light penetrates tissues at low levels, cells expressing this enzyme can be followed in living animals by external detection of the emitted light using low-light imaging systems.

A bioluminescence imaging system has been recently used to test the *in vivo* expression of NB transfected cells [45]. We used a reporter gene that code for a bioluminescent marker to label stably different NB cell lines and we monitored disease growth and metastasis following orthotopic implantation into recipients. The initial trafficking of the malignant cells through the body, as well as organ-specific homing and orthotopic expansion over time, as well as the visualization of the MRD after surgical removal of the primary mass and the response to NGR-targeted liposomal DOX therapy, have been readily visualized and quantified by highly sensitive, cooled CCD camera mounted in a light-tight specimen box (IVIS™; Xenogen).

Images were evaluated for BLI intensity over time (T_{21} and T_{44}). Treatment of NB-resected mice with TVT-DOX induced a partial arrest in primary tumor re-growth and possibly an inhibition of MRD, in 4 of 5 treated mice, while images from control buffer-treated NB-resected mice show tumor mass relapse and expansion in 4 of 5 mice. In NB-resected mice receiving TVT-DOX treatment, there was an increased life span compared to controls, with 2 of 5 animals still alive at 130 days after tumor challenge [46].

In some experiments, the visualization of MRD after surgical resection of the NB tumor, and also the response to TVT-DOX therapy, were quantified by a 1.5 Tesla magnetic resonance scanner (Philips Gyroscan NT-Intera) before and after gadolinium injection [46]. Images were obtained of the coronal and axial planes, perpendicular to the vertebral column of the animal. MRI was performed before and after i.v. injections of 0.5 mmol/kg gadolinium (MAGNEVIST®, gadopentetate dimeglumine).

To be highlighted is the fact that BLI and MRI are viable real-time, non invasive, quantitative and qualitative methods for monitoring the response to VTA therapy. But, while BLI was more sensitive than MRI for detecting early tumor responses to therapy, MRI was able to precisely identify focal MRD and appears to be more suited to the study of tumor growth *in vivo* and the effects of chemotherapy in experimental animal models [46]. Hence, we feel that MRI and BLI are complementary methods with promising roles in various types of preclinical research [56].

4. PATIENT-TAILORED TUMOR VASCULAR TARGETED THERAPIES

In the above described study, aminopeptidase N-targeted liposomes showed an enhanced anti-tumor and angiostatic effect against all the tumor animal models examined, and is a candidate for progression to clinical investigation. However, it must be born in mind that clinical trials based on the use of single, either pro- or anti-angiogenic, molecules can be more challenging than anticipated, and monotherapy with single angiogenesis inhibitor might not be sufficient to control cancer and the myriad of angiogenic factors produced by cancer cells. Phage display biopanning on viable cells is a powerful approach for identifying cell-specific peptides that mediate binding to individual tumor types [57]. This technology, based on the principle that bacteriophages can present specific binding ligands on their surface, has been used for discovering peptides that can specifically bind to organs, tumors, or cell types [32, 58].

In the near future, it may be possible to use phage display techniques on tumor patient specimens in order to develop novel ligand-targeted liposomal chemotherapeutic strategies that are based on the selective targeting of other novel molecular markers, expressed on the tumor vasculature or the tumor cell surface itself. Thus, a multiple target approach, based on a combination of anti-tumor and anti-vascular therapies, analogous to combination chemotherapy currently in widespread clinical use, could be expected to improve the therapeutic effects of nanomedicine drugs against many types of adult and pediatric solid tumors.

5. ACKNOWLEDGMENTS

Work supported by Fondazione Italiana per la Lotta al Neuroblastoma, Associazione Italiana per la Ricerca sul Cancro (AIRC, MFAG and IG) and Ministry of Health, Ricerca Finalizzata 2007. F.P., Fondazione Italiana per la Lotta al Neuroblastoma research fellow.

6. REFERENCES

1. Folkman J. Angiogenesis in cancer, vascular, rheumatoid and other disease. Nat Med 1995; 1(1): 27-31.
2. Risau W. Mechanisms of angiogenesis. Nature 1997; 386(6626): 671-674.
3. Ribatti D, Vacca A, Dammacco, F. The role of the vascular phase in solid tumor growth: a historical review. Neoplasia 1999; 1(4): 293-302.
4. Kleinman NR, Lewandowska K, Culp LA Tumour progression of human neuroblastoma cells tagged with a lacZ marker gene: earliest events at ectopic injection sites. Br J Cancer 1994: 69: 670-679.
5. Meitar D, Crawford SE, Rademaker, AW, Cohn SL. Tumor angiogenesis correlates with metastatic disease, N-myc amplification, and poor outcome in human neuroblastoma. J Clin Oncol 1996; 14(2): 405-414.
6. Ribatti D, Alessandri G, Vacca A, Iurlaro M, Ponzoni M. Human neuroblastoma cells produce extracellular matrix-degrading enzymes, induce endothelial cell proliferation and are angiogenic in vivo. Int J Cancer 1998; 77(3): 449-454.
7. Canete A, Navarro S, Bermudez J, Pellin A, Castel V, Llombart-Bosch, A. Angiogenesis in neuroblastoma: relationship to survival and other

prognostic factors in a cohort of neuroblastoma patients. J Clin Oncol 2000;18(1): 27-34.

8.   Eggert A, Ikegaki N, Kwiatkowski J, Zhao H, Brodeur GM, Himelstein, BP High-level expression of angiogenic factors is associated with advanced tumor stage in human neuroblastomas. Clin Cancer Res 2000; 6(5): 1900-1908.

9.   Ara T, Fukuzawa M, Kusafuka T, Komoto Y, Oue T, Inoue M, Okada, A. Immunohistochemical expression of MMP-2, MMP-9, and TIMP-2 in neuroblastoma: association with tumor progression and clinical outcome. J Pediatr Surg 1998; 33(8): 1272-1278.

10. Sakakibara M, Koizumi S, Saikawa Y, Wada H, Ichihara T, Sato H, Horita S, Mugishima H, Kaneko Y, Koike K. Membrane-type matrix metalloproteinase-1 expression and activation of gelatinase A as prognostic markers in advanced pediatric neuroblastoma. Cancer 1999; 85(1): 231-239.

11. Ribatti, D, Surico G, Vacca A, De Leonardis, F, Lastilla G, Montaldo PG, Rigillo N, Ponzoni M. Angiogenesis extent and expression of matrix metalloproteinase-2 and -9 correlate with progression in human neuroblastoma. Life Sci 2001; 68(10): 1161-1168.

12. Schweigerer L, Breit S, Wenzel A, Tsunamoto K, Ludwig R, Schwab, M. Augmented MYCN expression advances the malignant phenotype of human neuroblastoma cells: evidence for induction of autocrine growth factor activity. Cancer Res 1990; 50(14): 4411-4416.

13. Ribatti D, Raffaghello L, Pastorino F, Nico, B, Brignole C, Vacca A, Ponzoni M. In vivo angiogenic activity of neuroblastoma correlates with MYCN oncogene overexpression. Int J Cancer 2002; 102(4): 351-354.

14. Erdreich-Epstein A, Shimada H, Groshen S, Liu M, Metelitsa LS, Kim KS, Stins MF, Seeger RC, Durden DL. Integrins alpha(v)beta3 and alpha(v)beta5 are expressed by endothelium of high-risk neuroblastoma and their inhibition is associated with increased endogenous ceramide. Cancer Res 2000; 60(3): 712-721.

15. Huang D, Rutkowski JL, Brodeur GM, Chou PM, Kwiatkowski JL, Babbo A, Cohn SL. Schwann cell-conditioned medium inhibits angiogenesis. Cancer Res 2000; 60(21): 5966-5971.

16. Crawford SE, Stellmach V, Ranalli M, Huang, X, Huang L, Volpert O, De Vries GH, Abramson LP, Bouck, N. Pigment epithelium-derived factor (PEDF) in neuroblastoma: a multifunctional mediator of Schwann cell antitumor activity. J Cell Sci 2001; 114(24): 4421-4428.

17. Chlenski A, Liu S, Crawford SE, Volpert, OV, DeVries GH, Evangelista A, Yang Q, Salwen HR, Farrer R, Bray J, Cohn SL. SPARC is a key Schwannian-derived inhibitor controlling neuroblastoma tumor angiogenesis. Cancer Res 2002; 62(24): 7357-7363.

18. Leali D, Dell'Era P, Stabile H, Sennino B, Chambers AF, Naldini A, Sozzani S, Nico B, Ribatti D, Presta, M. Osteopontin (Eta-1) and fibroblast growth factor-2 cross-talk in angiogenesis. J Immunol 2003; 171(2): 1085-1093.

19. Takahashi F, Akutagawa S, Fukumoto H, Tsukiyama S, Ohe Y, Takahashi K, Fukuchi, Y, Saijo N, Nishio K Osteopontin induces angiogenesis of murine neuroblastoma cells in mice. Int J Cancer 2002; 98(5): 707-712.

20. Folkman, J. How is blood vessel growth regulated in normal and neoplastic tissue? G.H.A. Clowes memorial Award lecture. Cancer Res 1986; 46(2): 467-473.

21. Bergers G., Benjamin LE. Tumorigenesis and the angiogenic switch. Nat Rev Cancer 2003; 3(6): 401-410.

22. Teicher BA. Newer vascular targets. In: BA. Teicher, Ellis, LM (ed.), Antiangiogenic Agents in Cancer Therapy, Second Edition edition, Humana Press,Totowa, NJ: 2008; Vol., pp. 133-153.

23. Thorpe, P.E. Vascular targeting agents as cancer therapeutics. Clin Cancer Res, 2004, 10(2): 415-427.

24. Gabizon A, Catane R, Uziely B, Kaufman B, Safra T, Cohen R, Martin F, Huang A, Barenholz Y. Prolonged circulation time and enhanced accumulation in malignant exudates of doxorubicin encapsulated in polyethylene-glycol coated liposomes. Cancer Res 1994; 54(4): 987-992.

25   Allen TM. Ligand-targeted therapeutics in anticancer therapy. Nat Rev Cancer 2002; 2(10): 750-763.

26   Pastorino F, Marimpietri D, Brignole C, Di Paolo D, Pagnan G, Daga A, Piccardi F, Cilli, M, Allen TM, Ponzoni M. Ligand-targeted liposomal therapies of neuroblastoma. Curr Med Chem 2007; 14(29): 3070-3078.

27. Jain RK. Molecular regulation of vessel maturation. Nat Med 2003; 9(6): 685-693.

28. Nemeth JA, Nakada MT, Trikha M, Lang Z, Gordon MS, Jayson GC, Corringham R, Prabhakar U, Davis HM, Beckman RA. Alpha-v integrins as therapeutic targets in oncology. Cancer Invest 2007; 25(7): 632-646.

29. Rafii, S. and Lyden, D. Cancer. A few to flip the angiogenic switch. Science, 2008, 319(5860): 163-164.

30. Sato M, Arap W, Pasqualini, R. Molecular targets on blood vessels for cancer therapies in clinical trials. Oncology (Williston Park), 2007; 21(11): 1346-1352; discussion 1354-1345, 1367, 1370 passim.

31. Marchio S, Lahdenranta J, Schlingemann RO, Valdembri D, Wesseling P, Arap MA, Hajitou A, Ozawa MG, Trepel M, Giordano RJ, Nanus DM, Dijkman HB, Oosterwijk E, Sidman RL, Cooper MD, Bussolino F, Pasqualini R, Arap W. Aminopeptidase A is a functional target in angiogenic blood vessels. Cancer Cell 2004; 5(2): 151-162.

32. Sergeeva A, Kolonin MG, Molldrem JJ, Pasqualini R, Arap W. Display technologies: application for the discovery of drug and gene delivery agents. Adv Drug Deliv Rev 2006; 58(15): 1622-1654.

33. Pastorino F, Brignole C, Marimpietri D, Cilli M, Gambini C, Ribatti D, Longhi R, Allen TM, Corti A, Ponzoni M. Vascular damage and anti-angiogenic effects of tumor vessel-targeted liposomal chemotherapy. Cancer Res 2003; 63(21): 7400-7409.

34. Curnis F, Arrigoni G, Sacchi A, Fischetti L, Arap W, Pasqualini R, Corti A. Differential binding of drugs containing the NGR motif to CD13 isoforms in tumor vessels, epithelia, and myeloid cells. Cancer Res 2002; 62(3): 867-874.

35. O'Connell PJ, Gerkis V, d'Apice AJ. Variable O-glycosylation of CD13 (aminopeptidase N). J Biol Chem, 1991; 266(7): 4593-4597.

36. Colombo G, Curnis F, De Mori GM, Gasparri, A, Longoni C, Sacchi A, Longhi R, Corti A. Structure-activity relationships of linear and cyclic peptides containing the NGR tumor-homing motif. J Biol Chem 2002; 277(49): 47891-47897.

37. Klement G, Baruchel S, Rak J, Man S, Clark, K., Hicklin, D.J., Bohlen, P., and Kerbel, R.S. Continuous low-dose therapy with vinblastine and VEGF receptor-2 antibody induces sustained tumor regression without overt toxicity. J Clin Invest, 2000, 105(8): R15-24.

38. Jain RK. Normalizing tumor vasculature with anti-angiogenic therapy: a new paradigm for combination therapy. Nat Med 2001; 7(9): 987-989.

39. Jain RK. The next frontier of molecular medicine: delivery of therapeutics. Nat Med 1998; 4(6): 655-657.

40. Huang X, Molema G, King S, Watkins L, Edgington TS, Thorpe PE. Tumor infarction in mice by antibody-directed targeting of tissue factor to tumor vasculature. Science 1997; 275(5299): 547-550.

41. Moss TJ, Reynolds CP, Sather HN, Romansky SG, Hammond GD, Seeger RC. Prognostic value of immunocytologic detection of bone marrow metastases in neuroblastoma. N Engl J Med 1991; 324(4): 219-226.

42. Fidler IJ. Modulation of the organ microenvironment for treatment of cancer metastasis. J Natl Cancer Inst 1995; 87(21): 1588-1592.

43. Fidler, I.J. and Ellis, L.M. The implications of angiogenesis for the biology and therapy of cancer metastasis. Cell, 1994; 79(2): 185-188.

44. Khanna C, Jaboin JJ, Drakos E, Tsokos M, Thiele CJ. Biologically relevant orthotopic neuroblastoma xenograft models: primary adrenal tumor growth and spontaneous distant metastasis. In Vivo 2002; 16(2): 77-85.

45. Pastorino F, Brignole C, Di Paolo D, Nico B, Pezzolo A, Marimpietri D, Pagnan G, Piccardi F, Cilli M, Longhi R, Ribatti D, Corti A, Allen TM, Ponzoni M. Targeting liposomal chemotherapy via both tumor cell-specific and tumor vasculature-specific ligands potentiates therapeutic efficacy. Cancer Res 2006; 66(20): 10073-10082.

46. Pastorino F, Di Paolo D, Piccardi F, Nico B, Ribatti D, Daga A, Baio G, Neumaier CE, Brignole C, Loi M, Marimpietri D, Pagnan G, Cilli M, Lepekhin EA, Garde SV, Longhi R, Corti A, Allen TM, Wu JJ, Ponzoni M Enhanced antitumor efficacy of clinical-grade vasculature-targeted liposomal doxorubicin. Clin Cancer Res 2008; 14(22): 7320-7329.

47. Garde SV, Forte AJ, Ge M, Lepekhin EA, Panchal CJ, Rabbani SA, Wu JJ. Binding and internalization of NGR-peptide-targeted liposomal doxorubicin

48. (TVT-DOX) in CD13-expressing cells and its antitumor effects. Anticancer Drugs 2007; 18(10): 1189-1200.

48. Northfelt DW, Dezube BJ, Thommes JA, Levine R, Von Roenn JH, Dosik GM, Rios A, Krown SE, DuMond C, Mamelok RD. Efficacy of pegylated-liposomal doxorubicin in the treatment of AIDS-related Kaposi's sarcoma after failure of standard chemotherapy. J Clin Oncol 1997; 15(2): 653-659.

49. Gordon, A.N., Granai, C.O., Rose, P.G., Hainsworth, J., Lopez, A., Weissman, C., Rosales R, Sharpington T. Phase II study of liposomal doxorubicin in platinum- and paclitaxel-refractory epithelial ovarian cancer. J Clin Oncol 2000: 18(17): 3093-3100.

50. Joseph JM, Gross N, Lassau N, Rouffiac V, Opolon P, Laudani L, Auderset K, Geay JF, Muhlethaler-Mottet A, Vassal G. In vivo echographic evidence of tumoral vascularization and microenvironment interactions in metastatic orthotopic human neuroblastoma xenografts. Int J Cancer 2005; 113(6): 881-890.

51. Condeelis J, Segall JE. Intravital imaging of cell movement in tumours. Nat Rev Cancer 2003; 3(12): 921-930.

52. Ponce AM, Viglianti BL, Yu D, Yarmolenko PS, Michelich CR, Woo J, Bally MB, Dewhirst MW. Magnetic resonance imaging of temperature-sensitive liposome release: drug dose painting and antitumor effects. J Natl Cancer Inst 2007; 99(1): 53-63.

53. Edinger M, Cao YA, Verneris MR, Bachmann MH, Contag CH, Negrin RS. Revealing lymphoma growth and the efficacy of immune cell therapies using in vivo bioluminescence imaging. Blood 2003; 101(2): 640-648.

54. Armstrong SA, Kung AL, Mabon ME, Silverman LB, Stam RW, Den Boer ML, Pieters R, Kersey JH, Sallan SE, Fletcher JA, Golub TR, Griffin JD, Korsmeyer SJ. Inhibition of FLT3 in MLL. Validation of a therapeutic target identified by gene expression based classification. Cancer Cell 2003; 3(2): 173-183.

55. Xie X, Xia W, Li Z, Kuo HP, Liu Y, Li Z, Ding Q, Zhang S, Spohn B, Yang Y, Wei Y, Lang JY, Evans DB, Chiao PJ, Abbruzzese JL, Hung MC Targeted expression of BikDD eradicates pancreatic tumors in noninvasive imaging models. Cancer Cell 2007; 12(1): 52-65.

56. Clamp AR, Jayson G.C. The Role of Imaging in the Clinical Development of AntiAngiogenic Agents. In: B.A. Teicher, Ellis, L. M. (ed.), Antiangiogenic Agents in Cancer Therapy, Second Edition edition, Humana Press,Totowa, NJ: 2008; Vol., pp. 525-536.

57. Elayadi AN, Samli KN, Prudkin L, Liu YH, Bian A, Xie XJ, Wistuba, II, Roth, J.A., McGuire, MJ, Brown KC. A peptide selected by biopanning identifies the integrin alphavbeta6 as a prognostic biomarker for nonsmall cell lung cancer. Cancer Res 2007; 67(12): 5889-5895.

58. Pasqualini R, Ruoslahti E. Organ targeting in vivo using phage display peptide libraries. Nature 1996; 380(6572): 364-366.

CHAPTER 11

Tumor Targeting with Transgenic Endothelial Cells

Gerold Untergasser and Eberhard Gunsilius

Tumor Biology & Angiogenesis Lab, Department of Internal Medicine V, Medical University Innsbruck, TILAK & Oncotyrol, Innrain 66, 6020 Innsbruck, Austria

Correspondence to: Prof. Eberhard Gunsilius Tumor Biology & Angiogenesis Lab, Department of Internal Medicine V, Medical University Innsbruck, TILAK & Oncotyrol, Innrain 66, 6020 Innsbruck, Austria. Tel: 0043.512.50423255; Fax: 0043.51252199214778; Email: eberhard.gunsilius@i-med.ac.at

Abstract: The formation of tumor supporting vessels can be accomplished by the sprouting of preexisting vessels, i.e. the proliferation of resident endothelial cells (*angiogenesis*) or by *vasculogenesis*, i.e. the de novo formation of vessels by circulating endothelial progenitor cells (EPC) presumably deriving from the bone marrow. Cytokines and chemokines released by tumors and inflamed tissue have been shown to recruit EPC and other progenitor cells from the circulation to home to sites of active vessel and tumor growth. Therefore, EPC-based therapies might be used to target specifically malignant tumors. Incorporated autologous cells thereby function as "Trojan horses" and deliver enzymes for activation of cytotoxic agents or release antiangiogenic proteins. However, the extent of EPC incorporation and the precise mechanisms by which EPC contribute to neovessels or migrate and invade tumor tissue are still under investigation. Furthermore, cells used for therapeutic purposes, regardless of their origin, have to be produced under Good Manufacturing Practice (GMP) conditions and should be at least homogenous and unequivocally characterized to minimize potential risks of malignant transformation in individuals after transplantation. Thus, this review will summarize the current knowledge on EPC, their *ex-vivo* propagation, genetic modification and homing to tumors in preclinical trials.

1. INTRODUCTION

Tumors need sufficient nutrients and oxygen supply, otherwise tumor cells get acidic, hypoxic and necrotic. Thus, tumor growth is strongly dependent on the generation of new blood vessels [1]. Tumour blood vessels are generated by various mechanisms, such as cooption of the existing vascular network, expansion of the host vascular network by budding of endothelial sprouts (sprouting angiogenesis), remodelling and expansion of vessels by the insertion of interstitial tissue columns into the lumen of pre-existing vessels (intussusceptive angiogenesis) and homing of endothelial cell precursors (EPC; CEPs, angioblast-like cells) from the bone marrow or peripheral blood into the endothelial lining of neovessels (vasculogenesis) [2,3]. Bone marrow derived progenitor cells contribute significantly to neovascularization in a variety of tumors [4-6]. Despite significant contributions in animal systems the extent of incorporated EPCs into neovessels of malignant human tumors is still under investigation and strongly depending on the tumor-type studied [7].

EPCs might represent an ideal shuttle for a cell-based therapy targeting the expanding tumor, i.e. areas of hypoxia and inflammation. Specific targeting of tumors should be achieved since bone marrow

mononuclear cells and EPCs are mobilized and attracted from the circulation by a released cocktail of tumor-derived cytokines and chemokines. In particular VEGF [8] and SDF1 [9] produced under ischemic conditions can mobilize EPCs from the bone marrow and circulation to sites of active neovascularization. Genetically-modified EPCs can be used to deliver therapeutic proteins, such as secreted antiangiogenic proteins or enzymes for activation of cytotoxic agents into neovessels of the tumor [10,11]. Hitherto, this therapeutic attempt has been shown as proof of principle in different preclinical studies making use of murine tumor models or human tumor xenografts transplanted into immunocompromised mice [11-15]. Despite these promising results in preclinical animal models, we are still far away from a safe and specific cell-based therapy that can be used in a clinical setting. There are still stringent prerequisites for EPC based therapies in humans that need be reached or established, such as (i) a well characterized terminally differentiating cell-type that can be produced under GMP-conditions, (ii) a cell-type with high proliferative capacity for propagation and genetic modification, (iii) a save genetic modification system not causing transformation of cells and not inducing immune responses in the host, (iv) a genetic modification system allowing permanent and high expression of the target gene (v), a cell-type that can be mobilized by the chemokine-gradient and finally (vi) is able to home preferentially to the tumor and not to other organs.

2. SOURCES OF ENDOTHELIAL CELLS

BOEC or ECFC can be propagated from peripheral blood, cord blood and bone marrow aspirates after isolation of mononuclear cells, attachment to a collagen type-I matrix and stimulation with the two prominent angiogenic factors vascular growth factor (VEGF) and basic fibroblast growth factor (bFGF) [16,17]. BOEC can be easily propagated from peripheral blood samples within 1 month of propagation in adequate numbers required for cell therapy and importantly have a well characterized uniform endothelial cell phenotype (CD31$^+$, CD146$^+$, KDR$^+$, CD45$^-$, CD133$^-$, CD34$^-$). BOEC undergo regularly cellular senescence and show no chromosomal abnormalities and importantly still have the potential to home to the ischemic myocardium of

nude rats [18]. BOEC clones presumably originate from endothelial progenitor cells EPC also named circulating endothelial progenitors (CEP, see Fig. **1**). This cell type has been shown to differentiate from bone marrow progenitor cells and to incorporate into blood vessels of tumors [5,19]. Meanwhile, endothelial cells have also been differentiated *ex-vivo* from hematopoietic and mesenchymal stem cells and from tissue-resident stem cells. Moreover, monocytes have been shown to adhere on fibronectin-coated material and transdifferentiate under VEGF stimulation into "Hill colonies" [20] now named Colony Forming Unit Endothelial Cells (CFU-EC). Despite characteristics of monocytes (expression of CD14 and CD45) CFU-EC express endothelial surface markers, have a low proliferative capacity *in-vitro* and are still able to phagocyte bacteria [17]. This cell type does not incorporate in newly formed blood vessels, but homes to sites of ischemia [17]. In contrast, BOEC have been shown to incorporate in newly formed blood vessels of matrigel plugs in nude mice and retain a high proliferative potential [17]. EPC/CEP are very

Sources of EPC

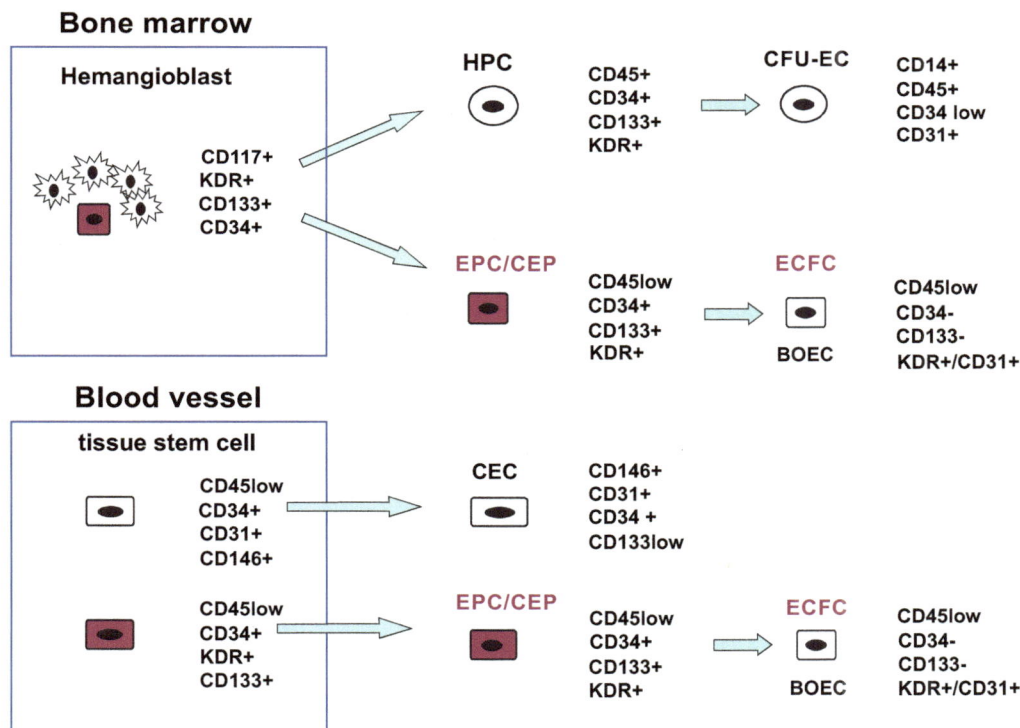

Fig. (1). There are various sources of endothelial cells or precursors for ex-vivo manipulation: (I) hematopoietic stem cells which are found in very rare numbers also in peripheral blood and to a higher extent in the bone-marrow, (II) circulating endothelial progenitor cells or" (EPC/CEP,) giving rise to "blood outgrowth endothelial cells" (BOEC) or "endothelial colony forming cells" (ECFC) under tissue culture conditions, (III) myeloid cells (CFU-EC) and (IV) circulating mature endothelial cells (CEC), derived from the endothelial layer of blood vessels. All cell types present in peripheral blood can differentiate towards an endothelial cell phenotype under appropriate culture conditions.

rare cell-types that can only be found at lowest frequencies in the circulation of healthy persons and tumor patients [21]. They can be identified by their complex phenotype $CD45^{low}$, $CD34^+$, $CD133^+$ and KDR^+. These markers are by no way specific for this cell-type and can be also found on subsets of hematopoietic stem cells [22] or tumor stem cells [23]. Hitherto, no single reliable marker for EPC has been discovered. Apart from the rare EPC cell-type, more abundant circulating endothelial cells (CEC) have been monitored in peripheral blood samples after damage of the vasculature [24]. CEC are mature endothelial cells expressing CD146 and therefore have a low proliferative potential. CEC are elevated in patients with advanced malignancies and vasculopathies [25] and monitoring of CEC has been proposed as surrogate marker for therapy-induced effects [26].

Based on essential premises for genetic modification and for use in cell-based therapies, i.e. (i) a characterized homogenous cell population, (ii) a high proliferative capacity and (iii) the capacity of terminal endothelial differentiation, BOEC seem the most appropriate cell-type for cell-based therpies targeting the tumor.

3. GENETIC MODIFICATION OF ENDOTHELIAL CELLS

Adenovirus

Adenoviruses can infect non-dividing cells (see Fig. 2). The adenoviral double stranded DNA is not incorporated into the host-genome and remains episomal as separate extra-chromosomal element in the

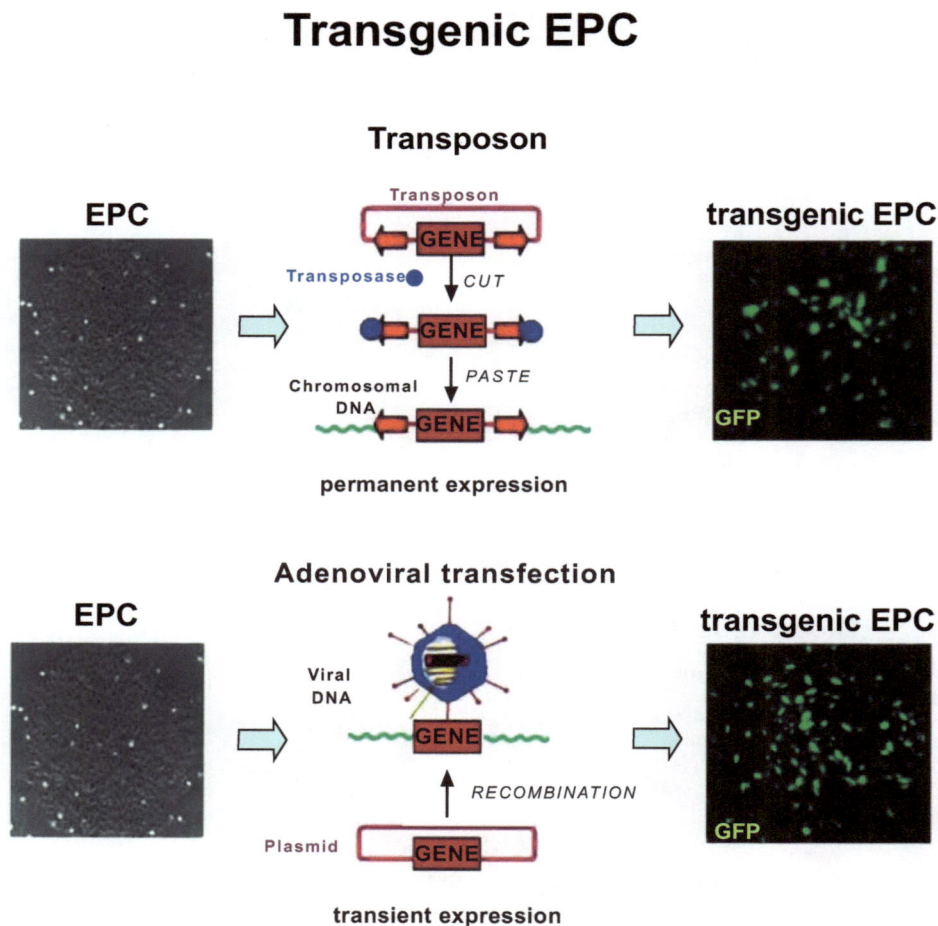

Fig. (2). Viral and non-viral systems for the genetic manipulation of endothelial cells. Recombinant adenoviruses can be generated by homologue recombination of the plasmid containing the gene of interest with the adenoviral DNA. These viruses are used to infect endothelial cells, that in turn transiently express the transgene GFP. The Sleeping Beauty (SB) transposon carrying the gene of interest is "cut" out of the plasmid vector by the engine of this machine (the transposase) and then "pasted" directly into the chromosome of endothelial cells, that in turn permanently express GFP.

nucleus of the target cells, i. e. cell loose the adenoviral DNA after mitotic division and DNA replication. Therefore, the episomal system avoids site effects due to genomic integration and activation /inactivation of oncogenes or tumor suppressor genes. The main disadvantage of the adenoviral systems is that the gene of interest is expressed only temporarily (transient, for a few days) and that repeated treatment during therapy would result in immune responses against viral components. Many types of endothelial cells, in particular confluent ones, express the required CAR receptor at high levels and therefore can easily be transfected [27]. Thus, adenovirus-based cancer gene therapy with less immunogenic virus types still has

potential to become one component of a multi-modality treatment approach to advanced cancer, along with surgery, radiotherapy, and chemotherapy [28].

Lentivirus

Lentiviruses are retroviruses that cause a stable incorporation of genes of interest into the host genome of dividing cells (integration). These integrating vector systems can deliver genetic material to a target cell with high efficiency enabling long-term expression of an encoded transgene. The use of lentiviral vectors offers multiple advantages in gene replacement therapy, because they combine efficient delivery, and ability to transduce proliferating and resting cells. They are less immunogenic than adenoviruses due to the absence of viral genes in the vector and no interference with pre-existing viral immunity. However, still innate and adaptive immune responses to the delivery vector have been reported [29]. Lentiviruses raise specific concerns on patient's safety, due to their possibilities to generate replication competent lentiviruses during vector production or *in vivo* due to recombination with infectious retroviruses such as human immunodeficiency virus (HIV).Moreover viruses can cause insertional mutagenesis due to lentivector proviral DNA integrations, potentially leading to oncogenesis; or they induce germline alteration and transmission of the transgene to the offspring;. To date, authorities in no country have formally approved the use of lentivectors for usage in patients [30].

Transposons

Transposable elements are non-viral gene delivery vehicles found ubiquitously in the nature. Transposon-based vectors have the capacity of stable genomic integration and long-lasting expression of transgenic constructs in a variety of mammalian cell-types [31]. For the genetic manipulation of EC and stem cells a transposon-based system called "sleeping-beauty" has been successfully used (own unpublished data and [32]). The Sleeping-beauty transposase is a member of the Tc1/mariner superfamily of transposable elements and induces a preferential insertion of the transposon into TA-rich sites of the host genome [33]. The transposon system offers a long-lasting, safe way to insert genes into the chromosomes of cells without use of any viral vectors. The transposon DNA can be designed to not harbor any viral sequences and therefore avoids immunologic reactions associated with viral vectors. Moreover, transposons show no preferences to insert in areas of transcriptional activity such as reported for most integrating viruses [34]. The sleeping beauty transposon technology has been patented by *Discovery Genomics Inc.* due to several safety advantages over viral vectors and is currently under investigation in preclinical trials in the United States [35]. However, due to a insertion preference of the transposon to intronic regions of the genome, it will be still necessary to carefully design and test clinical-grade transposons to avoid any unwanted side effects on RNA processing (i.e., alternative splicing) at the target site [34].

4. THERAPEUTIC GENES FOR ENDOTHELIAL CELL-BASED TUMOR TARGETING

Sucide Genes

"Suicide genes" are encoding proteins which convert non-toxic pro-drugs to toxic substances in transduced cells causing cell death of these cells. The herpes simplex thymidinekinase (HSV-TK), not normally expressed in mammalian cells, is a homodimer of approximately 30 kDa that effectively metabolizes gancyclovir and other nucleosides used in the treatment of viral disorders.. Gancyclovir is a nucleoside analogon that undergoes phosphorylation in the presence of HSV-TK. Gancyclovir-phosphates inhibit DNA replication by substitution for normal nucleosides in the DNA which leads to interruption of replication and cell death. A particularly attractive feature of utilizing HSV-TK to sensitize endothelial cells to gancyclovir is that, in addition to the killing of HSV-TK positive cells, HSV-TK negative cells in close proximity to the transduced cells are also rendered sensitive to gancyclovir and killed by exposure to the drug. This phenomenon has been designated a "bystander-effect".

Recently, HSV-TK/gancyclovir suicide gene therapy for has been studied in experimental glioblastoma animal models as well as in clinical trials. In these trials, genetically-modified murine fibroblasts overepressing the *HSV-TK* gene have been used to induce tumor necrosis and shrinkage [36]. Although the treatment was feasible and well tolerated, the encouraging results in animal models have so far not been reproduced in human glioblastoma.

Another system used cytosine deaminase (FCY1) which converts 5-fluorocytosine into 5-fluorouracil, a cytotoxic substance that next to endothelial cells also killed bystanding tumor cells via passive diffusion.

Cytokines and Antiangiogenic Proteins

Another option to destroy tumors is via cytokine based-gene therapy, where genes encoding local expressed immunostimulatory molecules are delivered by injected endothelial cells. GM-CSF, Interleukin-2 (IL-2) and Interleukin-12 (IL-12) have already been explored in a variety of animal models. GM-CSF augments the presentation of antigens, IL-2 is a stimulator for (anti-tumoral) T-cells and IL-12 augments the cytotoxic activity of various immune cells, including natural-killer cells [37,38].

Genes encoding antiangiogenic proteins might also be candidates for tumor targeting using transgenic endothelial cells. Thrombospondin-1, a member of the thrombospondin family, is a potent inhibitor of angiogenesis. Endostatin, a collagen type-18 fragment and endogenous inhibitor of angiogenesis causes endothelial cell apoptosis and has been tested already in preclinical and clinical models.

Tumor Targeting Using Transgenic Endothelial Cells

The systemic delivery of cytotoxic agents, immunotherapeutic substances and therapeutic genes to tumors is frequently hampered by their non-specificity for the target tissue. Systemic side effects occur and the amount of therapeutic "drug" that must be applied to get an antitumoral effect is often above the maximal tolerated dose. Therefore, targeted therapy using vehicles that show a tropism for tumors or tumor-associated tissues might be an interesting novel strategy. Since the work of Asahara et al. clearly demonstrating that cells with properties of endothelial progenitors from the blood of adult species are homing to sites of neovascularization [16] the concept of using endothelial cells or their progenitors as "trojan horses" to treat tumors has become an interesting concept. Several strategies for the equipment of endothelial cells with therapeutic genes are conceivable, assuming a more or less selective homing to malignant tumors. *Ex-vivo* expanded endothelial cells or their precursors can be genetically modified to express genes encoding for immunostimulatory proteinsor or antiangiogenic. Even regression of tumors using solely xenogenic endothelial cells exerting an immune-response has been described [39].

Moore at al. used CD34$^+$-cell derived human EPC (generated from human cord blood) to test their homing into an orthotopic glioblastoma in immuno-deficient SCID mice [40]. EPCs were labelled with a dye and injected intravenously. Indeed, they found up to 37-fold more EPC per histological section in the brain tumors compared to normal brain areas and to other organs (spleen, liver, lungs, kidneys), demonstrating a selective homing of systemically injected EPCs at least to brain tumors. These tumors are known to be highly vascularized and secrete high

amounts of VEGF. Over time the EPC became concentrated at the rim, the most proliferating area of the tumor. Interestingly, mature endothelial cells (HUVECs) also showed a tropism for brain tumors, although to a much lesser degree than EPCs. Of note, SCID mice tumor models harbor the problem that the homing behaviour of injected cells is far away from a syngenic model, as the tumor cells of human origin produce human chemotactic and pro-angiogenic mediators, which might primarily recruit syngenic human EPC.

Wei et al. showed that EPCs derived from mouse embryonic cells home preferentially to lung metastases after intravenous injection [41]. The number of labelled endothelial progenitors in other metastatic sites, such as liver and kidney was much lower, implicating a "first-pass effect" in the lung. Dye-labelled fibroblasts showed no homing to lung metastases. Next, they equipped *ex-vivo* expanded EPCs with a suicide gene-construct (cytosinedeaminase/UPRT) which converts the harmless prodrug 5-fluorocytosine (5-FC) into toxic 5-fluorouracil (5-FU). After systemic delivery of these transgenic EPCs were killed by 5-FU and also a bystander effect was observed, leading to eradication of metastases and to a longer survival of the treated mice.

The same group explored the usability of replicating oncolytic measles virus to treat malignant brain tumors in a mouse model. The attenuated measles virus of the Edmonston B vaccine strain infects cells preferentially by binding to CD46 (complement regulatory protein). Malignant cells including gliomas have a higher density of CD46 on their surface than normal cells. Importantly, BOEC also express CD46, so that these cells can be infected with the virus serving as a carrier to circumvent neutralization of virus particles by antibodies present in the blood. BOEC are relatively resistant to measles virus induced cell death. BOEC were infected with the measles virus and injected intratumorally into orthotopic brain tumors in a mouse model. When injected intravenously the virus containing BOEC were found accumulated in the brain tumors but not in surrounding brain tissue. After five injections the tumors were smaller than in control mice and the survival of the treated animals was slightly but significantly prolonged. An interesting observation was that numerous peritumorally injected BOEC containing virus particles migrated to the tumor (fibroblasts did not), accumulated there and also prolonged the survival of mice with U87 gliomas [42].

Ferrari et al. used CD34$^+$ cells (obtained from G-CSF stimulated human blood) or Sca1$^+$ cells (from mouse bone-marrow) transfected with the HSV-TK gene using retroviral gene transfer and transplanted these cells into sublethally irradiated tumor bearing mice. Genetically labelled CD34$^+$ cells or *ex-vivo* differentiated EPCs transplanted into sublethally irradiated tumor-bearing mice were found to migrate to and incorporate into the angiogenic vasculature of growing tumors. 10-25% of the CD31 positive cells isolated from the tumor vasculature were of of the donor phenotype (i.e. human). Interestingly, organs were only occasional infiltrated by human EPCs. Injection of human CD34$^+$ cells expressing the HSV-TK followed by treatment with gancyclovir resulted in a significant reduction in tumor growth compared to animals transplanted with GFP-expressing CD34$^+$ cells. Necrosis and apoptosis of tumor cells was found preferentially in the expanding border of the tumors. This area of the tumor also showed the highest number of EPCs incorporated into the tumor vasculature [11]. Similar results were obtained using mouse Sca1$^+$ cells.

We investigated the homing of modified human, *ex-vivo* expanded BOEC to human prostate xenotransplants in immune deficient mice. Circulating human CD34$^+$/CD133$^-$ cells were isolated, propagated, fluorescently labelled and injected into the blood stream of athymic nude mice bearing CRL-2505 prostate xenografts. BOEC homed to xenotransplants and comprised 1-3% of total tumor cells 5 days following injection as assessed by flow cytometry. Histological analysis revealed that BOEC were integrated throughout the developing neovasculature but preferentially accumulated in the peritumoral region. These data suggest that *ex-vivo* expanded EPC can contribute to vasculogenesis in prostate cancer [15].

In a next step, BOEC were infected with an adenovirus constructed to secrete a soluble form of the CSF-1 (colony stimulating factor-1, a macrophage stimulating protein) receptor CD115 that inhibits macrophage viability and migration *in vitro*. Tumor-associated macrophages (TAMs) are derived from a sub-population of circulating monocytes and are pro-angiogenic in hypoxic tumor regions. They promote remodelling of the extracellular matrix and secrete pro-angiogenic growth factors. The recruitment of TAMs to malignant tumors is mediated by CSF-1 which acts through the receptor tyrosine kinase CD115. Our assumption was that *ex-vivo* expanded and adenoviral-infected endothelial cells would migrate to human prostate tumors and there inhibit TAM mediated tumor development by secretion of the extracellular ligand binding domain of CD115. Indeed, after intracardial injection modified endothelial cells were found in the tumors, preferentially at their margins. We found a significantly decreased in the number of TAMs in the tumors and a reduction in the tumor volume, implicating that targeting stromal cell processes with modified endothelial cells has the potential to retard prostate tumor growth (unpublished data).

Dudeck et al. also used BOEC retrovirally transfected to express and secrete endostatin. Endostatin is a fragment of collagen type-18 that inhibits endothelial proliferation and angiogenesis and thereby leads to a retardation of the tumor growth [43]. The body distribution was studied using radiolabelled BOEC and revealed that cells accumulated within tumors but also to a lesser degree in various organs, such as liver, kidney, spleen and lung. Over time the number of BOEC in the lung decreased in comparison to other organs. BOEC were detectable up to 3 weeks after infection . Of note, the vessel count in tumors was more than four-fold higher in tumor bearing mice receiving BOEC compared to controls, implicating the support of tumor growth by increased angiogenesis mediated at least in part by systemically administered BOEC. The intravenous injection of transgenic BOEC secreting endostatin into mice bearing subcutaneous tumors led to retarded tumor growth. The tumor size was reduced by 28% in mice treated with endostatin transgenic BOEC. Moreover, the tumors had a lower vessel density compared to tumors of control BOEC-treated mice [44]. The use of BOEC which can be easily grown from peripheral blood renders this system particularly attractive for future studies in humans.

5. SUMMARY AND OUTLOOK

It is now clear that besides angiogenesis, i.e. the sprouting of new vessels from preexisting ones, another mechanism called vasculogenesis mediated by circulating cells with an endothelial phenotype is an machinery for generation of tumor blood vessels[45,46]. In the last years a compelling body of evidence has been generated supporting the homing of endothelial cells and/or their progenitors to sites where neovascularization takes place, e.g. to ischemic tissues and to malignant tumors. Whereas the administration of such cells for the treatment of limb ischemia or myocardial infarction is already tested in clinical trials [47], attempts to target malignant tumors are still in a preclinical stage.

The contribution of endothelial progenitor cells or other cells with an endothelial-like phenotype, either recruited from the bone-marrow or injected into the circulation, to tumor vascularization varies substantially depending on the animal model, the tumor type and the source of endothelial cells. In animals the range of endothelial cells contributing to tumor vascularization by vasculogenesis is between 0 and 100%. In humans suffering from cancer after allogeneic, sex-mismatched hematopoietic stem cell transplantation the amount of bone-marrow derived EC (i.e. derived from the mismatched graft) was estimated to be 4.8% [19], implicating that a targeted therapy using endothelial cells might be feasible also in humans. Very recently Reinisch et al. demonstrated that proliferating, functional and genomically stable human BOEC can be expanded to a relevant clinical quantity under GMP-compliant conditions in an xenoprotein-free system, a prerequisite for cell-based therapies in humans [48]. Novel imaging techniques allowing the detection of low amounts of injected cells *in vivo* in conjunction with GMP adherent culture techniques of autologous human endothelial cells or their precursors pave the way for early clinical studies on tumor targeting using transgenic endothelial cells in humans.

6. ACKNOWLEDGEMENTS

This work was supported by Oncotyrol, center for personalized medicine, www.oncotyrol.at

7. REFERENCES

1.   Folkman J, Bach M, Rowe JW, Davidoff F, Lambert P, Hirsch C, Goldberg A, Hiatt HH, Glass J, Henshaw E. Tumor Angiogenesis - Therapeutic Implications. New England Journal of Medicine 1971; 285(21): 1182-6.

2.   Risau W. Mechanisms of angiogenesis. Nature 1997; 386(6626): 671-674.

3.   Carmeliet P. Mechanisms of angiogenesis and arteriogenesis. Nat.Med. 2000; 6(4): 389-395.

4.   Lyden D, Hattori K, Dias S, Costa C, Blaikie P, Butros L, Chadburn A, Heissig B, Marks W, Witte L, Wu Y, Hicklin D, Zhu ZP, Hackett NR, Crystal RG, Moore MAS, Hajjar K A, Manova K, Benezra R, Rafii S. Impaired recruitment of bone-marrow-derived endothelial and hematopoietic precursor cells blocks tumor angiogenesis and growth. Nature Medicine 2001; 7(11): 1194-1201.

5.   Gunsilius E, Duba HC, Petzer AL, Kahler CM, Grunewald K, Stockhammer G, Gabl C, Dirnhofer S, Clausen J, Gastl G. Evidence from a leukaemia model for maintenance of vascular endothelium by bone-marrow-derived endothelial cells. Lancet 2000; 355(9216): 1688-1691.

6.   Rafii S, Lyden D, Benezra R, Hattori K, Heissig B. Vascular and haematopoietic stem cells: novel targets for anti-angiogenesis therapy? Nat.Rev.Cancer 2002; 2(11): 826-835.

7.   Peters BA, Diaz LA, Polyak K, Meszler L, Romans K, Guinan E. C, Antin JH, Myerson D, Hamilton SR, Vogelstein B, Kinzler KW, Lengauer C. Contribution of bone marrow-derived endothelial cells to human tumor vasculature. Nat.Med. 2005; 11(3): 261-262.

8.   Willett CG, Boucher Y, di Tomaso E, Duda DG, Munn LL, Tong RT, Chung DC, Sahani DV, Kalva SP, Kozin SV, Mino M, Cohen KS, Scadden DT, Hartford AC, Fischman AJ, Clark J, W.; Ryan, D. P.; Zhu, A. X.; Blaszkowsky, L. S.; Chen, H. X.; Shellito PC, Lauwers GY, Jain RK. Direct evidence that the VEGF-specific antibody bevacizumab has antivascular effects in human rectal cancer. Nat.Med. 2004; 10(2): 145-147.

9.   Abbott JD, Huang Y, Liu D, Hickey R, Krause DS, Giordano FJ. Stromal cell-derived factor-1alpha plays a critical role in stem cell recruitment to the heart after myocardial infarction but is not sufficient to induce homing in the absence of injury. Circulation 2004; 110(21): 3300-3305.

10. Rumpold H, Wolf D, Koeck R, Gunsilius E. Endothelial progenitor cells: a source for therapeutic vasculogenesis? J.Cell Mol.Med. 2004; 8(4): 509-518.

11. Ferrari N, Glod J, Lee J, Kobiler D, Fine HA. Bone marrow-derived, endothelial progenitor-like cells as angiogenesis-selective gene-targeting vectors. Gene Ther. 2003; 10(8): 647-656.

12. Davidoff AM, Ng CY, Brown P, Leary MA, Spurbeck WW, Zhou J, Horwitz E, Vanin EF, Nienhuis AW. Bone marrow-derived cells contribute to tumor neovasculature and, when modified to express an angiogenesis inhibitor, can restrict tumor growth in mice. Clin.Cancer Res. 2001; 7(9): 2870-2879.

13. De Palma M, Venneri MA, Roca C, Naldini L. Targeting exogenous genes to tumor angiogenesis by transplantation of genetically modified hematopoietic stem cells. Nat.Med. 2003; 9(6): 789-795.

14. Moore XL, Lu J, Sun L, Zhu CJ, Tan P, Wong MC. Endothelial progenitor cells' "homing" specificity to brain tumors. Gene Ther. 2004; 11(10): 811-818.

15. Lucas T, Untergasser G, Abraham D, Hofer E, Gunsilius E, Aharinejad S. Targeting human solid tumor xenografts with ex vivo expanded endothelial progenitor cells. FASEB 222. Abstr. 901.4. 2008.

16. Asahara T, Murohara T, Sullivan A, Silver M, van der Zee R, Li T, Witzenbichler B, Schatteman G, Isner JM. Isolation of putative progenitor endothelial cells for angiogenesis. Science 1997; 275(5302): 964-967.

17. Yoder MC, Mead LE, Prater D, Krier TR, Mroueh KN, Li F, Krasich R, Temm CJ, Prchal JT, Ingram DA. Re-defining endothelial progenitor cells via clonal analysis and hematopoietic stem/progenitor cell principals. Blood 2006.

18. Untergasser G, Koeck R, Wolf D, Rumpold H, Ott H, Debbage P, Koppelstaetter C, Gunsilius E. CD34+/CD133- circulating endothelial precursor cells (CEP): characterization, senescence and in vivo application. Exp.Gerontol. 2006; 41(6): 600-608.

19. Peters BA, Diaz LA, Polyak K, Meszler L, Romans K, Guinan EC, Antin JH, Myerson D, Hamilton SR, Vogelstein B, Kinzler KW, Lengauer C. Contribution of bone marrow-derived endothelial cells to human tumor vasculature. Nat.Med. 2005; 11(3): 261-262.

20. Hill JM, Zalos G, Halcox JP, Schenke WH, Waclawiw MA, Quyyumi AA, Finkel T. Circulating endothelial progenitor cells, vascular function, and cardiovascular risk. N.Engl.J.Med. 2003; 348(7): 593-600.

21. Steurer M, Kern J, Zitt M, Amberger A, Bauer M, Gastl G, Untergasser G, Gunsilius E. Quantification of circulating endothelial and progenitor cells: comparison of quantitative PCR and four-channel flow cytometry. BMC Res.Notes 2008; 1; 71.

22. Case J, Mead LE, Bessler WK, Prater D, White HA, Saadatzadeh MR, Bhavsar JR, Yoder MC, Haneline LS, Ingram DA. Human CD34+AC133+VEGFR-2+ cells are not endothelial progenitor cells but distinct, primitive hematopoietic progenitors. Exp.Hematol. 2007; 35(7): 1109-1118.

23. Singh SK, Clarke ID, Terasaki M, Bonn VE, Hawkins C, Squire J, Dirks PB. Identification of a cancer stem cell in human brain tumors. Cancer Res. 2003; 63(18): 5821-5828.

24. Strijbos MH, Gratama JW, Kraan J, Lamers CH, den Bakker MA, Sleijfer S. Circulating endothelial cells in oncology: pitfalls and promises. Br.J.Cancer 2008; 98(11): 1731-1735.

25. Blann AD, Woywodt A, Bertolini F, Bull TM, Buyon JP, Clancy RM, Haubitz M, Hebbel RP, Lip GY, Mancuso P, Sampol J, Solovey A, Dignat-George F. Circulating endothelial cells. Biomarker of vascular disease. Thromb.Haemost. 2005; 93(2): 228-235.

26. Duda DG, Cohen KS, di Tomaso E, Au P, Klein RJ, Scadden DT, Willett CG, Jain RK. Differential CD146 expression on circulating versus tissue endothelial cells in rectal cancer patients: implications for circulating endothelial and progenitor cells as biomarkers for antiangiogenic therapy. J.Clin.Oncol. 2006; 24(9): 1449-1453.

27. Carson SD, Hobbs JT, Tracy SM, Chapman NM. Expression of the coxsackievirus and adenovirus receptor in cultured human umbilical vein endothelial cells: regulation in response to cell density. J.Virol. 1999; 73(8): 7077-7079.

28. Shirakawa T. The current status of adenovirus-based cancer gene therapy. Mol.Cells 2008; 25(4): 462-466.

29. Follenzi A, Santambrogio L, Annoni A. Immune responses to lentiviral vectors. Curr.Gene Ther. 2007; 7(5): 306-315.

30. Connolly JB. Lentiviruses in gene therapy clinical research. Gene Ther. 2002; 9(24): 1730-1734.

31. Liu G, Aronovich EL, Cui Z, Whitley CB, Hackett PB. Excision of Sleeping Beauty transposons: parameters and applications to gene therapy. J.Gene Med. 2004; 6(5): 574-583.

32. Tolar J, Osborn M, Bell S, McElmurry R, Xia L, Riddle M, Panoskaltsis-Mortari A, Jiang Y, McIvor RS, Contag CH, Yant SR, Kay MA, Verfaillie CM, Blazar BR. Real-time in vivo imaging of stem cells following transgenesis by transposition. Mol.Ther. 2005; 12(1): 42-48.

33. Liu G, Geurts AM, Yae K, Srinivasan AR, Fahrenkrug SC, Largaespada DA, Takeda J, Horie K, Olson WK, Hackett PB. Target-site preferences of Sleeping Beauty transposons. J.Mol.Biol. 2005; 346(1): 161-173.

34. Yant SR, Wu X, Huang Y, Garrison B, Burgess SM, Kay MA. High-resolution genome-wide mapping of transposon integration in mammals. Mol.Cell Biol. 2005; 25(6): 2085-2094.

35. Williams DA. Sleeping beauty vector system moves toward human trials in the United States. Mol.Ther. 2008; 16(9): 1515-1516.

36. Stockhammer G, Brotchi J, Leblanc R, Bernstein M, Schackert G, Weber F, Ostertag C, Mulder NH, Mellstedt H, Seiler R, Yonekawa Y, Twerdy K, Kostron H, De Witte O, Lambermont M, Velu T, Laneuville P, Villemure JG, Rutka JT, Warnke P, Laseur M, Mooij JJ, Boethius J, Mariani L, Gianella-Borradori A. Gene therapy for glioblastoma correction of gliobestome. multiform: in vivo tumor

37. transduction with the herpes simplex thymidine kinase gene followed by ganciclovir. J.Mol.Med. 1997; 75(4): 300-304.

37. DiMeco F, Rhines LD, Hanes J, Tyler BM, Brat D, Torchiana E, Guarnieri M, Colombo MP, Pardoll DM, Finocchiaro G, Brem H, Olivi A. Paracrine delivery of IL-12 against intracranial 9L gliosarcoma in rats. J.Neurosurg. 2000; 92(3): 419-427.

38. Faber C, Terao E, Morga E, Heuschling P. Interleukin-4 enhances the in vitro precursor cell recruitment for tumor-specific T lymphocytes in patients with glioblastoma. J.Immunother. 2000; 23(1): 11-16.

39. Wei YQ, Wang QR, Zhao X, Yang L, Tian L, Lu Y, Kang B, Lu CJ, Huang MJ, Lou YY, Xiao F, He QM, Shu JM, Xie XJ, Mao YQ, Lei S, Luo F, Zhou LQ, Liu CE, Zhou H, Jiang Y, Peng F, Yuan LP, Li Q, Wu Y, Liu JY. Immunotherapy of tumors with xenogeneic endothelial cells as a vaccine. Nat.Med. 2000; 6(10): 1160-1166.

40. Moore XL, Lu J, Sun L, Zhu CJ, Tan P, Wong MC. Endothelial progenitor cells' "homing" specificity to brain tumors. Gene Ther. 2004; 11(10): 811-818.

41. Wei J, Blum S, Unger M, Jarmy G, Lamparter M, Geishauser A, Vlastos GA, Chan G, Fischer KD, Rattat D, Debatin KM, Hatzopoulos AK, Beltinger C. Embryonic endothelial progenitor cells armed with a suicide gene target hypoxic lung metastases after intravenous delivery. Cancer Cell 2004; 5(5): 477-488.

42. Wei J, Wahl J, Nakamura T, Stiller D, Mertens T, Debatin KM, Beltinger C. Targeted release of oncolytic measles virus by blood outgrowth endothelial cells in situ inhibits orthotopic gliomas. Gene Ther. 2007; 14(22): 1573-1586.

43. O'Reilly MS, Boehm T, Shing Y, Fukai N, Vasios G, Lane WS, Flynn E, Birkhead JR, Olsen BR, Folkman J. Endostatin: an endogenous inhibitor of angiogenesis and tumor growth. Cell 1997; 88(2): 277-285.

44. Dudek AZ, Bodempudi V, Welsh BW, Jasinski P, Griffin RJ, Milbauer L, Hebbel RP. Systemic inhibition of tumour angiogenesis by endothelial cell-based gene therapy. Br.J.Cancer 2007; 97(4): 513-522.

45. Asahara T, Masuda H, Takahashi T, Kalka C, Pastore C, Silver M, Kearne M, Magner M, Isner JM. Bone marrow origin of endothelial progenitor cells responsible for postnatal vasculogenesis in physiological and pathological neovascularization. Circ.Res. 1999; 85(3): 221-228.

46. Lyden D, Hattori K, Dias S, Costa C, Blaikie P, Butros L, Chadburn A, Heissig B, Marks W, Witte L, Wu Y, Hicklin D, Zhu Z, Hackett NR, Crystal RG, Moore MA, Hajjar KA, Manova K, Benezra R, Rafii S. Impaired recruitment of bone-marrow-derived endothelial and hematopoietic precursor cells blocks tumor angiogenesis and growth. Nat.Med. 2001; 7(11): 1194-1201.

47. Dimmeler S, Burchfield J, Zeiher AM. Cell-based therapy of myocardial infarction. Arterioscler.Thromb.Vasc.Biol. 2008; 28(2): 208-216.

48.   Reinisch A, Hofmann NA, Obenauf AC, Kashofer K, Rohde E, Schallmoser K, Thaler D, Fruehwirth M, Linkesch W, Speicher MR, Strunk D. Making Functional Endothelial Progenitors: Humanized Large-Scale Animal Serum-Free Propagated Adult Blood-Derived Endothelial Colony-Forming Cells Assemble Stable Perfused Vessels in Vivo. Blood 2008, 112(11), Abstr. 1882.

Tumor Vascular Disrupting Agents

Gillan Tozer and Chyso Kanthou

Tumor Microcirculation Group, Section of Oncology, School of Medicine & Biomedical Sciences, University of Sheffield, Beech Hill Road, Sheffield S10 2RX, UK

Address correspondence to: Professor Gillian Tozer, Tumor Microcirculation Group, Section of Oncology, School of Medicine & Biomedical Sciences, University of Sheffield, Beech Hill Road, Sheffield. S10 2RX, UK Tel: +44 114 2712423; Fax: +44 114 2713314; Email: g.tozer@sheffield.ac.uk

Abstract: Tumor vascular disrupting agents (VDAs) are characterized by their ability to produce a very rapid and selective shut-down of tumor blood flow sufficient to induce extensive secondary tumor cell death. This effect is brought about by efficacy against established tumor blood vessels, making their mode of action conceptually distinct from that of the anti-angiogenic agents. Three main groups of VDAs are currently in clinical trial, consisting of DMXAA (5, 6-dimethylxanthenone-4-acetic acid), tubulin binding agents including the combretastatins and junctional protein inhibitors. These agents have different primary targets but produce similar morphological and functional effects on the tumor vasculature. The signaling pathways that mediate these effects are only partially understood but, in the case of disodium combretastatin A-4 3-0-phosphate (CA-4-P), undoubtedly involve activation of the small GTP-ase Rho and Rho kinase. Innate and induced resistance mechanisms need to be investigated in order to provide new targets for improving the efficacy of VDAs, especially in combination with conventional cancer treatments. Here, we review the developmental status of, and mechanisms of action and resistance to, currently available VDAs.

1. INTRODUCTION

Tumor vascular disrupting agents or VDAs are designed to target *established* tumor blood vessels, with the aim of shutting down tumor blood flow and inducing extensive secondary tumor cell death. This approach is conceptually distinct from anti-angiogenic therapy, which aims to prevent the development of neovasculature, although individual agents may possess both vascular disrupting and anti-angiogenic properties. Distinct molecular signatures associated with the tumor vasculature are being developed as therapeutic targets for tumor vascular disruption [1, 2]. In addition, several classes of low molecular weight drugs have been found to possess innate tumor vascular disrupting properties and a number of these are now in clinical trial. Deciphering the mechanisms of action and bases for treatment resistance of these agents should provide novel pathways for further drug development in this area.

2. DMXAA

DMXAA (5, 6-dimethylxanthenone-4-acetic acid) is a derivative of flavone-8-acetic acid that causes rapid vascular shut-down in a range of pre-clinical tumor models. DMXAA entered Phase I clinical trial via the

Cancer Research Campaign, now Cancer Research UK, in 1995 [3], and is the most advanced of the VDAs in clinical development. It is being further developed, as ASA404, by Novartis, under license from Antisoma plc (UK). Following a successful randomized Phase II clinical trial of ASA404 in combination with carboplatin and paclitaxel for advanced previously untreated non-small cell lung cancer, this compound is now in Phase III trial for this condition. Results of the Phase II trial showed an increase in patient survival from 8.8 months, for chemotherapy alone, to 14.0 months, with the addition of DMXAA [4]. Clinical evaluation in other tumor types is also on-going (http: //www.novartisoncology. com/).

3. COMBRETASTATINS AND OTHER TUBULIN-BINDING AGENTS

Microtubule-depolymerising tubulin-binding agents are by far the largest group of VDAs in clinical development (Table **1**).

The potent anti-cancer agents, vincristine and vinblastine, have tumor vascular disrupting effects in animal tumors but at doses higher than clinically achievable [5, 6]. The combretastatins bind β-tubulin at a different site from vincristine/vinblastine and have

Table 1. Tubulin binding VDAs in clinical trial.

Drug	Web-site	Drug type
Zybrestat™	http://www.oxigene.com/	CA-4-P, a combretastatin prodrug
OXI4503	http://www.oxigene.com/	CA-1-P, a combretastatin prodrug
ZD6126	http://www.astrazeneca.com/	colchicine analogue prodrug
AVE8062	http://www.sanofi-aventis.com/	synthetic combretastatin prodrug
ABT-751	http://www.abbott.com/	sulfonamide β-tubulin inhibitor
TZT-1027 (soblidotin)	http://www.aska-pharma.co.jp/	Synthetic derivative of dolastatin-10, a marine organism
Trisenox™	http://www.trisenox.com/	arsenic trioxide
NPI-2358	http://www.nereuspharm.com/	extract from marine fungus
MPC-6827 (Azixa™)	http://www.myriad.com/	4-arylaminoquinazoline β-tubulin inhibitor
CYT997	http://www.cytopia.com.au/	Orally active α-tubulin inhibitor
BCN105	http://www.bionomics.com.au/	Synthetic tubulin binding agent

structural similarity to the classic tubulin-binding agent, colchicine, which itself disrupts tumor blood vessels but is too toxic for clinical use, probably because of its pseudo-irreversible binding to tubulin [5, 7]. The combretastatins were originally isolated from the Cape Bushwillow tree, *Combretum caffrum* [8]. The lead compound is CA-4-P (disodium combretastatin A-4 3-*0*-phosphate), which is a stable pro-drug for the active compound, CA-4 [9]. Based on pre-clinical data demonstrating selective tumor blood flow shut-down (Fig. **1** [10-12], CA-4-P entered clinical trial in the UK and USA in 1998 and is now being developed as CA4 Prodrug/fosbretabulin/ Zybrestat™ by OXiGENE Inc. (http://www.oxigene.com/).

A Phase II/III trial of CA-4-P, in combination with chemotherapy, for anaplastic thyroid cancer is on-going. Phase II trials are also running for CA-4-P, in gynaecological tumor s and non-squamous cell non-small cell lung cancer. The latter trial includes the anti-angiogenic agent, bevacizumab (Avastin™), in the standard chemotherapy arm. Interestingly, a Phase I clinical study, in advanced solid tumor s, showed that addition of bevacizumab helped sustain the vascular shut-down observed for CA-4-P alone [13]. A sodium phosphate pro-drug of combretastatin A-1, CA-1-P

[14] (OXiGENE compound OXI4503) [15-18], is also in Phase I clinical trial. This compound was more potent than CA-4-P, in pre-clinical studies. In addition, there are numerous synthetic analogues of the combretastatins. For example, the Sanofi-Aventis compound AVE8062, licensed from Ajinomoto Co., Inc., is a pro-drug for a combretastatin derivative, which is cleaved by aminopeptidases, to form the active drug [19-22]. AVE8062 is in Phase III clinical trial for sarcoma and non-small cell lung cancer (http://en.sanofi-aventis.com/Aventis).

Apart from the combretastatins, other tubulin binding agents have potential as VDAs. A pro-drug analogue of colchicine, N-acetylcolchinol-O-phosphate (ZD6126), has reached Phase II clinical trials [23] (http://www.angiogene.co.uk/) and other agents are at earlier stages of development (Table **1**).

4. JUNCTIONAL PROTEIN INHIBITORS

Monoclonal antibodies targeted to the vascular cell-cell junction-associated protein, VE-cadherin, are active against the established tumor vasculature [24]. N-cadherin is also involved with the structural integrity of blood vessels and its down-regulation

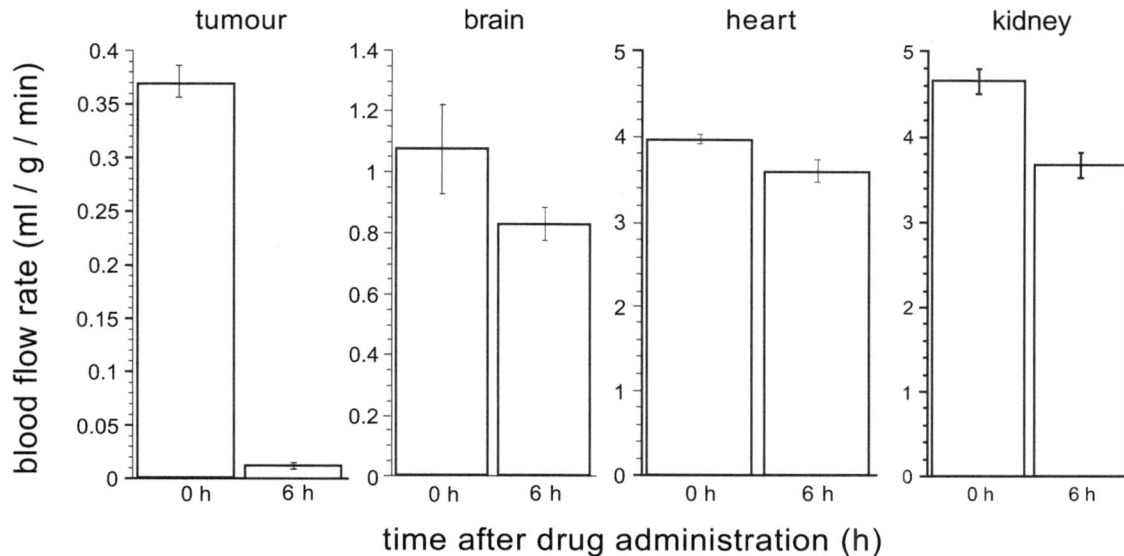

Fig. (1). Blood flow rate in the P22 rat sarcoma versus normal tissues of the BDIX rat in control (0h) and CA-4-P (30 mg/kg) treated (6h) rats. Blood flow rate was estimated from tissue uptake of intravenously administered, radiolabelled iodo-antipyrine.

prevents cell aggregation and induces apoptosis [25]. The peptide N-cadherin inhibitor, ADH-1, developed by Adherex, entered clinical trial in 2006 and is now in Phase II development, with evidence of haemorrhage in treated tumors (http://www.adherex.com/). Low molecular weight antagonists are currently under development.

5. CELLULAR EVENTS

The hall-mark of VDAs is their very rapid effects on tumor blood vessels. For instance, CA-4-P and DMXAA cause a significant decrease in tumor blood flow within minutes of drug exposure, with maximum effects between 1 and 6 hours [26, 27]. For CA-4-P, these rapid effects are paralleled *in vitro*, by re-modeling of the endothelial cytoskeleton, triggered by disruption of interphase microtubules [28]. Endothelial cells are particularly sensitive to CA-4-P and similar compounds. Effects predominantly consist of increased development of actin stress fibers, actinomyosin contractility, rounding up of cells, formation of focal adhesions, disruption of cell-cell junctions involving both VE- and N-cadherin, and increase in monolayer permeability [28, 29]. Additionally, in a sub-population of cells, F-actin accumulates around the surface of severely contracted cells in the form of surface blebs. Signalling pathways associated with these changes involve the small GTP-ase, RhoA, and Rho kinase and stress-activated protein kinase-2/p38 (SAPK/p38) [28, 30]. We have recently confirmed the importance of Rho kinase *in vivo* by

using a small molecule inhibitor, which blocked CA-4-P-induced necrosis in a colorectal xenografted tumor model (unpublished data).

The primary target of DMXAA is unknown. Cytoskeletal effects in endothelial cells are confined to the actin skeleton, involving partial dissolution of actin filaments [31]. Unlike CA-4-P, DMXAA causes significant intratumoral increases in the activity of tumor necrosis factor alpha (TNF) [32]. However, the time-course of blood flow shut-down in animal models was not consistent with TNF induction, leading to the concept that DMXAA causes its vascular effects by both indirect action via induced cytokines and direct action on tumor endothelial cells. This theory was substantiated on discovering that tumor vascular damage was attenuated but not blocked, in tumors growing in TNF receptor-1-deficient mice, following DMXAA treatment [33]. *In vitro* studies have strongly suggested that DMXAA induces TNF in conjunction with a co-stimulator [34]. TNF acts as a vascular disrupting agent in its own right [35], and modifies the actin cytoskeleton and permeability through the Rho/Rac pathway [36]. DMXAA directly stimulates various signaling pathways *in vitro*, including the SAPK/p38 pathway, inhibition of which prevents some of the *in vitro* effects of the drug [37]. In addition, DMXAA has been shown to directly stimulate mouse dendritic cells *in vitro*, with subsequent proinflammatory cytokine release [38]. Dendritic cells, especially tumor-associated macrophages, are a likely important source of increased levels of TNF and nitric oxide (NO) in treated tumors. In the same study, administration of DMXAA to tumor-bearing mice, led to stimulation of dendritic cells in tumor-draining lymph nodes by 24h after treatment and a subsequent increase in numbers of CD8+ T cells in the animals' spleens, which correlated with tumor response. Stimulation of the specific activator of the TANK-binding kinase 1 (TBK1)-interferon (IFN) regulatory factor 3 (IRF-3) signaling pathway, in murine macrophages, has also been observed *in vitro*, implicating interferon in DMXAA's mechanism of action [39, 40]. Although not able to account for the early tumor vascular effects of DMXAA, these studies illustrate the complex series of events that dictates ultimate tumor response to VDAs. The interesting finding that non-steroidal anti-inflammatory drugs, such as diclofenac and salicylate, significantly increased the tumor growth retarding effects of DMXAA *in vivo* may relate to the finding that DMXAA-induced IFN-beta expression in macrophages was inhibited by salicylate [41]. This implies a protective role for activated macrophages in treated tumors, which requires further investigation and may relate to important pro-angiogenic roles of this cell type in the tumor microenvironment [42].

6. IN VIVO MECHANISMS: VASCULAR SHUT-DOWN

The rapid vascular shut-down elicited by VDAs is most likely attributed to direct effects on various vascular components. A rapid increase in tumor vascular permeability has been reported in animal models following administration of both CA-4-P [43] and DMXAA [44], which is consistent with *in vitro* effects on the endothelial actin cytoskeleton and junctional proteins [28]. VE-cadherin antagonists, when combined with CA-4-P *in vivo*, also synergised in disrupting tumor blood vessels [29]. An increase in vascular permeability to macromolecules may increase viscous resistance to flow in tumor blood vessels, as proteins leak into the interstitium. Geometric resistance to blood flow also may increase, as a result of associated endothelial cell changes. Tumor supplying arterioles constrict in response to CA-4-P and AVE8062 [45], with a consequent decrease in flow, most likely as a direct contraction of vascular smooth muscle cells in response to Rho kinase activation, mediated by phosphorylation of myosin light chain, as observed for CA-4-P in endothelial cells [28]. Tumor intersitial fluid pressure decreases following CA-4-P or ZD6126 administration [46, 47] and this may reflect a decrease in intra-vascular pressure down-stream from the constricted arterioles. A temporary imbalance between IFP and intravascular pressure could contribute to collapse of sinusoidal tumor blood vessels. As blood flow falls below a critical level, red cells stack to form rouleaux, thus increasing blood stagnation, as observed by intravital microscopy of tumors following CA-4-P treatment

[26]. Sustained vascular damage leads to hemorrhage and coagulation, within the first few hours of drug exposure [48]. That coagulation is not a triggering event for blood flow shut-down was shown for AVE8062, where anti-coagulants had no effect on the initial tumor vascular response to the drug [49]. Activation of platelets causes the release of serotonin, which can be detected indirectly via its principal hepatic metabolite, 5-HIAA (5-hydroxyindole acetic acid). Increases in plasma 5-HIAA concentrations have been observed following DMXAA, colchicine and vinblastine treatment [50], as well as with CA-4-P (Baguley, personal communication). In addition to coagulation, platelets may contribute to blood flow shut-down via effects of serotonin, which acts on G-protein coupled receptors to induce actin stress fibre formation [51] and reduce tumor blood flow [52].

Tumor infiltration by immune effector cells, such as neutrophils and macrophages occurs within hours of VDA exposure [53] (and unpublished results). Production of damaging reactive oxygen species by neutrophils, following interaction with vascular endothelial cells, may contribute to VDA-induced vascular damage and it has been suggested that both DMXAA [38] and CA-4-P [54] enhance the immune response to implanted tumor s. However, pro-angiogenic tumor -associated macrophages may also contribute to tumor re-vascularization after VDA treatment and so the net effect of immune effector cells on treatment outcome remains to be resolved.

VDAs can affect endothelial cell proliferation and migration and are cytotoxic to endothelial cells *in vitro*. Therefore, if drug exposures *in vivo* are sufficient, they can be anti-angiogenic as well as vascular disrupting and endothelial cell death can contribute to vascular damage, although it is not a pre-requisite, as often assumed. It is also worth noting that tumor cells are variably sensitive to the cytotoxic effects of CA-4-P, so that direct tumor cell killing may contribute to treatment outcome under some circumstances. Endothelial cell death can occur via various mechanisms. For CA-4-P, extensive damage to interphase microtubules can lead to a relatively early cell death, where the blebbing morphology described above is an early manifestation [28]. Using electron microscopy, a recent study demonstrated endothelial cell blebbing in tumor microvessels *in vivo* [55]. Disruption of VE-cadherin-associated cell-cell junctions is also associated with a cell death pathway mediated by inhibition of PI3K/Akt signaling [29]. In proliferating endothelial cells, CA-4-P induces an apoptosis-like cell death resulting from damage to mitotic spindles, which are at least as sensitive to the drug as interphase microtubules [56]. This type of cell death is associated with accumulation of cells at G2/M in the cell cycle and thus requires prolonged drug exposures for effects to be manifested. It is therefore not a factor in the initial CA-4-P-induced vascular shut-down, although it may contribute to its extent. In contrast, apoptosis is manifested earlier for DMXAA; a 10-fold increase in TUNEL staining of endothelial cells within solid tumors in mice was reported within 30 minutes of DMXAA administration [57]. Additionally, CA-1-P (Oxi4503), was found to induce endothelial apoptosis by 1 hour after treatment, in a hemangioendothelioma model [58]. This may relate to the formation of reactive quinone intermediates on CA-1-P metabolism [59] and a reactive metabolite detected following *in vivo* administration of CA-1-P but not CA-4-P [60].

7. INNATE RESISTANCE

The susceptibility of most solid tumor s to vascular disrupting therapy is most likely linked to well-known characteristics of the tumor microcirculation, which distinguish it from normal tissues. Tumors commonly present with regions of hypoxia and necrosis, which suggests that their blood supply is barely adequate to support tumor growth. Indeed, blood flow is spatially and temporally heterogeneous, arising from disorganized vascular architecture and stresses from the expanding tissue surrounding it. Poorly flowing vessels are likely to require less intervention to induce shut-down than more efficient vessels. Morphologically too, tumor blood vessels are abnormal. They often appear sinusoidal, with very thin vascular walls comprised of irregularly shaped endothelial cells, poor cell-cell contact, abnormal

basement membrane and variable distribution of pericytes, which often make poor contact with endothelial cells. These characteristics contribute to high vascular permeability to macromolecules and high interstitial fluid pressure, which may in turn contribute to tumor susceptibility to VDAs.

Although most solid tumor s do respond to VDAs, the extent of response, in pre-clinical models, is variable and the reasons for some tumor s displaying innate resistance is not entirely clear. Responses have been documented in carcinomas and sarcomas, tumor s transplanted in both sub-cutaneous and orthotopic sites, spontaneous primary tumor s and metastases [12, 61-64]. Knowledge of the factors that dictate innate resistance or susceptibility will enable appropriate selection of patients for VDA treatment and provide avenues for further research into methods of targeting the established tumor vasculature. Resistance may occur at the tissue or cellular level and putative factors dictating resistance are shown in Table **2**.

There is evidence that vascular response to CA-4-P positively correlates with tumor vascular permeability to macromolecules [65] and this may relate to level of interstitial fluid pressure. However, the relationship between vascular permeability and IFP is not straightforward and another study has reported that the amount of tumor cell kill obtained with ZD6126 is negatively correlated with pre-treatment IFP [46]. The reasons for this association are unclear but may relate to pharmacokinetics, with poor drug access in tumor s

Table 2. Putative factors dictating tumor susceptibility to VDAs and their potential effects. *relevant for cell death pathway associated with mitosis; **relevant for tubulin bindng agents only.

Factor	Effect
High proliferation rate of endothelial cells*	Sensitizes to cell killing effects
Unique endothelial expression of tubulin sub-types, mutations, post-translational changes or microtubule-associated proteins**	May influence microtubule disruption
Defective cell-cell junctions	Sensitizes to further disruption
Hypoxia, hypoxia-reoxygenation, hypoglycaemia	Influences signalling events
Regional blood flow instabilities	Sensitizes to further disruption
High vascular permeability ± high interstitial fluid pressure	Increases viscous flow resistance / vascular shut-down in response to arteriolar constriction
Poor pericyte function	Reduces blood vessel stability following endothelial damage
Self-trapping of VDA	Increases drug exposure

with high IFP [46]. We have recently shown that a splice variant of VEGF-A, VEGF188, in a mouse model, is uniquely associated with pericyte recruitment to tumor blood vessels [66]. Tumor s that expressed only this single isoform of VEGF-A were resistant to CA-4-P treatment, suggesting that pericyte support of tumor blood vessels is an important cause of tumor resistance to VDAs.

At the cellular level, theories for explaining innate differences in resistance to the combretastatins have centred around differences between endothelial cell proliferation rates, tubulin isotypes and post-translational modifications (Table **2**). However, these theories remain to be investigated and are not relevant for other VDAs such as DMXAA.

Tumor response to all current VDAs is characterized by resistance of the tumor rim. This intra-tumor variation in innate resistance is treatment limiting and warrants separate consideration.

8. RESISTANCE OF THE TUMOR RIM

A single, well-tolerated dose of a VDA can kill over 90% of tumor cells, in animal models. However, tumor cells repopulate from a peripheral rim of surviving cells and these have proved exceptionally difficult to eradicate, to the extent that none of the current VDAs are curative as single agents, even in repeated dosing schedules. Both animal and human studies have shown that the vascular effects of CA-4-P are more profound at the tumor centre than at the periphery (Fig. **2**) [67]. Intravital microscopy showed sustained, albeit sluggish blood flow at the periphery of tumor s following CA-4-P treatment, at times when blood was completely static or blood vessels had

collapsed in the centre [26]. The basis for this regional difference in response is unclear. The vascular bed of tumor s is typically rarefied towards the centre, with smaller vessels, at a lower density, than at the periphery. These vessels may be innately sensitive to VDAs or the vascular reserve at the periphery may provide alternative pathways to blood flow, even when some of the vessels are shut-down. IFP is also typically low in the peripheral rim of tumor s, rising steeply towards the centre [68] and this may provide some protection against vascular shut-down at the periphery.

Despite resistance of the tumor rim to VDAs, their combined use with certain conventional and novel treatment approaches is showing promise, with spatial co-operation of the combined treatments likely to be an important contributory factor. Other reasons for success of combined treatments include additive effects of independent targets, independent toxicities and potentiating effects. Clearly, the primary target of VDAs is different from that of conventional cytotoxics and so it is hoped that VDAs will be effective against some tumor cells that survive conventional treatment alone. Conventional chemotherapy and radiotherapy are more effective against highly proliferative and well-oxygenated tumor cells, which often reside at the tumor periphery, therefore providing some degree of spatial co-operation. In addition, blood flow is often more efficient at the tumor periphery than the centre, providing better tumor cell exposure to blood-borne agents in this region.

A clear rationale for combining VDAs with conventional treatment has been substantiated in results obtained from pre-clinical studies. Good tumor responses have been reported for combination with

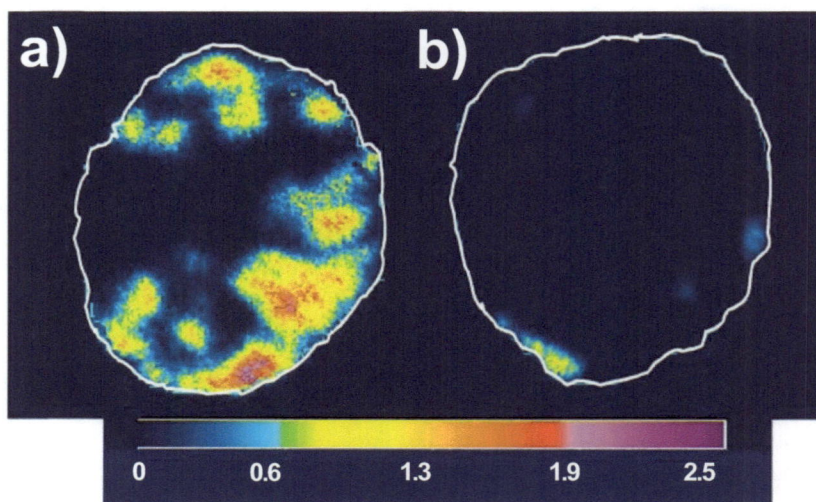

Fig. (2). Pseudo-colour images of distribution of blood flow rate in the P22 rat sarcoma following no treatment (a) and at 24h after CA-4-P (100 mg/kg) (b). Blood flow rate was estimated from tumor uptake of intravenously administered radiolabelled iodo-antipyrine. Autoradiography was used for measuring tissue dstribution of radioactivity. Note minimal blood flow in the majority of the tumor in (b) but resistance of the tumor rim.

radiotherapy and cytotoxic drugs, most notably platinum drugs and taxanes [69, 70] and there is some evidence that this can be achieved without any increase in toxicity [71]. Optimum scheduling is a complex issue for addition of VDAs to conventional treatments. It has generally been found that VDAs are best scheduled *after* a dose of radiation, in order to avoid VDA-induced tumor hypoxia affecting sensitivity of tumor cells to subsequent radiation doses. A recent study also showed that AVE8062 (AC7700) was best, scheduled 48h rather than 2h, after a single 5Gy dose of radiation [72]. This was attributed to the VDA preventing the growth-promoting increase in tumor blood flow that is often seen following radiation treatment. It is also inadvisable to schedule chemotherapeutic drugs within hour's post-VDA treatment, when blood flow is reduced and tumor regions are inaccessible to blood-borne drugs. One study showed that the effects of ZD6126 were compromised if given within a day after administration of the microtubule-stabilizing drug, paclitaxel [73]. However, it may be possible to harness VDA-induced blood flow shut-down following chemotherapy, so that chemotherapeutic drugs are 'trapped' in tumor tissue. Self-trapping of the VDA in tumor tissue has also been reported [12] and this phenomenon would add to the intrinsic tumor sensitivity to these agents. Drug trapping could play an important role in some of the reported benefits of combined treatments but it is not the only factor, as illustrated in one study, where 5-fluorouracil (5-FU) was combined with CA-4-P, with a beneficial effect on tumor growth, in the absence of any corresponding increases in tumor levels of 5-FU [74]. In radiotherapy, tumor blood vessels are prone to damage and these radiation-damaged vessels may be particularly sensitive to VDA treatment, accounting for some of the benefit of the combined approach. There is some evidence that CA-4-P and ZD6126 have a particular impact on the hypoxic tumor cell population but the mechanisms behind this effect need further investigation [75]. Recently, the clinical combination of radiotherapy and CA-4-P, in a palliative setting, has shown some benefit, in terms of vascular effects, as estimated by contrast-enhanced dynamic CT [76].

Novel biological anti-cancer agents may provide significant spatial co-operation with VDAs, by targeting the VDA-resistant tumor rim. For instance, antibodies targeted to epitopes on the surface of tumor cells are often seen to accumulate around the tumor periphery, with poor tumor penetration. This is likely to result from both poor delivery (blood flow) and poor extravasation (convective transport) at the tumor centre. In animal models, good therapeutic outcomes have been reported for the combination of radioimmunotherapy with both DMXAA and CA-4-P [64, 77].

Novel drug delivery systems may also impact on the resistant tumor rim. Liposome-based nano-particles tend to accumulate at the tumor rim for the same reasons as antibodies. One study described the development of nano-particles, with CA-4 incorporated into the pegylated lipid envelope and doxorubicin in the core [78]. This was designed to ensure preferential release of doxorubicin only after trapping of the nano-particles in tumor tissue following CA-4-induced vascular shut-down. Liposome encapsulation of ZD6126, with or without integrin targeting was also found to be beneficial. This was most likely due to an increased plasma half-life and altered tissue distribution of the drug and its active metabolite, with no influence of the targeting moiety [79]. Encapsulation of CA-4 in integrin-targeted liposomes, for targeting irradiated blood vessels, has also been tested [80]. This method has potential for improving the combination of VDAs and radiotherapy.

9. INDUCED RESISTANCE

VDA treatment induces tumor blood flow reduction and subsequent hypoxia [81], which may be accompanied by re-oxygenation. Hypoxia and reactive oxygen species are well-known stimuli for pro-angiogenic gene expression and it follows that rapid renewal of tumor angiogenesis following VDA treatment is likely to be a major source of induced treatment resistance. Increased expression of both VEGF and/or bFGF has been reported in xenografted tumor s following CA-4-P and CA-1-P administration [58, 82]. The expression of hypoxia-inducible factor-1 (HIF-1) was also found to increase in endothelial cells treated with CA-4-P, even under aerobic conditions [83]. In addition, the number of circulating endothelial progenitor cells in mice was found to increase following treatment with both these agents, which contributed to tumor re-vascularization [84]. Infiltration of VDA-treated tumor s by bone-marrow-derived immature monocytes, which can differentiate into mature F4/80+ tumor -associated macrophages, may also influence tumor re-vascularisation via production of pro-angiogenic cytokines, growth factors and proteases [42] and contribute to resistance. These considerations are consistent with good therapeutic results in animal models for combination of VDAs with anti-angiogenic agents, such as the VEGF receptor tyrosine kinase inhibitor, ZD6474 [85], bevacizumab [86] and nitric oxide inhibitors [12]. Another possibility is the combination of VDAs with hypoxia-targeted approaches such as the use of bioreductive cytotoxic drugs that are activated under hypoxic conditions [52, 87].

The cellular components of blood vessels are less susceptible than tumor cells to the mutations that give rise to drug resistance. However, VDAs may indirectly influence resistance of tumor cells to associated chemotherapy via their effects on tumor oxygenation and nutrient supply. For instance, CA-4-P increased the tumor cell expression of glucose-regulated protein, GRP78, in an animal model [88]. GRP78 is an endoplastic reticulum associated chaperone molecule associated with drug resistance that is up-regulated by severe glucose depletion, anoxia and acidosis.

10. TOXICITY

Using contrast-enhanced magnetic resonance imaging, Several Phase I/II clinical trials of DMXAA and CA-4-P demonstrated reduced tumor perfusion, within short times of drug administration, confirming pre-clinical results [67, 89]. As expected, toxicity was different from that experienced by patients undergoing conventional chemotherapy. The most common adverse events for DMXAA included reversible confusion, tremor, slurred speech and visual disturbance [3, 90]. Most common adverse events for CA-4-P were mild (Grade 1 or 2) nausea, vomiting, headache, fatigue and tumor pain. Dose-limiting toxicities included dyspnea, myocardial ischaemia and reversible motor neuropathy [91-93].

Cardiovascular side-effects of VDAs have been the main concern in clinical trials. For CA-4-P, hypertension preceded three cases of reversible myocardial effects, which contributed to establishing the maximum tolerated dose in man. Hypertension was also observed in rats [12], which most likely arises from widespread vasoconstriction in normal tissues. Administration of vasodilators with CA-4-P or ZD6126, in animal models, was found to alleviate cardiovascular effects, without affecting tumor vascular disruption [94, 95], suggesting that this may alleviate some of the clinical problems, along-side careful screening of potential patients for cardiovascular conditions.

11. CONCLUSIONS

DMXAA and CA-4-P are the lead compounds of a promising group of VDAs, which are conceptually distinct from the anti-angiogenic agents and should provide valuable augmentation of conventional cancer therapy. The vascular effects of VDAs are primarily characterized by a rapid and selective shut-down of tumor blood vessels. Further research is needed to determine the factors dictating susceptibility of blood vessels to VDAs and methods for overcoming induced resistance.

12. ACKNOWLEDGEMENTS

We would like to thank all our colleagues, past and present, at the Gray Cancer Institute, London, UK and University of Sheffield, Sheffield, UK, for their contribution to our research that forms part of this review. The authors' research was supported by a programme grant from Cancer Research UK. Professor Tozer is currently a member of an ASA404 Advisory Board for Novartis Oncology.

13. REFERENCES

1. Neri D, Bicknell R. Tumor vascular targeting. Nat Rev Cancer 2005; 5(6): 436-46.
2. Schliemann C, Neri D. Antibody-based targeting of the tumor vasculature. Biochim Biophys Acta 2007; 1776(2): 175-92.
3. Jameson MB, Thompson PI, Baguley BC, et al. Clinical aspects of a phase I trial of 5,6-dimethylxanthenone-4-acetic acid (DMXAA), a novel antivascular agent. Br J Cancer 2003; 88(12): 1844-50.
4. McKeage MJ, Von Pawel J, Reck M, et al. Randomised phase II study of ASA404 combined with carboplatin and paclitaxel in previously untreated advanced non-small cell lung cancer. Br J Cancer 2008; 99(12): 2006-12.
5. Baguley BC, Holdaway KM, Thomsen LL, et al. Inhibition of growth of colon 38 adenocarcinoma by vinblastine and colchicine: evidence for a vascular mechanism. Eur J Cancer 1991; 27: 482-487.
6. Hill SA, Lonergan SJ, Denekamp J, et al. Vinca alkaloids: anti-vascular effects in a murine tumor . Eur J Cancer 1993; 9: 1320-1324.
7. Lin CM, Ho HH, Pettit GR, et al. Antimitotic natural products combretastatin A-4 and combretastatin A-2: studies on the mechanism of their inhibition of the binding of colchicine to tubulin. Biochemistry 1989; 28: 6984-6991.
8. Pettit GR, Cragg GM, Singh SB. Antineoplastic agents, 122. Constituents of Combretum caffrum. J Nat Prod 1987; 50: 386-391.
9. Pettit GR, Temple C, Narayanan VL,et al. Antineoplastic agents 322. Synthesis of combretastatin A-4 prodrugs. Anticancer Drug Des. 1995; 10: 299-309.
10. Chaplin DJ, Pettit GR, Parkins CS, et al. Antivascular approaches to solid tumor therapy: evaluation of tubulin binding agents. Br. J. Cancer 1996; 74 (Suppl. XXVII): S86-S88.
11. Dark GD, Hill SA, Prise VE, et al. Combretastatin A-4, an agent that displays potent and selective toxicity toward tumor vasculature. Cancer Res. 1997; 57: 1829-1834.
12. Tozer GM, Prise VE, Wilson J, et al. Combretastatin A-4 phosphate as a tumor vascular-targeting agent: early effects in tumors and normal tissues. Cancer Res. 1999; 59: 1626-1634.
13. Nathan PD, Judson I, Padhani A, et al. A Phase I Study of the Safety, Tolerability and Antitumor Activity of Escalating Doses of Combretastatin A4 Phosphate (CA4P) Given in Combination with Bevacizumab to Subjects with Advanced Solid Tumors – Final results. J Clin Oncol 2008; 26(Suppl): 3550.
14. Pettit GR, Lippert III JW. Antineoplastic agents 429. Syntheses of the combretastatin A-1 and combretastatin B-1 prodrugs. Anticancer Drug Des 2000; 15: 203-216.

15. Holwell SE, Bibby MC. Activity of combretastatin A1 phosphate in murine models of liver metastasis. Br J Cancer 2001; 85 Supp 1-34.

16. Hill SA, Tozer GM, Chaplin DJ. Preclinical evaluation of the antitumor activity of the novel vascular targeting agent Oxi 4503. Anticancer Res 2002; 22: 1453-1458.

17. Holwell SE, Cooper PA, Grosios K, et al. Combretastatin A-1 phosphate a novel tubulin-binding agent with in vivo vascular effects in experimental tumor s. Anticancer Res 2002; 22: 707-711.

18. Hua J, Sheng Y, Pinney KG, et al. Oxi4503, a novel vascular targeting agent: effects on blood flow and antitumor activity in comparison to combretastatin A-4 phosphate. Anticancer Res 2003; 23(2B): 1433-1440.

19. Hori K, Saito S Nihei Y, et al. Antitumor effects due to irreversible stoppage of tumor tissue blood flow: evaluation of a novel combretastatin A-4 derivative, AC7700. Jpn J Cancer Res 1999; 90: 1026-1038.

20. Nihei Y, Suga Y, Morinaga Y. A novel combretastatin A-4 derivative, AC-7700, shows marked antitumor activity against advanced solid tumors and orthotopically transplanted tumors. Jpn J Cancer Res 1999; 90: 1016-1025.

21. Hori K, Saito S, Sato Y. Stoppage of blood flow in 3-methylcholanthrene-induced primary tumor due to a novel combretastatin A-4 derivative, AC7700, and its antitumor effect. Med Sci Monit 2001; 7: 26-33.

22. Hori K, Saito S, Kubota K. A novel combretastatin A-4 derivative, AC7700, strongly stanches tumor blood flow and inhibits growth of tumor s developing in various tissues and organs. Br J Cancer 2002; 86(10): 1604-1614.

23. Davis PD, Hill SA, Galbraith SM, et al. J. In ZD6126: a new agent causing selective damage of tumor vasculature, 91st Annual Meeting of the American Association for Cancer Research, San Francisco, 2000; p 329.

24. Corada M, Zanetta L, Orsenigo F, et al. A monoclonal antibody to vascular endothelial-cadherin inhibits tumor angiogenesis without side effects on endothelial permeability. Blood 2002; 100(3): 905-911.

25. Blaschuk OW, Rowlands TM. Cadherins as modulators of angiogenesis and the structural integrity of blood vessels. Cancer Metastasis Rev 2000; 19(1-2): 1-5.

26. Tozer GM, Prise VE, Wilson J, et al. Mechanisms associated with tumor vascular shut-down induced by combretastatin A-4 phosphate: intravital microscopy and measurement of vascular permeability. Cancer Res 2001; 61: 6413-6422.

27. Chen G, Horsman MR, Pedersen M, et al. The effect of combretastatin A4 disodium phosphate and 5,6-dimethylxanthenone-4-acetic acid on water diffusion and blood perfusion in tumor s. Acta Oncol 2008; 47(6): 1071-1076.

28. Kanthou C, Tozer GM. The tumor vascular targeting agent combretastatin A-4-phosphate induces reorganization of the actin cytoskeleton and early membrane blebbing in human endothelial cells. Blood 2002; 99: 2060-2069.

29. Vincent L, Kermani P, Young LM, et al. Combretastatin A4 phosphate induces rapid regression of tumor neovessels and growth through interference with vascular endothelial-cadherin signaling. J Clin Invest 2005; 115(11): 2992-3006.

30. Kanthou C, Tozer GM. Tumor targeting by microtubule-depolymerizing vascular disrupting agents. Exp Opin Ther Targets 2007; 11: 1443-1457.

31. Tozer GM, Kanthou C, Baguley BC. Disrupting tumor blood vessels. Nat Rev Cancer 2005; 5(6): 423-35.

32. Ching LM, Goldsmith D, Joseph WR, et al. Induction of intratumoral tumor necrosis factor (TNF) synthesis and hemorrhagic necrosis by 5,6-dimethylxanthenone-4-acetic acid (DMXAA) in TNF knockout mice. Cancer Res 1999: 59 (14): 3304-7.

33. Zhao L, Ching LM, Kestell P, et al. The antitumor activity of 5, 6-dimethylxanthenone-4-acetic acid (DMXAA) in TNF receptor-1 knockout mice. Br J Cancer 2002; 87(4): 465-470.

34. Wang LC, Reddy CB, Baguley BC, et al. Induction of tumor necrosis factor and interferon-gamma in cultured murine splenocytes by the antivascular agent DMXAA and its metabolites. Biochem Pharmacol 2004; 67(5)937-945.

35. Kallinowski F, Schaefer C, Tyler G, et al. In vivo targets of recombinant human tumor necrosis factor-α: blood flow, oxygen consumption and growth of isotransplanted rat tumor s. Br. J. Cancer 1989; 60: 555-560.

36. Wojciak-Stothard B, Ridley AJ. Rho GTPases and the regulation of endothelial permeability. Vascul Pharmacol 2002; 39(4-5): 187-199.

37. Zhao L, Marshall ES, Kelland LR, et al. Evidence for the involvement of p38 MAP kinase in the action of the vascular disrupting agent 5,6-dimethylxanthenone-4-acetic acid (DMXAA). Invest New Drugs 2007; 25(3): 271-276.

38. Wallace A, LaRosa DF, Kapoor V, et al. The vascular disrupting agent, DMXAA, directly activates dendritic cells through a MyD88-independent mechanism and generates antitumor cytotoxic T lymphocytes. Cancer Res 2007; 67(14): 7011-7019.

39. Roberts ZJ, Goutagny N, Perera PY, et al. The chemotherapeutic agent DMXAA potently and specifically activates the TBK1-IRF-3 signaling axis. J Exp Med 2007; 204(7): 1559-1569.

40. Roberts ZJ, Ching LM, Vogel SN. IFN-beta-dependent inhibition of tumor growth by the vascular disrupting agent 5,6-dimethylxanthenone-4-acetic acid (DMXAA). J Interferon Cytokine Res 2008; 28(3): 133-139.

41. Wang LC, Ching LM, Paxton J W, et al. Enhancement of the action of the antivascular drug 5,6-dimethylxanthenone-4-acetic acid (DMXAA; ASA404) by non-steroidal anti-inflammatory drugs. Invest New Drugs 2008.

42. Murdoch C, Muthana M, Coffelt SB, et al. The role of myeloid cells in the promotion of tumor angiogenesis. Nat Rev Cancer 2008; 8(8): 618-631.

43. Reyes-Aldasoro CC, Wilson I, Prise VE, et al. Estimation of Apparent Tumor Vascular Permeability from Multiphoton Fluorescence Microscopic Images of P22 Rat Sarcomas In Vivo. Microcirculation 2008; 15: 65-79.

44.   Chung F, Liu J, Ching LM, et al. Consequences of increased vascular permeability induced by treatment of mice with 5,6-dimethylxanthenone-4-acetic acid (DMXAA) and thalidomide. Cancer Chemother Pharmacol 2008; 61(3): 497-502.

45.   Hori K, Saito S. Microvascular mechanisms by which the combretastatin A-4 derivative AC7700 (AVE8062) induces tumor blood flow stasis. Br J Cancer 2003; 89(7): 1334-1344.

46.   Skliarenko JV, Lunt SJ, Gordon ML, et al. Effects of the vascular disrupting agent ZD6126 on interstitial fluid pressure and cell survival in tumors. Cancer Res 2006; 66(4): 2074-2080.

47.   Ley CD, Horsman MR, Kristjansen PE. Early effects of combretastatin-A4 disodium phosphate on tumor perfusion and interstitial fluid pressure. Neoplasia 2007; 9(2): 108-112.

48.   Prise VE, Honess DJ, Stratford MRL, et al. The vascular response of tumor and normal tissues in the rat to the vascular targeting agent, combretastatin A-4-phosphate, at clinically relevant doses. Int J Oncol 2002; 21: 717-726.

49.   Nihei Y, Suzuki M, Okano A, et al. Evaluation of antivascular and antimitotic effects of tubulin binding agents in solid tumor therapy. Jpn J Cancer Res 1999; 90: 1387-1396.

50.   Baguley BC, Zhuang L, Kestell, P. Increased plasma serotonin following treatment with flavone-8-acetic acid, 5,6-dimethylxanthenone-4-acetic acid, vinblastine, and colchicine: relation to vascular effects. Oncol Res 1997; 9(2): 55-60.

51.   Alexander JS, Hechtman HB, Shepro, D. Serotonin induced actin polymerization and association with cytoskeletal elements in cultured bovine aortic endothelium. Biochem Biophys Res Commun 1987; 143(1): 152-158.

52.   Lash CJ, Li AE, Rutland M, et al. Enhancement of the anti-tumor effects of the antivascular agent 5,6-dimethylxanthenone-4-acetic acid (DMXAA) by combination with 5-hydroxytryptamine and bioreductive drugs. Br J Cancer 1998; 78(4): 439-445.

53.   Parkins CS, Holder AJ, Hill SA, et al. Determinants of anti-vascular action by combretastatin A-4 phosphate: role of nitric oxide. Br J Cancer 2000; 83: 811-816.

54.   Badn W, Kalliomaki S, Widegren B, et al. Low-dose combretastatin A4 phosphate enhances the immune response of tumor hosts to experimental colon carcinoma. Clin Cancer Res 2006; 12(15): 4714-4719.

55.   Yeung SC, She M, Yang H, et al. Combination chemotherapy including combretastatin A4 phosphate and paclitaxel is effective against anaplastic thyroid cancer in a nude mouse xenograft model. J Clin Endocrinol Metab 2007; 92(8): 2902-2909.

56.   Kanthou C, Greco O, Stratford A, et al. The tubulin-binding agent combretastatin A-4-phosphate arrests endothelial cells in mitosis and induces mitotic cell death. Am J Pathol 2004; 165(4): 1401-1411.

57.   Ching LM, Cao Z, Kieda C, et al. Induction of endothelial cell apoptosis by the antivascular agent 5,6-Dimethylxanthenone-4-acetic acid. Br J Cancer 2002; 86(12)1937-1942.

58.   Sheng Y, Hua J, Pinney KG, et al. Combretastatin family member OXI4503 induces tumor vascular collapse through the induction of endothelial apoptosis. Int J Cancer 2004; 111(4): 604-610.

59.   Folkes LK, Christlieb M, Madej E, et al. Oxidative Metabolism of Combretastatin A-1 Produces Quinone Intermediates with the Potential To Bind to Nucleophiles and To Enhance Oxidative Stress via Free Radicals. Chem Res Toxicol 2007; 20: 1885-1894.

60.   Kirwan IG, Loadman PM, Swaine DJ, et al. Comparative preclinical pharmacokinetic and metabolic studies of the combretastatin prodrugs combretastatin A4 phosphate and A1 phosphate. Clin Cancer Res 2004; 10(4): 1446-1453.

61.   Horsman M, Ehrnrooth E, Ladekarl M, et al. The effect of combretastatin A-4 disodium phosphate in a C3H mouse mammary carcinoma and a variety of murine spontaneous tumors. Int. J. Radiat. Oncol. Biol. Phys. 1998; 42: 895-898.

62.   Chaplin DJ, Pettit GR, Hill SA. Anti-vascular approaches to solid tumor therapy: evaluation of combretastatin A4 phosphate. Anticancer Res 1999; 19: 189-196.

63.   Grosios K, Holwell SE, McGown AT, et al. In vivo and in vitro evaluation of combretastatin A-4 and its sodium phosphate prodrug. Br. J. Cancer 1999; 81: 1318-1327.

64.   Pedley RB, Hill SA, Boxer GM, et al. Eradication of colorectal xenografts by combined radioimmunotherapy and combretastatin a-4 3-O-phosphate. Cancer Res 2001; 61(12)4716-4722.

65.   Beauregard DA, Hill SA, Chaplin DJ, et al. The susceptibility of tumors to the antivascular drug combretastatin A4 phosphate correlates with vascular permeability. Cancer Res 2001; 61(18): 6811-6815.

66.   Tozer GM, Akerman S, Cross NA, et al. Blood vessel maturation and response to vascular-disrupting therapy in single vascular endothelial growth factor-A isoform-producing tumors. Cancer Res 2008; 68(7); 2301-2311.

67.   Galbraith SM, Maxwell RJ, Lodge MA, et al. Combretastatin A4 phosphate has tumor antivascular activity in rat and man as demonstrated by dynamic magnetic resonance imaging. J Clin Oncol 2003; 21(15)2831-2842.

68.   Boucher Y, Baxter LT, Jain RK. Interstitial pressure gradients in tissue-isolated and subcutaneous tumors: implications for therapy. Cancer Res. 1990; 50: 4478-4484.

69.   Murata R, Siemann DW, Overgaard J, et al. Interaction between combretastatin A-4 disodium phosphate and radiation in murine tumors. Radiother Oncol 2001; 60(2): 155-161.

70.   Siemann DW, Rojiani AM. Enhancement of radiation therapy by the novel vascular targeting agent ZD6126. Int J Radiat Oncol Biol Phys 2002; 53(1); 164-171.

71.   Horsman MR, Siemann DW. Pathophysiologic effects of vascular-targeting agents and the implications for combination with conventional therapies. Cancer Res 2006; 66(24): 11520-11539.

72.   Hori K, Furumoto S, Kubota K. Tumor blood flow interruption after radiotherapy strongly inhibits tumor regrowth. Cancer Sci 2008; 99(7): 1485-1491.

73. Martinelli M, Bonezzi K, Riccardi E, et al. Sequence dependent antitumor efficacy of the vascular disrupting agent ZD6126 in combination with paclitaxel. Br J Cancer 2007; 97(7): 888-894.

74. Grosios K, Loadman PM, Swaine DJ, et al. Combination chemotherapy with combretastatin A-4 phosphate and 5-fluorouracil in an experimental murine colon adenocarcinoma. Anticancer Research 2000; 20: 229-234.

75. Li L, Rojiani A, Siemann D. Targeting the tumor vasculature with combretastatin A-4 disodium phosphate: effects on radiation therapy. Int J Radiat Oncol Biol Phys 1998; 42: 899-903.

76. Ng QS, Goh V, Carnell D, et al. Tumor antivascular effects of radiotherapy combined with combretastatin a4 phosphate in human non-small-cell lung cancer. Int J Radiat Oncol Biol Phys 2007; 67(5): 1375-1380.

77. Pedley RB, Boden JA, Boden R, et al. Ablation of colorectal xenografts with combined radioimmunotherapy and tumor blood flow-modifying agents. Cancer Res 1996; 56(14): 3293-3300.

78. Sengupta S, Eavarone D, Capila I, et al. Temporal targeting of tumor cells and neovasculature with a nanoscale delivery system. Nature 2005; 436(7050)568-572.

79. Fens MH, Hill KJ, Issa J,et al. Liposomal encapsulation enhances the antitumor efficacy of the vascular disrupting agent ZD6126 in murine B16.F10 melanoma. Br J Cancer 2008; 99(8); 1256-1264.

80. Pattillo CB, Sari-Sarraf F, Nallamothu R, et al. Targeting of the antivascular drug combretastatin to irradiated tumors results in tumor growth delay. Pharm Res 2005; 22(7)1117-1120.

81. El-Emir E, Boxer GM, Petrie IA, et al. Tumor parameters affected by combretastatin A-4 phosphate therapy in a human colorectal xenograft model in nude mice. Eur J Cancer 2005; 41(5): 799-806.

82. Boehle AS, Sipos B, Kliche U, et al. Combretastatin A-4 prodrug inhibits growth of human non-small cell lung cancer in a murine xenotransplant model. Ann Thorac Surg 2001; 71: 1657-1665.

83. Dachs GU, Steele AJ, Coralli C, et al. Anti-vascular agent Combretastatin A-4-P modulates hypoxia inducible factor-1 and gene expression. BMC Cancer 2006; 6: 280-291.

84. Shaked Y, Ciarrocchi A, Franco M, et al. Therapy-induced acute recruitment of circulating endothelial progenitor cells to tumors. Science 2006; 313(5794): 1785-1787.

85. Siemann DW, Shi W. Efficacy of combined antiangiogenic and vascular disrupting agents in treatment of solid tumors. Int J Radiat Oncol Biol Phys 2004; 60(4): 1233-1240.

86. Siemann DW, Shi W. Dual targeting of tumor vasculature: combining Avastin and vascular disrupting agents (CA4P or OXi4503). Anticancer Res 2008; 28(4B): 2027-2031.

87. Tozer GM, Kanthou C, Lewis G, et al. Tumor vascular disrupting agents: combating treatment resistance. Br J Radiol 2008; 81(Spec No): S12-20.

88. Dong D, Ko B, Baumeister P, et al. Vascular targeting and antiangiogenesis agents induce drug resistance effector GRP78 within the tumor microenvironment. Cancer Res 2005; 65(13): 5785-5791.

89. Galbraith SM, Rustin GJ, Lodge M A, et al. Effects of 5,6-dimethylxanthenone-4-acetic acid on human tumor microcirculation assessed by dynamic contrast-enhanced magnetic resonance imaging. J Clin Oncol 2002; 20(18): 3826-3840.

90. Rustin GJ, Bradley C, Galbraith S, et al. 5,6-dimethylxanthenone-4-acetic acid (DMXAA), a novel antivascular agent: phase I clinical and pharmacokinetic study. Br J Cancer 2003; 88(8)1160-1167.

91. Dowlati A, Robertson K, Cooney M, et al. A phase I pharmacokinetic and translational study of the novel vascular targeting agent combretastatin a-4 phosphate on a single-dose intravenous schedule in patients with advanced cancer. Cancer Res 2002; 62(12): 3408-3416.

92. Rustin GJ, Galbraith SM, Anderson H, et al. Phase I clinical trial of weekly combretastatin A4 phosphate: clinical and pharmacokinetic results. J Clin Oncol 2003; 21(15)2815-2822.

93. Cooney MM, Radivoyevitch T, Dowlati A, et al. Cardiovascular safety profile of combretastatin a4 phosphate in a single-dose phase I study in patients with advanced cancer. Clin Cancer Res 2004; 10(1 Pt 1): 96-100.

94. Honess DJ, Hylands F, Chaplin DJ, et al. In Combretastatin-A-4-P induced hypertension can be controlled with conventional antihypertensive therapy in a rat model without compromising the reduction in tumor blood flow, AACR 96th Annual Meeting 2005, Anaheim, Orange County, CA, U.S.A., 2005: p 704.

95. Gould S, Westwood FR, Curwen JO, et al. Effect of pretreatment with atenolol and nifedipine on ZD6126-induced cardiac toxicity in rats. J Natl Cancer Inst 2007; 99(22): 1724-1728.

CHAPTER 13

Inhibitors of Angiogenesis Based on Thrombospondin-1

Giulia Taraboletti and Katiuscia Bonezzi

Tumor Angiogenesis Unit, Department of Oncology, Mario Negri Institute for Pharmacological Research, Bergamo, Italy

Address correspondence to: Giulia Taraboletti, Department of Oncology, Mario Negri Institute for Pharmacological Research, via Gavazzeni, 11, 24126 Bergamo, Italy; Tel: (39)-035-319888; Fax: (39)-035-319331; Email: taraboletti@marionegri.it

Abstract: Angiogenesis-driven pathologies, including cancer, are sustained by a preponderance of angiogenic factors over endogenous inhibitors of new-vessel formation. Restoring this balance represents a logical therapeutic strategy to treat these pathologies. Therefore, endogenous inhibitors of angiogenesis, and in particular thrombospondin-1 (TSP-1), are a powerful source of potential antiangiogenic tools. Different therapeutic approaches have been proposed to exploit the antiangiogenic properties of TSP-1, including TSP-1 fragments, synthetic peptides and peptidomimetics, gene therapy strategies and agents that up-regulate TSP-1 expression. This review focuses on the possibility of exploiting TSP-1 for the design of antiangiogenic agents, with particular reference on their use in antineoplastic therapies.

1. INTRODUCTION

The formation of new blood vessels is a highly controlled process, particularly in adults. Endogenous inhibitors of angiogenesis are Nature's response to the need for efficient negative control of this process. It is therefore reasonable to consider these agents as optimal inhibitors, and to exploit them for the design of therapies aimed at blocking angiogenesis-driven pathologies, including - but not limited to - tumor progression and metastasis [1]. The role of thrombospondins (TSP) in tumor angiogenesis and progression has been clearly indicated by preclinical studies (reviewed in [2]), particularly by tumorigenicity experiments in mice with tissue-specific overexpression of TSP-1 [3, 4]. Loss of TSP-1 production is considered determinant in the "angiogenic switch" that releases tumors from the dormant state to an angiogenic, malignant disease, and over-expression of TSP-1 reduces primary tumor growth and angiogenesis in preclinical models [5-11].

Thrombospondin-1 (TSP-1) was the first identified endogenous inhibitor of angiogenesis [12, 13]. Of the five members that constitute the TSP family in mammals, TSP-1 and TSP-2 (forming group A, homotrimeric TSPs) are very similar in domain organization. Although TSP-1 and TSP-2 have different patterns of expression in different tissues during development and in adulthood, they share the ability to inhibit angiogenesis.

Each TSP-1 monomer consists of an N-terminal globular domain, followed by the coiled-coil oligomerization domain, a von Willebrand Factor type C, procollagen domain, three properdin-like type I repeats, and a signature domain comprising three epidermal growth factor (EGF)-like type II repeats, the calcium-binding wire - type III repeats, and the lectin-like C-terminal globular domain (Fig. **1**) [14].

Unlike many other endogenous inhibitors of angiogenesis, which are fragments of larger molecules with no intrinsic antiangiogenic activity, TSP-1 is active both as a whole molecule and as fragments. Its

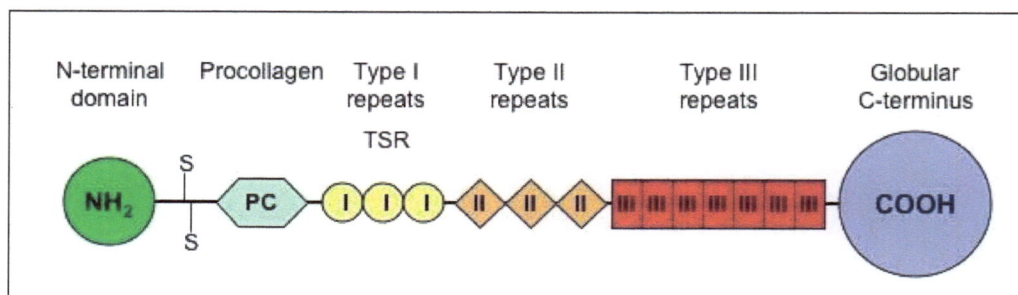

Fig. (1). Modular structure of the TSP-1 monomer.

effect on angiogenesis is extremely complex and context-dependent. Like other matricellular proteins, it is composed of a succession of different functional domains, each able to specifically interact with cell receptors, soluble cytokines and growth factors, extracellular matrix components, and proteases. The local presence of these receptors/ligands and the bioavailability of each TSP-1 domain will therefore dictate the pattern of molecular interactions, hence the biological effect of TSP-1 in a given biological setting. Although TSP-1 is commonly considered an inhibitor of angiogenesis, it can also stimulate it, through biologically active pro-angiogenic domains, mostly mapped in the N-terminal domain [15-20]. Thus, TSP-based antiangiogenic therapies could be designed either to mimic the molecule's antiangiogenic properties or to antagonize its pro-angiogenic activity.

TSP-1 can affect angiogenesis both directly and indirectly. As a direct inhibitor, it interacts with specific receptors on endothelial cells to affect cell viability and functions related to angiogenesis. As an indirect inhibitor, it binds to and influences the activity/bioavailability of various mediators of angiogenesis, such as angiogenic factors, cytokines and proteases.

Although this review will mostly focus on the effects of TSP on endothelial cells, TSP-1 is also active on other cell types involved in angiogenesis, including smooth muscle cells, monocytes/macrophages and T cells [21, 22].

Here we focus on TSP-1 and tumor-associated angiogenesis. A brief description of membrane receptors or soluble TSP-1 ligands is provided, followed by a list of active sequences and the evidence that these TSP-peptides are *bona fide* inhibitors of angiogenesis and tumor growth.

2. "DRUGGABLE" TSP-1 RECEPTORS AND LIGANDS

TSP-1 interacts with a variety of receptors on the surface of endothelial cells, eliciting both anti- and pro-angiogenic responses. Therapeutic exploitation could therefore by achieved by TSP-1 mimetics in the first case, and by antagonists in the latter.

Membrane Receptors

CD36, the first TSP-1 membrane receptor identified [23, 24], is an 88 kDa glycoprotein expressed by platelets and many cell types, including microvascular but not large-vessel endothelial cells [25].

The TSP-1/CD36 interaction occurs between the conserved CLESH-1 domain in CD36 and the type I repeats in TSP-1 [26]. Homology searches indicate that the TSP-1 recognition motif of CD36 is found in several molecules, within and outside the CD36

family, including lysosomal integral membrane protein II (LIMPII) [27] and HIV envelope gp120 [28]. On the other hand, a large family of proteins - the TSR-superfamily - contains sequences similar to the type I repeats [29]. It is therefore plausible that the CLESH/TSR pattern of recognition extends beyond the CD36/TSP-1 system and is implicated in different molecular networks and biological processes.

CD36 mediates the inhibitory effects of TSP-1 on FGF-2-induced endothelial cell migration, morphological organization [26, 30] and angiogenesis in the cornea assay [31]. By preventing free fatty acids uptake by CD36, TSP-1 causes inhibition of eNOS and therefore the NO-dependent response [32]. TSP-1 binding to CD36 induces endothelial cell apoptosis through the sequential activation of p59fyn, caspase-3 and p38 MAPK [31]. Apoptosis ultimately involves death receptors, the Fas/FasL (CD95/CD95L) or the TNFa/TNF-R1 systems, with possible differences in endothelial cell types and stimuli [33, 34].

Interestingly, the TSP-1/CD36 interaction affects the activity/expression of other receptors involved in angiogenesis. TSP-1, via CD36, down-modulates vascular endothelial growth factor (VEGF) receptor 2 (VEGFR-2) [30]. CD36 is also constitutively associated with ß1 integrin in endothelial cells [30], with interesting implications for the mechanisms of the anti-motility activity of TSP-1 and the possibility of cooperative antiangiogenic activity between integrin antagonists and CD36-binding sequences of TSP-1.

CD47, also known as IAP (integrin-associated protein), was initially identified as the cell membrane receptor for the adhesive sequence 4N1 (KRFYVVMWKK) in the C-terminal G domain of TSP-1, mediating TSP-1-induced cell spreading [35, 36]. CD47 forms a signaling complex with αvß3 and other integrins (reviewed in [21, 37]). The soluble 4N1 peptide reportedly inhibits tube formation, though not proliferation, of capillary endothelial cells, and FGF-2-induced neovascularization in the cornea assay [38].

The TSP-1/CD47 interaction is important in the inhibition of nitric oxide (NO) by TSP-1. Although both CD47 and CD36 contribute to NO regulation by TSP-1, only CD47 has proved necessary for this effect, since ligation of CD36 was unable to block NO signaling in cells lacking CD47 [32]. Regulation of NO signaling by TSP-1 has important consequences on the regulation not only of angiogenesis, but also of tumor blood flow, hence potentially on the activity of vasoactive and vascular targeting agents [39].

The N-terminal domain of TSP-1, mostly responsible for the pro-angiogenic activity of the molecule [17-20], binds **heparin and related molecules**, such as heparansulfate proteoglycans and sulfatides. The N-terminal domain of TSP-1 interacts with syndecan-4 to stimulate endothelial cell tubulogenesis and protect cells from apoptosis [40]. Syndecan-4 binds two TSP-

1 peptides bearing the consensus motifs for binding to glycosaminoglycans, Hep I (aa 17-35) and Hep II (aa 78-94). Hep II also comprises the binding sequence for $\alpha6$ integrin, pointing to cooperation between the two ligands in the regulation of endothelial cell activity by TSP-1.

The Hep I peptide in the heparin-binding domain of TSP-1 also signals through a receptor co-complex involving calreticulin and low-density lipoprotein receptor (**LDLR**)-related protein (**LRP**) to stimulate endothelial cell motility and focal adhesion disassembly through activation of the PI3K signaling pathway [41]. These molecules are endocytic receptors for TSP-1 [42]. The interaction of TSP-1 with VLDLR or LRP-1 and endocytosis of the TSP-VEGF complex contribute to the CD36-independent inhibition of VEGF activity by TSP-1 and have been proposed as the mechanism of the homeostatic activity of TSP in preserving the quiescence of normal endothelium [43, 44]. In addition, LRP-1 reportedly mediates TSP-2-dependent internalization of MMP-2 [45, 46].

TSP interacts with several **integrins** expressed by endothelial cells and involved in angiogenesis, including $\alpha3\beta1$, $\alpha4\beta1$, $\alpha5\beta1$, $\alpha6\beta1$, $\alpha9\beta1$, and $\alpha v\beta3$. Binding sites for $\beta1$ integrins have been mapped in the N-terminal domain [19, 47, 48], the second and third type I repeats [49, 50] and the type II repeats (the latter reportedly not recognized by endothelial cells) [49]. Independently of whether the interaction between the intact TSP-1 and $\beta1$ integrins elicited pro- or anti-angiogenic functions in endothelial cells, preclinical studies indicate that small TSP-1 peptides containing the integrin binding site, as well as disintegrins or anti-integrin antibodies, can be used to block endothelial cell pro-angiogenic functions such as adhesion, proliferation, survival, wound healing, motility and angiogenesis in the chorioallantoic membrane (CAM) assay [18, 19, 51]. Interaction of TSP-1 or a peptide comprising the entire type I repeats with $\beta1$ integrins inhibited VEGF-induced migration through a PI3k-dependent mechanism [50].

The integrin-recognition RGD sequence is present in the type III repeats of TSP-1, and interacts with $\alpha v\beta3$ and $\alpha5\beta1$ integrins [52]. Although cryptic in calcium loaded TSP-1, under certain conditions this sequence can mediate the pro-adhesive property of TSP-1 for endothelial cells [52]. The role of this sequence in angiogenesis still needs to be clarified.

The usefulness of integrins as targets for antiangiogenic and antineoplastic therapies is still debated. Nonetheless, integrin antagonists have shown antiangiogenic and antineoplastic activity in preclinical studies, and some are currently undergoing clinical evaluation for cancer treatment (reviewed in [53, 54]). The use of integrin ligands for target-specific delivery of imaging or therapeutic agents is another possible means of exploiting integrin-binding

sequences, including integrin recognizing TSP peptides.

Soluble Ligands

Consistent with its matricellular nature, TSP-1 binds and influences the activity/bioavailability of different mediators of angiogenesis, such as angiogenic factors, cytokines and proteases [2, 55, 56].

TSP-1 binds to **angiogenic factors** including FGF-2, VEGF, HGF, PDGF, and the viral protein tat [57-61]. We found that TSP-1 bound FGF-2 with high affinity - in the nanomolar range, similar to the affinity of the growth factor for heparin [58], and the binding site was located within the type III repeats [60]. Heparin prevented the TSP-1/FGF-2 interaction [58, 60], suggesting that negatively charged residues of TSP-1 bound the heparin-recognizing region of FGF-2. Indeed, TSP-1 prevented FGF-2 binding to heparan sulfate proteoglycans in the extracellular matrix and on the surface of endothelial cells, where they constitute the low-affinity receptors [59]. As a consequence, TSP-1 and the type III repeats prevent FGF-2 binding to cells and long-term internalization, and deplete the extracellular matrix of stored FGF-2, an important event in the regulation of FGF-2 location and bioavailability [58, 59]. TSP-1 also affects the interaction with the matrix of two other heparin-binding angiogenic factors, VEGF and HGF [57, 59]

The FGF-2/TSP-1 interaction is modulated by calcium ions, since low calcium concentrations are required for binding [60], suggesting that, as for other active sites in the type III repeats, the FGF-2 binding site is not exposed in calcium-replete TSP-1, and its exposure/availability is regulated by environmental conditions.

TSP-1 binds VEGF [44, 62, 63]. The VEGF-binding domain is conceivably located in the type I repeats of TSP-1, since the TSR in connective tissue growth factor (CTGF) binds specifically to $VEGF_{165}$, preventing its binding to endothelial cells, and inhibiting VEGF-induced tube formation *in vitro* and angiogenesis *in vivo* in the Matrigel assay [63]. TSP-1 binding to VEGF inhibits VEGF association with the extracellular matrix [59]. TSP-1 has also been reported to influence VEGF internalization through LRP-1, acting as a regulator of ovarian angiogenesis and follicle development [44].

Tumors in mice that lack TSP-1 in the mammary gland have a high level of bioactive, receptor-associated VEGF [3]. Direct interaction of TSP-1 with the growth factor, or indirect mechanisms involving MMP-9 might contribute to the regulation of VEGF bioavailability by TSP-1.

TSP-1 is an important regulator of **protease** activity, as it binds and inhibits the activity of matrix metalloproteinases (MMP), urokinase plasminogen activator, plasmin, neutrophil elastase and cathepsin G

[64, 65]. Since proteases are critical regulators of angiogenesis – by directly promoting endothelial cell invasive processes and by releasing angiogenic factors stored in the extracellular matrix - this activity has profound effects on the whole angiogenic process.

TSP-1 was originally reported to stimulate the expression of MMP-9 by endothelial cells, promoting their ability to invade and form tubes in collagen gel culture [66]. In line with these findings, we found that the angiogenic N-terminal domain of TSP- increased the release of MMP-9 and MMP-2 and reduced TIMP-2 expression by endothelial cells, whereas the antiangiogenic 140kDa TSP-1 fragment boosted TIMP-2 expression [17]. TSP-1 has been shown to suppress the enzymatic activation of proMMP-9 by MMP-3, regulating the levels of active MMP-9 in tumors [3]. TSP-1 and TSP-2 also interact with MMP-2 [45, 46, 67]. The TSP-2 N-terminal domain binds to MMP-2, and promotes the clearance of extracellular MMP-2 through endocytosis by the scavenger receptor LRP [45, 46].

TSP-1, but not other TSPs, binds and activates **TGFß** through sequences located in the type I repeats [68, 69]. This activation influences angiogenesis in a complex manner. In some experimental models, TGFß activation was implicated in the antineoplastic and antimetastatic activity of the type I repeats {Yee, 2009 #359}.

3. EXPLOITABLE TSP-1 SEQUENCES

Given TSP-1's multiple roles in angiogenesis, it is not surprising that different active TSP-1 sequences have been described. Their identification and functional analysis has sometimes been difficult and controversial, mostly because of the proximity of active sequences (for example in the "crowded" type I repeats) and the formation of a complex network of interactions between TSP-1 receptor/ligands (e.g. CD36 and ß1 integrins, or CD47 and αvß3 integrin, or αvß3 integrin and VEGFR-2 [30, 71]). This situation - typical of matricellular proteins - leads to the formation of large multi-molecular complexes in the pericellular space, which tune downstream signaling, hence also the final cell response to the environment. With such a complexity of physical and functional associations, it becomes extremely difficult to isolate a single signal/sequence. However, it is clear that the activity of each sequence is context-dependent, as it varies with the environmental conditions and the predominant angiogenic stimuli. Nonetheless, each active TSP-1 sequence represents a potential prototype for the development of angiogenesis inhibitors.

Type I Repeats (TSR)

The TSR, commonly considered the main antiangiogenic site of TSP-1, is also present in several

other proteins outside the TSP family, often enabling them to inhibit angiogenesis [29, 72].

Among a number of recombinant fragments covering most of the TSP-1 molecule, only the fragments containing the second and third type I repeats prevented endothelial cell proliferation and angiogenesis in the CAM assay [20]. Chronic treatment with the type I repeats reduced tumor growth and angiogenesis in an orthotopic pancreatic xenograft [73, 74] and in a model of polyoma middle T transgenic mice {Yee, 2009 #359}.

As mentioned above, different peptides within this relatively small region are active in inhibiting angiogenesis, though none of them is singly as potent as the entire molecule.

A 19-residue Mal II peptide, derived from the second type I repeat, has been used as a template for designing antiangiogenic ABT-510 (see below). Although not active in the native configuration, D-enantiomer residue substitutions gave the peptide strong, CD36-dependent antiangiogenic activity [75]. The 7-mer GVITRIR was identified as the minimal active sequence [75]. The adjacent sequence CSVTCG, first considered the binding site for CD36 [76], was later shown to be dispensable for the antiangiogenic activity of TSP-1 [26] and, according to the analysis of the TSR crystal structure, not readily available as the two cysteines are involved in separate disulfide bonds [77].

A tryptophan-rich motif containing the heparin-binding consensus sequence WSPW (WSHWSxPWS) inhibited endothelial cell proliferation and motility, induced endothelial cell apoptosis, and inhibited FGF-2 induced angiogenesis in the CAM assay [20, 78, 79]. Retro-inverso peptides of this sequence inhibited the growth of MDA-MB-435 carcinoma in the mammary fat pad of nude mice [20, 80].

The type I repeats is also involved in the recognition and activation of TGFß, a critical regulator of tumor growth. The tryptophan-rich motif binds TGFß, which is then activated through the KRFK sequence [68, 69].

Von Willebrand Factor Type C/procollagen Domain

Peptides from the pro-collagen region of TSP-1, particularly the NGVQYRN sequence, inhibited angiogenesis *in vivo* in the rat cornea assay, and in a mouse polyvinyl sponge model [81] but not in the CAM [20]. Differences in the assay conditions or species used might account for these conflicting findings.

C-Terminal Cassette/Signature Domain

The region comprising the type II repeats, the type III repeats and the C-terminal globular end is the most conserved region in the TSP family [82]. Its structural/functional properties are affected by calcium. The cooperative binding of calcium ions is the main feature of the type III repeats, and profoundly affects the structure and availability of active sequences in the whole cassette.

The type III repeats contains a cryptic integrin interacting sequence RGD [83], two sequences that bind cathepsin G and neutrophil elastase [64], binding sites for collagen V, and attachment sites for neutrophils [84] and sickle red blood cells [85]. The CD47 recognition sequence, located in the C-terminal globular end, is also involved in angiogenesis [38].

We described a recombinant fragment containing the entire region of the type III repeats that bound FGF-2, prevented FGF-2 binding to endothelial cells and inhibited FGF-2-induced endothelial cell proliferation *in vitro* and angiogenesis in the CAM assay [60], indicating the possibility of exploiting this TSP-1 region for antiangiogenic therapies.

Many of the active sequences in the C-terminal cassette, such as the RGD sequence and the binding sites for FGF-2, CD47, neutrophil elastase and cathepsin G, are not exposed in physiological conditions, and become exposed only after drastic structural changes induced by a low calcium concentration, ligands, or reduction of disulfide bonds, indicating the importance of the environmental conditions in the bioavailability and activity of these sites [60, 64, 83, 86].

4. THERAPEUTIC STRATEGIES

Different therapeutic approaches have been proposed to exploit the antiangiogenic properties of TSP-1, all essentially aimed at raising the concentration of TSP-1, or selected TSP peptides, in order to switch the balance between angiogenic factors and inhibitors in favor of the latter.

Peptides and Peptido-Mimetics

As described above, the antiangiogenic and antineoplastic activity of synthetic peptides based on the active sequences of TSP-1 indicated the feasibility of developing TSP-1 peptides as antiangiogenic /antineoplastic agents.

The advantages of synthetic peptides over large molecules include lower immunogenicity, and the possibility of introducing modifications during synthesis. Limitations are the short half-life *in vivo*, potential low stability and sensitivity to proteases, and immunogenicity in larger peptides [87].

Several chemical modifications can improve peptide stability, bioavailability, potency, tumor targeting ability, and PK/PD. Examples are the use of non-natural amino-acids, cyclization, linkage to proteins,

retro-inverso analogues, or polysucrose conjugates [20, 75, 80, 87]. Worth considering is the possibility of rationally designing inhibitory peptides and non-peptidic small molecules to mimic the desired amino acid sequence, with better activity and/or PK/PD properties [87].

Bioinformatics tools have been used to identify and analyze potential antiangiogenic sequences from endogenous proteins containing the TSR motifs. Several peptides have been identified, either from proteins related to TSP [88] or derived from proteins of the CCN family [89]. They all had antiangiogenic properties, as they inhibited endothelial cell proliferation and motility in a CD36-dependent manner [72].

Using a different approach, the structures of many endogenous inhibitors of angiogenesis have been compared, with the aim of finding common structural motifs. TSP-1 type I repeats, PF4, endostatin, angiostatin, and gamma IFN-inducible protein 10, all share a common structure involving an antiparallel ß-sheet and a preponderance of positively charged and hydrophobic residues. Peptides have been designed to mimic this structure, leading to the development of the antiangiogenic peptide anginex, and non-peptide derivatives [90].

These studies have laid the basis for the design of peptidic or non-peptidic mimetics of TSP with greater activity or more drug-like properties.

Two TSP-1-based peptido-mimetics developed as antiangiogenic agents for antineoplastic therapy have reached clinical trials so far: ABT510 and CVX-045.

ABT-510. This modified nonapeptide was the first TSP-1-based antiangiogenic compound to be developed and to reach clinical experimentation. It is based on the 7-mer active sequence GVITRIR in the second type I repeat. The N- and C- terminally capped version of the GVITRIR enantiomer substituting D-isoleucine for the first L-Ile residue [75] with the additional introduction of the non-natural amino acid norvaline in place of the first Arg, and addition of sarcosine at the N-terminus and proline ethylamide at the C-terminus, resulted in peptides ABT-526 (formerly known as DI-TSP) and the more soluble ABT-510 (DI-TSP1a, with D-allo-isoleucine instead of D-isoleucine) [91, 92]. These peptides had favorable potency, solubility and PD/PK profile [92].

Both peptides inhibited microvascular endothelial cell motility and proliferation, induced apoptosis in a CD36 dependent manner, up-regulated endothelial CD95L/FasL and inhibited angiogenesis *in vivo*, in the rat cornea model and in the mouse Matrigel assays [91-94]. Although more potent than the original GV(DI)TRIR in inducing caspase activation in vascular cells, ABT-510 was less potent in inhibiting CD36 fatty acid translocase activity, suggesting that ABT-510 might have different activities from TSP-1 and might act through other receptors or pathways [95].

ABT-510 and ABT-526 inhibited tumor growth and reduced microvessel density in preclinical tumor models, including syngeneic and xenograft gliomas [93], orthotopic bladder cancer [91], the Lewis lung carcinoma [92], a ras-dependent and VEGF-independent tumor model [96], and orthotopic ovarian carcinoma xenografts [97]. ABT-510-induced vessel normalization has been reported [97]. The peptides inhibited B16F10 experimental metastasis, affecting both the number and size of lung colonies [91], and reduced secondary dissemination from ovarian cancer xenografts [97]. ABT-510 induced apoptosis of CD36-expressing tumor cells [97], suggesting a double effect on both the vascular and tumor compartments.

Preclinical studies have highlighted the potentiation of the antineoplastic efficacy of ABT-510 in combination with conventional chemotherapy [94, 98] or another antiangiogenic agent, the histone deacetylase inhibitor valproic acid [99].

ABT-510 and ABT-526 have shown promising activity in the treatment of canine cancer where, as single agents, they induced some objective responses and disease stabilization [100]. There was evidence of cooperative activity between ABT-526 and chemotherapy (lomustine) in prolonging response in pet dogs with relapsed non-Hodgkin's lymphoma, with no signs of additional toxicity [101].

Phase I clinical studies indicated that ABT-510, 20-260 mg daily (as a single dose or split for twice/day administration) for several months, was safe and had a good toxicity profile. After subcutaneous bolus injection ABT-510 was rapidly absorbed and eliminated, with a half-life of approximately 1 hour [102]. At all the doses tested, the potential therapeutic threshold was achieved - defined as plasma concentration higher than 100 ng/mL for at least 3 hours per day, resulting in 75% of maximum efficacy in preclinical murine models. MTD could not be defined [102]. Like other angiogenesis inhibitors, ABT-510 showed little clinical activity as a single agent on renal cell carcinoma, soft tissue sarcoma and melanoma [103-105], suggesting potential clinical use in combination regimens. The safety of ABT-510 in combination with chemotherapeutics, such as gemcitabine and cisplatin, and 5-FU/leucovorin, was indicated by the good tolerability and lack of significant PK interactions [106, 107]. ABT-510 has been tested in a number of phase I and II clinical trials in lymphoma, renal cell carcinoma, soft tissue sarcoma, non-small cell lung carcinoma, and metastatic melanoma.

CVX-045 is a fusion molecule, produced by covalently attaching two TSP-1 mimetic nonamer peptides to the Fab binding site of a humanized scaffold antibody. This interesting approach has proved successful, since the compound retains the activity of the TSP peptides and the advantageous PK of antibodies. CVX-045 reduced tumor growth in xenograft models, as either single treatment or in combination with 5FU, CPT-11 or sunitinib [108, 109]. A phase I trial for CVX-045 found no dose-limiting toxicities but some possibly drug-related adverse events. Biologic activity was indicated by changes in tumor blood flow observed by MRI analysis [110, 111].

Gene Therapy

The efficacy of antiangiogenic therapies depends on sustained levels of the inhibitors. Gene therapy approaches have therefore been proposed to provide continuous delivery of antiangiogenic factors. Viral and non-viral vectors have been proposed for the delivery of TSP-1. Recombinant adeno-associated virus-mediated delivery of the three TSP-1 type I repeats resulted in the expression of the transgene in normal tissues, reduced VEGF-induced angiogenesis, and reduced tumor growth and microvessel density both locally and at distant sites [112].

Fibroblasts retrovirally transduced to produce high levels of TSP-2 and embedded in polymer scaffolds were used as a cell-based strategy to ensure continuous *in vivo* production of TSP-2. The resulting high levels of the inhibitor inhibited angiogenesis and tumor growth in different models [113], proving the feasibility of this strategy.

Up-Regulators of TSP Synthesis: Targeting Regulatory Mechanisms Controlling TSP-1 Expression

The genetic control of TSP-1 production by tumor cells has been investigated with the aim of clarifying the mechanisms of the "angiogenic switch" associated with tumor progression. A number of oncogenes and oncosuppressor genes that influence TSP-1 expression have been identified, including p53, p73 [115], c-jun, Myc, H-ras and K-ras, usually with oncogenesis suppressing and oncosuppressor genes stimulating TSP-1 expression [114]. Inactivation of p53 by mutation or allelic loss results in a decrease in TSP-1 production [116, 117]. Therapeutic strategies aimed at restoring p53, such as topical delivery of p53 DNA to the lung, have proved able to increase TSP-1 expression, reducing lung tumor burden and microvessel density and prolonging the survival of tumor-bearing mice [118].

Agents that stimulate TSP-1 production can be used to inhibit angiogenesis. Known angiogenesis inhibitors act by raising TSP-1 levels. TSP-1 stimulatory agents include the peroxisome proliferator-activated receptor (PPAR)α agonist fenofibrate [119], thrichostatin-A [120], and differentiating factors such as retinoic acid [121]. Inhibitors of DNA methyltransferases and histone deacetylases have been reported to increase the expression of epigenetically silenced genes, including TSP-1, in tumor conditioned endothelial cells [122].

Attention has recently shifted to the role of **microRNAs** (miRNAs) in the angiogenic activity of oncogenes or angiogenic factors through the regulation of TSP-1 expression [123, 124]. Expression of TSP-1 is negatively controlled by the c-Myc regulated cluster miRNA-17-92, over-expressed in many human cancers and stimulated by VEGF [123, 124]. Within the miR-17-92 cluster, miR-18a has been indicated as responsible for TSP-1 regulation in endothelial cells [123] and miR-19 in a model of Myc and Ras-transformed colonocytes [124]. Inhibition of miR-17-92 resulted in increased TSP-1 expression and reduced VEGF-induced endothelial cell proliferation, migration and morphogenesis. In an *in vivo* model, endothelial cell specific inactivation of Dicer, the terminal endonuclease responsible for the generation of miRNAs, increased TSP-1 expression and reduced VEGF- and tumor- induced angiogenesis and tumor growth [123]. Interestingly, down-regulation of miR-17-92 might be the mechanism of the c-Myc-mediated increased expression of TSP-1 caused by the cytotoxic drug 5-FU [125].

Besides the important information on the role of miRNAs in angiogenesis, these study lay the ground for development of antiangiogenic strategies based on modulation of miRNA expression/activity.

An interesting case is the observation that TSP-1 expression is regulated by viral - rather than host - miRNAs. The poor expression of TSP-1 in Kaposi's sarcoma [126] has been associated with the expression in the host cells of miRNAs encoded by Kaposi's sarcoma-associated herpes virus [127]. This regulation of host cellular gene expression by viral miRNAs casts useful light on the pathogenesis of diseases such as Kaposi's sarcoma, and might indicate targeting viral miRNAs as a new therapeutic strategy.

An increase in TSP-1 production has been indicated as the mechanism of the antiangiogenic activity of **metronomic chemotherapy**, i.e. frequent low doses of chemotherapeutic agents, as a way of optimizing their antiangiogenic properties. The antiangiogenic and antineoplastic activity of metronomic, low-dose cyclophosphamide was associated with increased levels of TSP-1, and was lost in TSP-1-null mice [128, 129]. Similarly, TSP-1 was induced in colon cancer models after treatment with 5-FU [125], in rat prostate tumors treated with cyclophosphamide, doxorubicin or paclitaxel [130], and in HT-29 colon cancer xenografts treated with metronomic, but not MTV irinotecan [131]. Low-dose metronomic irinotecan raised plasma levels of TSP-1 and TSP-1 gene expression in PBMC in patients with metastatic colorectal cancer [132].

5.   FURTHER   ISSUES   AND CONSIDERATIONS

TSP-1 in Non-Oncologic Angiogenesis-Driven Pathologies

This review has focused on TSP-1-based antiangiogenic therapies for development as antineoplastic agents. However, angiogenesis inhibitors, including TSP-1-based compounds, have broad application in a variety of angiogenesis-driven pathologies, such as rheumatoid arthritis, inflammatory bowel disease, and the prevention of graft rejection. A peptide from the type III repeats containing the binding site for neutrophils and netrophil elastase, reduced neovascularization, leukocyte infiltration and thickening of the joint synovial lining, in a rat model of erosive arthritis [133]. ABT-510 has been proposed as an adjuvant agent in the therapy of inflammatory bowel disease, where it mimics the protective effect of TSP-1 [134], and in combination with immunosuppressive therapies to prevent chronic graft rejection [135].

Unpredictable Effects

TSP-1 can have multiple and sometimes dichotomous effects on tumor progression. Not always is its production beneficial: in some cases, it can actually promote tumor progression, particularly when TSP-1 is associated with tumor cell differentiation status. In a model of squamous cell carcinoma the presence of TSP-1 correlated with malignant behavior, whereas antisense-mediated inhibition of TSP-1 expression resulted in less tumorigenic clones, that gave raise to more differentiated tumors *in vivo* [136].

TSP-1 has direct effects on tumor cells, often stimulating pro-malignant functions such as motility and invasiveness [137]. In a model of mammary tumors in polyoma middle T transgenic mice, endogenous TSP-1 had a protective effect against primary tumor growth, but potentiated lung metastasis by promoting tumor cell migration {Yee, 2009 #359}. These unpredictable effects might be avoided by using selective TSP-1 domains.

CEP/CEC

Another property of TSP-1 potentially contributing to its antiangiogenic activity is the ability to reduce the mobilization of viable circulating endothelial cells (CEC) and putative endothelial progenitor cells (CEP), associated with angiogenic responsiveness. TSP-1 null mice had five times higher levels of CEC and CEP than the parental mice. Treatment of these mice with ABT-510 brought CEC and CEP back to control levels [138]. In addition, ABT-510 normalized the high levels of CEC and CEP in four tumor mouse models syngeneic in different strains [138] and in dogs with tumors [100]. A suggestion of a decrease or stabilization in the number of CEC, correlated with prolonged disease stabilization, was reported in patients treated with ABT-510, although the clinical data provide no conclusive evidence of activity on CEP in these patients [105, 106, 139]. The extent and clinical relevance of TSP-1-induced changes in CEC/CEP levels still need further investigation.

TSP-1 Based Therapeutics in Combination Therapies

The optimal antineoplastic use of antiangiogenic compounds is in combination with conventional therapies. The general aim is to achieve simultaneous double targeting of the transformed cells and the tumor stroma compartment. Besides this two-compartment action, the greater activity of combination therapies comes from a more complex effect of the antiangiogenic compound on the PK/PD properties of the chemotherapeutics.

Preclinical studies have indicated the advantageous antineoplastic activity of combination therapies with TSP-1-based agents and chemotherapeutics. TSP-1 boosted the antineoplastic activity of irinotecan on HT-29 colon xenografts [140]. ABT-510 potentiated the activity of chemotherapy in experimental models [94, 98].

A strong rationale for combining chemotherapy with TSP-1 derived agents is the chemo-sensitizing activity of TSP-1. Transcriptional down-regulation of TSP-1 by Txr1 makes prostate cancer cells resistant to paclitaxel, but the addition of exogenous TSP-1 partially reverses resistance and increases paclitaxel-induced apoptosis [141]. The effect was mediated by CD47 and appeared to be specific for paclitaxel, indicating the possibility of exploiting TSP-1-derived CD47 binding peptido mimetics in combination therapies - at least with taxanes - to enhance cytotoxicity.

The possibility of combining TSP-1 based agents with other antiangiogenic strategies is suggested by the lower TSP-1 levels in patients after treatment with bevacizumab, possibly as a feedback mechanism [142, 143]. This hypothesis is supported by the increased antineoplastic activity of ABT-510 when combined with an antiangiogenic agent [99].

Besides chemotherapy, a promising strategy is to combine TSP-1-based inhibitors with agents that increase the expression of TSP-1 targets (e.g. CD36 or CD95). For example, agonists of peroxisome proliferator-activated receptor gamma (PPARgamma) enhance CD36 expression in endothelial cells, boosting the efficacy of ABT510 on angiogenesis and tumor growth [144]. PPARgamma agonists might therefore potentiate the activity of TSP-1-based agents or of therapies that act through TSP-1, such as metronomic therapy.

TSP-1 and ABT-510 induce apoptosis by increasing FasL/CD95L. Several cytotoxic agents, including cyclophosphamide, cisplatin, docetaxel and doxorubicin induce the expression of CD95 by endothelial cells *in vitro* and *in vivo* at low, non-cytotoxic doses, therefore complementing the activity of ABT-510 in experimental *in vivo* models [94, 98].

Through its effect on endothelial cells, TSP-1 increases the antitumor efficacy of radiation therapy in human melanoma xenografts [145]. Conversely, by inhibiting the cytoprotective activity of nitric oxide (NO) through signaling via CD47, endogenous TSP-1 has radiosensitizing activity, limiting the survival of irradiated soft tissues. TSP-1/CD47 antagonists might thus be used to protect normal tissue from damage caused by radiotherapy, particularly since the lack of TSP-1 does not appear to limit tumor response to radiation [146].

TSP-1 as a Chemopreventive Agent

There is currently much interest in the development of agents to prevent the onset of tumorigenesis, and inhibitors of angiogenesis have been proposed as chemopreventive compounds. TSP-1 is particularly suited for this application. Targeted over-expression of TSP-1 in the skin of mice reduced chronic UV skin damages [147] and prevented the early malignant stages of chemical-induced skin tumorigenesis [4], suggesting the potential for TSP-based chemoprevention therapies.

Resistance to TSP-1-Based Antiangiogenic Therapies

Escape or resistance to therapy is a recognized problem in the clinical use of angiogenesis inhibitors. The presence of TSP-1 in the stroma of human tumors, sometimes correlated with a poor prognosis [148], is indicative of the tumor's ability to override TSP-1 antiangiogenic action.

Several general mechanisms of resistance/escape, common to most antiangiogenic agents, are applicable to TSP-1. They include increased production of angiogenic factors ("angiogenic rescue"), vascular mimicry, host vessel cooption, and selection of angiogenesis-independent tumor cell clones [149]. In addition, mechanisms of resistance specific to TSP-1 have been identified.

In an *in vivo* experimental model of TSP-1 overproduction by the tumor stroma, resistance to the antiangiogenic activity of TSP-1 was due to selection of tumor cells that produced high levels of angiogenic factors or adapted to proliferate in response to TSP-1-activated TGFß [150, 151].

Modulation of expression of the endothelial cell targets of TSP-1 is another mechanism of escape to TSP-1. Plasminogen activator inhibitor-1 (PAI-1) prevents plasmin-induced release of a soluble, pro-apoptotic FasL fragment, protecting endothelial cells from apoptosis, therefore representing a potential mechanism of resistance to the FasL-mediated pro-apoptotic activity of TSP-1 [152].

PMA or other PKC agonists inhibit the expression of CD36 by microvascular endothelial cells [25]. VEGF and withdrawal of shear stress reduce CD36 expression in endothelial cells, and sprouting capillaries have a low expression of the receptor [153]. Although interesting, this needs further confirmation as the modulation of CD36 expression was observed in HUVEC, previously reported not to express CD36.

As mentioned above, several molecules contain CLESH-1 homology motifs that mediate CD36 binding to TSP-1. One of these, the circulating histidin-rich glycoprotein (HRGP), binds TSP-1 and acts as a soluble decoy to block the anti-angiogenic activity of TSP-1. Therefore HRPG, and possibly other CLESH containing proteins, offer a potential mechanism of resistance to the antiangiogenic effects of TSP-1 [154].

6. CONCLUSIONS

Exploiting endogenous inhibitors of angiogenesis holds out promise for antiangiogenic drug design. The entire molecule, isolated active peptides, the receptors/ligands involved, signaling pathways and mechanisms of action are all potential areas for drug development. In the case of TSP-1, the agents developed so far - particularly ABT-510 - have shown promising activity, but clearly much still needs to be done to improve their properties, particularly in terms of PK and PD. Among other possible approaches, the rational design of peptidic and non-peptidic mimetics of TSP-1 might lead to improved antiangiogenic compounds.

7. ACKNOWLEDGEMENTS

The authors thank Jack Henkin for information on ABT-510 and for helpful comments on the manuscript. Studies from our laboratory are supported by grants from the Italian Association for Cancer Research (AIRC), Cariplo Foundation, European Union FP7 Health-F2-2008-201342, and the Italian Ministry of Health, Contract No. onc_ord 25/07.

8. REFERENCES

1.   Nyberg P, Xie L, Kalluri R. Endogenous inhibitors of angiogenesis. Cancer Res 2005; 65(10): 3967-3979.
2.   Armstrong LC, Bornstein P. Thrombospondins 1 and 2 function as inhibitors of angiogenesis. Matrix Biol 2003; 22(1): 63-71.
3.   Rodriguez-Manzaneque JC, Lane TF, Ortega MA, Hynes RO, Lawler J, Iruela-Arispe ML. Thrombospondin-1 suppresses spontaneous tumor growth and inhibits activation of matrix metalloproteinase-9 and mobilization of vascular endothelial growth factor. Proc Natl Acad Sci U S A 2001; 98(22): 12485-12490.
4.   Hawighorst T, Oura H, Streit M, Janes L, Nguyen L, Brown LF, Oliver G, Jackson DG, Detmar M. Thrombospondin-1 selectively inhibits early-stage carcinogenesis and angiogenesis but not tumor lymphangiogenesis and lymphatic metastasis in transgenic mice. Oncogene 2002; 21(52): 7945-7956.
5.   Bouck N, Stellmach V, Hsu SC. How tumors become angiogenic. Advanced in Cancer Research 1996; 69: 135-174.
6.   Volpert OV, Alani RM. Wiring the angiogenic switch: Ras, Myc, and Thrombospondin-1. Cancer Cell 2003; 3(3): 199-200.
7.   Holmgren L, Jackson G, Arbiser J. p53 induces angiogenesis-restricted dormancy in a mouse fibrosarcoma. Oncogene 1998; 17(7): 819-824.
8.   Weinstat-Saslow DL, Zabrenetzky VS, VanHoutte K, Frazier WA, Roberts DD, Steeg PS. Transfection of thrombospondin 1 complementary DNA into a human breast carcinoma cell line reduces primary tumor growth, metastatic potential, and angiogenesis. Cancer Res 1994; 54: 6504-6511.
9.   Almog N, Henke V, Flores L, Hlatky L, Kung AL, Wright RD, Berger R, Hutchinson L, Naumov GN, Bender E, Akslen LA, Achilles EG, Folkman J. Prolonged dormancy of human liposarcoma is associated with impaired tumor angiogenesis. FASEB J 2006; 20(7): 947-949.
10.   Kragh M, Quistorff B, Tenan M, Van Meir EG, Kristjansen PE. Overexpression of thrombospondin-1 reduces growth and vascular index but not perfusion in glioblastoma. Cancer Res 2002; 62(4): 1191-1195.
11.   Streit M, Velasco P, Brown LF, Skobe M, Richard L, Riccardi L, Lawler J, Detmar M. Overexpression of thrombospondin-1 decreases angiogenesis and inhibits the growth of human cutaneous squamous cell carcinomas. Am J Pathol 1999; 155(2): 441-452.
12.   Good DJ, Polverini PJ, Rastinejad F, Le Beau MM, Lemons RS, Frazier WA, Bouck NP. A tumor suppressor-dependent inhibitor of angiogenesis is immunologically and functionally indistinguishable from a fragment of thrombospondin. Proc.Natl.Acad.Sci.USA 1990; 87: 6624-6628.
13.   Taraboletti G, Roberts D, Liotta LA, Giavazzi R. Platelet thrombospondin modulates endothelial cell adhesion, motility, and growth: a potential angiogenesis regulatory factor. J Cell Biol 1990; 111(2): 765-772.
14.   Carlson CB, Lawler J, Mosher DF. Structures of thrombospondins. Cell Mol Life Sci 2008; 65(5): 672-686.
15.   Nicosia RF, Tuszynski GP. Matrix-bound thrombospondin promotes angiogenesis in vitro. J Cell Biol 1994; 124: 183-193.
16.   BenEzra D, Griffin BW, Maftzir G, Aharonov O. Thrombospondin and in vivo angiogenesis induced by basic fibroblast growth factor or

lipopolysaccharide. Invest Ophtalmol Vis Sci 1993; 34: 3601-3608.

17. Taraboletti G, Morbidelli L, Donnini S, Parenti A, Granger HJ, Giavazzi R, Ziche M. The heparin binding 25 kDa fragment of thrombospondin-1 promotes angiogenesis and modulates gelatinase and TIMP-2 production in endothelial cells. Faseb J 2000; 14(12): 1674-1676.

18. Chandrasekaran L, He CZ, Al-Barazi H, Krutzsch HC, Iruela-Arispe ML, Roberts DD. Cell contact-dependent activation of alpha3beta1 integrin modulates endothelial cell responses to thrombospondin-1. Mol Biol Cell 2000; 11(9): 2885-2900.

19. Calzada MJ, Zhou L, Sipes JM, Zhang J, Krutzsch HC, Iruela-Arispe ML, Annis DS, Mosher DF, Roberts DD. Alpha4beta1 integrin mediates selective endothelial cell responses to thrombospondins 1 and 2 in vitro and modulates angiogenesis in vivo. Circ Res 2004; 94(4): 462-470.

20. Iruela-Arispe ML, Lombardo M, Krutzsch HC, Lawler J, Roberts DD. Inhibition of angiogenesis by thrombospondin-1 is mediated by 2 independent regions within the type 1 repeats. Circulation 1999; 100(13): 1423-1431.

21. Brown EJ, Frazier WA. Integrin-associated protein (CD47) and its ligands. Trends Cell Biol 2001; 11(3): 130-135.

22. Kuznetsova SA, Roberts DD. Functional regulation of T lymphocytes by modulatory extracellular matrix proteins. Int J Biochem Cell Biol 2004; 36(6): 1126-1134.

23. Asch AS, Barnwell J, Silverstein RL, Nachman RL. Isolation of the thrombospondin membrane receptor. J Clin Invest 1987; 79: 1054-1061.

24. Febbraio M, Hajjar DP, Silverstein RL. CD36: a class B scavenger receptor involved in angiogenesis, atherosclerosis, inflammation, and lipid metabolism. J Clin Invest 2001; 108(6): 785-791.

25. Swerlick RA, Lee KH, Wick TM, Lawley TJ. Human dermal microvascular endothelial but not human umbilical vein endothelial cells express CD36 in vivo and in vitro. J Immunol 1992; 148(1): 78-83.

26. Dawson DW, Pearce SF, Zhong R, Silverstein RL, Frazier WA, Bouck NP. CD36 mediates the In vitro inhibitory effects of thrombospondin-1 on endothelial cells. J Cell Biol 1997; 138(3): 707-717.

27. Crombie R, Silverstein R. Lysosomal integral membrane protein II binds thrombospondin-1. Structure-function homology with the cell adhesion molecule CD36 defines a conserved recognition motif. J Biol Chem 1998; 273(9): 4855-4863.

28. Crombie R, Silverstein RL, MacLow C, Pearce SF, Nachman RL, Laurence J. Identification of a CD36-related thrombospondin 1-binding domain in HIV-1 envelope glycoprotein gp120: relationship to HIV-1-specific inhibitory factors in human saliva. J Exp Med 1998; 187(1): 25-35.

29. Tucker RP. The thrombospondin type 1 repeat superfamily. Int J Biochem Cell Biol 2004; 36(6): 969-974.

30. Primo L, Ferrandi C, Roca C, Marchio S, di Blasio L, Alessio M, Bussolino F. Identification of CD36

31. molecular features required for its in vitro angiostatic activity. FASEB J 2005; 19(12): 1713-1715.

31. Jimenez B, Volpert OV, Crawford SE, Febbraio M, Silverstein RL, Bouck N. Signals leading to apoptosis-dependent inhibition of neovascularization by thrombospondin-1. Nat Med 2000; 6(1): 41-48.

32. Isenberg JS, Ridnour LA, Dimitry J, Frazier WA, Wink DA, Roberts DD. CD47 is necessary for inhibition of nitric oxide-stimulated vascular cell responses by thrombospondin-1. J Biol Chem 2006; 281(36): 26069-26080.

33. Volpert OV, Zaichuk T, Zhou W, Reiher F, Ferguson TA, Stuart PM, Amin M, Bouck NP. Inducer-stimulated Fas targets activated endothelium for destruction by anti-angiogenic thrombospondin-1 and pigment epithelium-derived factor. Nat Med 2002; 8(4): 349-357.

34. Rege TA, Stewart J, Jr., Dranka B, Benveniste EN, Silverstein RL, Gladson CL. Thrombospondin-1-induced apoptosis of brain microvascular endothelial cells can be mediated by TNF-R1. J Cell Physiol 2009; 218(1): 94-103.

35. Gao AG, Lindberg FP, Dimitry JM, Brown EJ, Frazier WA. Thrombospondin modulates alpha v beta 3 function through integrin-associated protein. J Cell Biol 1996; 135(2): 533-544.

36. Gao AG, Lindberg FP, Finn MB, Blystone SD, Brown EJ, Frazier WA. Integrin-associated protein is a receptor for the C-terminal domain of thrombospondin. J Biol Chem 1996; 271(1): 21-24.

37. Isenberg JS, Roberts DD, Frazier WA. CD47: a new target in cardiovascular therapy. Arterioscler Thromb Vasc Biol 2008; 28(4): 615-621.

38. Kanda S, Shono T, Tomasini-Johansson B, Klint P, Saito Y. Role of thrombospondin-1-derived peptide, 4N1K, in FGF-2-induced angiogenesis. Exp Cell Res 1999; 252(2): 262-272.

39. Isenberg JS, Hyodo F, Ridnour LA, Shannon CS, Wink DA, Krishna MC, Roberts DD. Thrombospondin 1 and vasoactive agents indirectly alter tumor blood flow. Neoplasia 2008; 10(8): 886-896.

40. Nunes SS, Outeiro-Bernstein MA, Juliano L, Vardiero F, Nader HB, Woods A, Legrand C, Morandi V. Syndecan-4 contributes to endothelial tubulogenesis through interactions with two motifs inside the pro-angiogenic N-terminal domain of thrombospondin-1. J Cell Physiol 2008; 214(3): 828-837.

41. Orr AW, Elzie CA, Kucik DF, Murphy-Ullrich JE. Thrombospondin signaling through the calreticulin/LDL receptor-related protein co-complex stimulates random and directed cell migration. J Cell Sci 2003; 116(Pt 14): 2917-2927.

42. Godyna S, Liau G, Popa I, Stefansson S, Argraves WS. Identification of the low density lipoprotein receptor-related protein (LRP) as an endocytic receptor for thrombospondin-1. J Cell Biol 1995; 129(5): 1403-1410.

43. Oganesian A, Armstrong LC, Migliorini MM, Strickland DK, Bornstein P. Thrombospondins use the VLDL receptor and a nonapoptotic pathway to inhibit cell division in microvascular endothelial cells. Mol Biol Cell 2008; 19(2): 563-571.

44.   Greenaway J, Lawler J, Moorehead R, Bornstein P, Lamarre J, Petrik J. Thrombospondin-1 inhibits VEGF levels in the ovary directly by binding and internalization via the low density lipoprotein receptor-related protein-1 (LRP-1). J Cell Physiol 2007; 210(3): 807-818.

45.   Fears CY, Grammer JR, Stewart JE, Jr., Annis DS, Mosher DF, Bornstein P, Gladson CL. Low-density lipoprotein receptor-related protein contributes to the antiangiogenic activity of thrombospondin-2 in a murine glioma model. Cancer Res 2005; 65(20): 9338-9346.

46.   Yang Z, Strickland DK, Bornstein P. Extracellular matrix metalloproteinase 2 levels are regulated by the low density lipoprotein-related scavenger receptor and thrombospondin 2. J Biol Chem 2001; 276(11): 8403-8408.

47.   Krutzsch HC, Choe BJ, Sipes JM, Guo N, Roberts DD. Identification of an alpha(3)beta(1) integrin recognition sequence in thrombospondin-1. J Biol Chem 1999; 274(34): 24080-24086.

48.   Calzada MJ, Sipes JM, Krutzsch HC, Yurchenco PD, Annis DS, Mosher DF, Roberts DD. Recognition of the N-terminal modules of thrombospondin-1 and thrombospondin-2 by alpha6beta1 integrin. J Biol Chem 2003; 278(42): 40679-40687.

49.   Calzada MJ, Annis DS, Zeng B, Marcinkiewicz C, Banas B, Lawler J, Mosher DF, Roberts DD. Identification of novel beta1 integrin binding sites in the type 1 and type 2 repeats of thrombospondin-1. J Biol Chem 2004; 279(40): 41734-41743.

50.   Short SM, Derrien A, Narsimhan RP, Lawler J, Ingber DE, Zetter BR. Inhibition of endothelial cell migration by thrombospondin-1 type-1 repeats is mediated by beta1 integrins. J Cell Biol 2005; 168(4): 643-653.

51.   Staniszewska I, Zaveri S, Del Valle L, Oliva I, Rothman VL, Croul SE, Roberts DD, Mosher DF, Tuszynski GP, Marcinkiewicz C. Interaction of alpha9beta1 integrin with thrombospondin-1 promotes angiogenesis. Circ Res 2007; 100(9): 1308-1316.

52.   Lawler J, Weinstein R, Hynes RO. Cell attachment to thrombospondin: the role of Arg-Gly-Asp, calcium, and integrin receptors. J Cell Biol 1988; 107: 2351-2361.

53.   Avraamides CJ, Garmy-Susini B, Varner JA. Integrins in angiogenesis and lymphangiogenesis. Nat Rev Cancer 2008; 8(8): 604-617.

54.   Silva R, D'Amico G, Hodivala-Dilke KM, Reynolds LE. Integrins: the keys to unlocking angiogenesis. Arterioscler Thromb Vasc Biol 2008; 28(10): 1703-1713.

55.   Rusnati M, Presta M. Extracellular angiogenic growth factor interactions: an angiogenesis interactome survey. Endothelium 2006; 13(2): 93-111.

56.   Kazerounian S, Yee KO, Lawler J. Thrombospondins in cancer. Cell Mol Life Sci 2008; 65(5): 700-712.

57.   Lamszus K, Joseph A, Jin L, Yao Y, Chowdhury S, Fuchs A, Polverini PJ, Goldberg ID, Rosen EM. Scatter factor binds to thrombospondin and other extracellular matrix components. Am J Pathol 1996; 149(3): 805-819.

58.   Taraboletti G, Belotti D, Borsotti P, Vergani V, Rusnati M, Presta M, Giavazzi R. The 140-kilodalton antiangiogenic fragment of thrombospondin-1 binds to basic fibroblast growth factor. Cell Growth Differ 1997; 8(4): 471-479.

59.   Margosio B, Marchetti D, Vergani V, Giavazzi R, Rusnati M, Presta M, Taraboletti G. Thrombospondin 1 as a scavenger for matrix-associated fibroblast growth factor 2. Blood 2003; 102(13): 4399-4406.

60.   Margosio B, Rusnati M, Bonezzi K, Cordes BL, Annis DS, Urbinati C, Giavazzi R, Presta M, Ribatti D, Mosher DF, Taraboletti G. Fibroblast growth factor-2 binding to the thrombospondin-1 type III repeats, a novel antiangiogenic domain. Int J Biochem Cell Biol 2008; 40(4): 700-709.

61.   Rusnati M, Taraboletti G, Urbinati C, Tulipano G, Giuliani R, Molinari-Tosatti MP, Sennino B, Giacca M, Tyagi M, Albini A, Noonan D, Giavazzi R, Presta M. Thrombospondin-1/HIV-1 tat protein interaction: modulation of the biological activity of extracellular Tat. Faseb J 2000; 14(13): 1917-1930.

62.   Gupta K, Gupta P, Wild R, Ramakrishnan S, Hebbel RP. Binding and displacement of vascular endothelial growth factor (VEGF) by thrombospondin: Effect on human microvascular endothelial cell proliferation and angiogenesis. Angiogenesis 1999; 3: 147-158.

63.   Inoki I, Shiomi T, Hashimoto G, Enomoto H, Nakamura H, Makino K, Ikeda E, Takata S, Kobayashi K, Okada Y. Connective tissue growth factor binds vascular endothelial growth factor (VEGF) and inhibits VEGF-induced angiogenesis. Faseb J 2002; 16(2): 219-221.

64.   Hogg PJ. Thrombospondin 1 as an enzyme inhibitor. Thrombosis and Haemostasis 1994; 72: 787-792.

65.   Iruela-Arispe ML, Luque A, Lee N. Thrombospondin modules and angiogenesis. Int J Biochem Cell Biol 2004; 36(6): 1070-1078.

66.   Qian X, Wang TN, Rothman VL, Nicosia RF, Tuszynski GP. Thrombospondin-1 modulates angiogenesis in vitro by up-regulation of matrix metalloproteinase-9 in endothelial cells. Exp Cell Res 1997; 235(2): 403-412.

67.   Bein K, Simons M. Thrombospondin type 1 repeats interact with matrix metalloproteinase 2. Regulation of metalloproteinase activity. J Biol Chem 2000; 275(41): 32167-32173.

68.   Schultz-Cherry S, Chen H, Mosher DF, Misenheimer TM, Krutzsch HC, Roberts DD, Murphy-Ullrich JE. Regulation of transforming growth factor-b activation by discrete sequences of thrombospondin 1. J Biol Chem 1995; 270: 7304-7310.

69.   Young GD, Murphy-Ullrich JE. The tryptophan-rich motifs of the thrombospondin type 1 repeats bind VLAL motifs in the latent transforming growth factor-beta complex. J Biol Chem 2004; 279(46): 47633-47642.

70.   Yee KO, Connolly CM, Duquette M, Kazerounian S, Washington R, Lawler J. The effect of thrombospondin-1 on breast cancer metastasis. Breast Cancer Res Treat 2009; 114(1): 85-96.

71. Borges E, Jan Y, Ruoslahti E. Platelet-derived growth factor receptor beta and vascular endothelial growth factor receptor 2 bind to the beta 3 integrin through its extracellular domain. J Biol Chem 2000; 275(51): 39867-39873.

72. Karagiannis ED, Popel AS. A systematic methodology for proteome-wide identification of peptides inhibiting the proliferation and migration of endothelial cells. Proc Natl Acad Sci U S A 2008; 105(37): 13775-13780.

73. Zhang X, Galardi E, Duquette M, Delic M, Lawler J, Parangi S. Antiangiogenic treatment with the three thrombospondin-1 type 1 repeats recombinant protein in an orthotopic human pancreatic cancer model. Clin Cancer Res 2005; 11(6): 2337-2344.

74. Zhang X, Connolly C, Duquette M, Lawler J, Parangi S. Continuous administration of the three thrombospondin-1 type 1 repeats recombinant protein improves the potency of therapy in an orthotopic human pancreatic cancer model. Cancer Lett 2007; 247(1): 143-149.

75. Dawson DW, Volpert OV, Pearce SF, Schneider AJ, Silverstein RL, Henkin J, Bouck NP. Three distinct D-amino acid substitutions confer potent antiangiogenic activity on an inactive peptide derived from a thrombospondin-1 type 1 repeat. Mol Pharmacol 1999; 55(2): 332-338.

76. Asch AS, Silbiger S, Heimer E, Nachman RL. Thrombospondin sequence motif (CSVTCG) is responsible for CD36 binding. Biochem Biophys Res Commun 1992; 182(3): 1208-1217.

77. Tan K, Duquette M, Liu JH, Dong Y, Zhang R, Joachimiak A, Lawler J, Wang JH. Crystal structure of the TSP-1 type 1 repeats: a novel layered fold and its biological implication. J Cell Biol 2002; 159(2): 373-782.

78. Vogel T, Guo N, Krutzsch HC, Blake DA, Hartman J, Mendelovitz S, Panet A, Roberts DD. Modulation of endothelial cell proliferation, adhesion, and motility by recombinant heparin-binding domain and synthetic peptides from the type I repeats of thrombospondin. J Cell Biochem 1993; 53: 74-84.

79. Guo N, Krutzsch HC, Inman JK, Roberts DD. Thrombospondin 1 and type I repeat peptides of thrombospondin 1 specifically induce apoptosis of endothelial cells. Cancer Res 1997; 57(9): 1735-1742.

80. Guo NH, Krutzsch HC, Inman JK, Shannon CS, Roberts DD. Antiproliferative and antitumor activities of D-reverse peptides derived from the second type-1 repeat of thrombospondin-1. J Pept Res 1997; 50(3): 210-21.

81. Tolsma SS, Volpert OV, Good DJ, Frazier WA, Polverini PJ, Bouck N. Peptides derived from two separate domains of the matrix protein thrombospondin-1 have anti-angiogenic activity. J Cell Biol 1993; 122(2): 497-511.

82. Adams JC. Functions of the conserved thrombospondin carboxy-terminal cassette in cell-extracellular matrix interactions and signaling. Int J Biochem Cell Biol 2004; 36(6): 1102-1114.

83. Kvansakul M, Adams JC, Hohenester E. Structure of a thrombospondin C-terminal fragment reveals a novel calcium core in the type 3 repeats. Embo J 2004; 23(6): 1223-1233.

84. Majluf-Cruz A, Manns JM, Uknis AB, Yang X, Colman RW, Harris RB, Frazier W, Lawler J, DeLa Cadena RA. Residues F16-G33 and A784-N823 within platelet thrombospondin-1 play a major role in binding human neutrophils: evaluation by two novel binding assays. J Lab Clin Med 2000; 136(4): 292-302.

85. Watkins NA, Du LM, Scott JP, Ouwehand WH, Hillery CA. Single-chain antibody fragments derived from a human synthetic phage-display library bind thrombospondin and inhibit sickle cell adhesion. Blood 2003; 102(2): 718-724.

86. Carlson CB, Bernstein DA, Annis DS, Misenheimer TM, Hannah BL, Mosher DF, Keck JL. Structure of the calcium-rich signature domain of human thrombospondin-2. Nat Struct Mol Biol 2005; 12(10): 910-914.

87. Sulochana KN, Ge R. Developing antiangiogenic peptide drugs for angiogenesis-related diseases. Curr Pharm Des 2007; 13(20): 2074-2086.

88. Karagiannis ED, Popel AS. Anti-angiogenic peptides identified in thrombospondin type I domains. Biochem Biophys Res Commun 2007; 359(1): 63-69.

89. Karagiannis ED, Popel AS. Peptides derived from type I thrombospondin repeat-containing proteins of the CCN family inhibit proliferation and migration of endothelial cells. Int J Biochem Cell Biol 2007; 39(12): 2314-2323.

90. Griffioen AW, van der Schaft DW, Barendsz-Janson AF, Cox A, Struijker Boudier HA, Hillen HF, Mayo KH. Anginex, a designed peptide that inhibits angiogenesis. Biochem J 2001; 354(Pt 2): 233-242.

91. Reiher FK, Volpert OV, Jimenez B, Crawford SE, Dinney CP, Henkin J, Haviv F, Bouck NP, Campbell SC. Inhibition of tumor growth by systemic treatment with thrombospondin-1 peptide mimetics. Int J Cancer 2002; 98(5): 682-689.

92. Haviv F, Bradley MF, Kalvin DM, Schneider AJ, Davidson DJ, Majest SM, McKay LM, Haskell CJ, Bell RL, Nguyen B, Marsh KC, Surber BW, Uchic JT, Ferrero J, Wang YC, Leal J, Record RD, Hodde J, Badylak SF, Lesniewski RR, Henkin J. Thrombospondin-1 mimetic peptide inhibitors of angiogenesis and tumor growth: design, synthesis, and optimization of pharmacokinetics and biological activities. J Med Chem 2005; 48(8): 2838-2346.

93. Anderson JC, Grammer JR, Wang W, Nabors LB, Henkin J, Stewart JE, Jr., Gladson CL. ABT-510, a modified type 1 repeat peptide of thrombospondin, inhibits malignant glioma growth in vivo by inhibiting angiogenesis. Cancer Biol Ther 2007; 6(3): 454-462.

94. Quesada AJ, Nelius T, Yap R, Zaichuk TA, Alfranca A, Filleur S, Volpert OV, Redondo JM. In vivo upregulation of CD95 and CD95L causes synergistic inhibition of angiogenesis by TSP1 peptide and metronomic doxorubicin treatment. Cell Death Differ 2005; 12(6): 649-658.

95. Isenberg JS, Yu C, Roberts DD. Differential effects of ABT-510 and a CD36-binding peptide derived from the type 1 repeats of thrombospondin-1 on fatty

acid uptake, nitric oxide signaling, and caspase activation in vascular cells. Biochem Pharmacol 2008; 75(4): 875-882.

96. Viloria-Petit A, Miquerol L, Yu JL, Gertsenstein M, Sheehan C, May L, Henkin J, Lobe C, Nagy A, Kerbel RS, Rak J. Contrasting effects of VEGF gene disruption in embryonic stem cell-derived versus oncogene-induced tumors. EMBO J 2003; 22(16): 4091-4102.

97. Greenaway J, Henkin J, Lawler J, Moorehead R, Petrik J. ABT-510 induces tumor cell apoptosis and inhibits ovarian tumor growth in an orthotopic, syngeneic model of epithelial ovarian cancer. Mol Cancer Ther 2009; 8(1): 64-74.

98. Yap R, Veliceasa D, Emmenegger U, Kerbel RS, McKay LM, Henkin J, Volpert OV. Metronomic low-dose chemotherapy boosts CD95-dependent antiangiogenic effect of the thrombospondin peptide ABT-510: a complementation antiangiogenic strategy. Clin Cancer Res 2005; 11(18): 6678-6685.

99. Yang Q, Tian Y, Liu S, Zeine R, Chlenski A, Salwen HR, Henkin J, Cohn SL. Thrombospondin-1 peptide ABT-510 combined with valproic acid is an effective antiangiogenesis strategy in neuroblastoma. Cancer Res 2007; 67(4): 1716-1724.

100. Rusk A, McKeegan E, Haviv F, Majest S, Henkin J, Khanna C. Preclinical evaluation of antiangiogenic thrombospondin-1 peptide mimetics, ABT-526 and ABT-510, in companion dogs with naturally occurring cancers. Clin Cancer Res 2006; 12(24): 7444-7455.

101. Rusk A, Cozzi E, Stebbins M, Vail D, Graham J, Valli V, Henkin J, Sharpee R, Khanna C. Cooperative activity of cytotoxic chemotherapy with antiangiogenic thrombospondin-I peptides, ABT-526 in pet dogs with relapsed lymphoma. Clin Cancer Res 2006; 12(24): 7456-7464.

102. Hoekstra R, de Vos FY, Eskens FA, Gietema JA, van der Gaast A, Groen HJ, Knight RA, Carr RA, Humerickhouse RA, Verweij J, de Vries EG. Phase I safety, pharmacokinetic, and pharmacodynamic study of the thrombospondin-1-mimetic angiogenesis inhibitor ABT-510 in patients with advanced cancer. J Clin Oncol 2005; 23(22): 5188-5197.

103. Ebbinghaus S, Hussain M, Tannir N, Gordon M, Desai AA, Knight RA, Humerickhouse RA, Qian J, Gordon GB, Figlin R. Phase 2 study of ABT-510 in patients with previously untreated advanced renal cell carcinoma. Clin Cancer Res 2007; 13(22 Pt 1): 6689-6695.

104. Baker LH, Rowinsky EK, Mendelson D, Humerickhouse RA, Knight RA, Qian J, Carr RA, Gordon GB, Demetri GD. Randomized, phase II study of the thrombospondin-1-mimetic angiogenesis inhibitor ABT-510 in patients with advanced soft tissue sarcoma. J Clin Oncol 2008; 26(34): 5583-5588.

105. Markovic SN, Suman VJ, Rao RA, Ingle JN, Kaur JS, Erickson LA, Pitot HC, Croghan GA, McWilliams RR, Merchan J, Kottschade LA, Nevala WK, Uhl CB, Allred J, Creagan ET. A phase II study of ABT-510 (thrombospondin-1 analog) for the

treatment of metastatic melanoma. Am J Clin Oncol 2007; 30(3): 303-309.

106. Gietema JA, Hoekstra R, de Vos FY, Uges DR, van der Gaast A, Groen HJ, Loos WJ, Knight RA, Carr RA, Humerickhouse RA, Eskens FA. A phase I study assessing the safety and pharmacokinetics of the thrombospondin-1-mimetic angiogenesis inhibitor ABT-510 with gemcitabine and cisplatin in patients with solid tumors. Ann Oncol 2006; 17(8): 1320-1327.

107. Hoekstra R, de Vos FY, Eskens FA, de Vries EG, Uges DR, Knight R, Carr RA, Humerickhouse R, Verweij J, Gietema JA. Phase I study of the thrombospondin-1-mimetic angiogenesis inhibitor ABT-510 with 5-fluorouracil and leucovorin: a safe combination. Eur J Cancer 2006; 42(4): 467-472.

108. Pirie-Shepherd SR, Leedom TA, Do J, Huang H, Lingna L, Lai J, Johnson K, Osothprarop T, Rizzo JD, Doppalapudi VR, Lappe RW, Bradshaw C, Roberts S, Levin NJ, Woodnutt G *CVX.045: a novel thrombospondin-1 (TSP-1) mimetic CovX-Body(TM) that potentiates chemotherapy and targeted therapy in preclinical xenograft models*, 99th Annual meeting of the American Association for Cancer Research, San Diego, CA, AACR: San Diego, CA, 2008; p Abstract nr 1114.

109. Levin NJ, Leedom TA, Doppalapudi VR, Li L, Lai J, Johnson K, Rizzo JD, Lappe RW, Bradshaw CW, Woodnutt G. CVX-045: a novel thrombospondin-1 (TSP-1) mimetic CovX-Body that potentiates chemotherapy in preclinical colon cancer models. J Clin Oncol 2007; 25: 14011.

110. Mendelson DS, Dinolfa M, Cohen RB, Rosen LS, Gordon MS, Byrnes B, Bear I, Schoenfeld SL. First-in-human dose escalation safety and pharmacocynetic (PK) trial of a novel intravenous (IV) thrombospondin-1 (TSP-1) mimetic humanized monoclonal CovX Body (CVX-045) in patients (pts) with advanced solid tumors. J Clin Oncol 2008; 26(15S): 3524.

111. Molckovsky A, Siu LL. First-in-class, first-in-human phase I results of targeted agents: Highlights of the 2008 American Society of Clinical Oncology meeting. J Hematol Oncol 2008; 1(1): 20.

112. Zhang X, Xu J, Lawler J, Terwilliger E, Parangi S. Adeno-associated virus-mediated antiangiogenic gene therapy with thrombospondin-1 type 1 repeats and endostatin. Clin Cancer Res 2007; 13(13): 3968-3976.

113. Streit M, Stephen AE, Hawighorst T, Matsuda K, Lange-Asschenfeldt B, Brown LF, Vacanti JP, Detmar M. Systemic inhibition of tumor growth and angiogenesis by thrombospondin-2 using cell-based antiangiogenic gene therapy. Cancer Res 2002; 62(7): 2004-2012.

114. Ren B, Yee KO, Lawler J, Khosravi-Far R. Regulation of tumor angiogenesis by thrombospondin-1. Biochim Biophys Acta 2006; 1765(2): 178-188.

115. Vikhanskaya F, Bani MR, Borsotti P, Ghilardi C, Ceruti R, Ghisleni G, Marabese M, Giavazzi R, Broggini M, Taraboletti G. p73 overexpression increases VEGF and reduces thrombospondin-1

production: implications for tumor angiogenesis. Oncogene 2001; 20(50): 7293-7300.

116. Dameron KM, Volpert OV, Tainsky MA, Bouck N. Control of angiogenesis in fibroblasts by p53 regulation of thrombospondin-1. Science 1994; 265(5178): 1582-1584.

117. Dameron KM, Volpert OV, Tainsky MA, Bouck N. The p53 tumor suppressor gene inhibits angiogenesis by stimulating the production of thrombospondin. Cold Spring Harb Symp Quant Biol 1994; 59: 483-489.

118. Gautam A, Densmore CL, Melton S, Golunski E, Waldrep JC. Aerosol delivery of PEI-p53 complexes inhibits B16-F10 lung metastases through regulation of angiogenesis. Cancer Gene Ther 2002; 9(1): 28-36.

119. Panigrahy D, Kaipainen A, Huang S, Butterfield CE, Barnes CM, Fannon M, Laforme AM, Chaponis DM, Folkman J, Kieran MW. PPARalpha agonist fenofibrate suppresses tumor growth through direct and indirect angiogenesis inhibition. Proc Natl Acad Sci U S A 2008; 105(3): 985-990.

120. Kang JH, Kim SA, Chang SY, Hong S, Hong KJ. Inhibition of trichostatin A-induced antiangiogenesis by small-interfering RNA for thrombospondin-1. Exp Mol Med 2007; 39(3): 402-411.

121. Castle VP, Ou X, O'Shea S, Dixit VM. Induction of thrombospondin 1 by retinoic acid is important during differentiation of neuroblastoma cells. J Clin Invest 1992; 90(5): 1857-1863.

122. Hellebrekers DM, Jair KW, Vire E, Eguchi S, Hoebers NT, Fraga MF, Esteller M, Fuks F, Baylin SB, van Engeland M, Griffioen AW. Angiostatic activity of DNA methyltransferase inhibitors. Mol Cancer Ther 2006; 5(2): 467-475.

123. Suarez Y, Fernandez-Hernando C, Yu J, Gerber SA, Harrison KD, Pober JS, Iruela-Arispe ML, Merkenschlager M, Sessa WC. Dicer-dependent endothelial microRNAs are necessary for postnatal angiogenesis. Proc Natl Acad Sci U S A 2008; 105(37): 14082-14087.

124. Dews M, Homayouni A, Yu D, Murphy D, Sevignani C, Wentzel E, Furth EE, Lee WM, Enders GH, Mendell JT, Thomas-Tikhonenko A. Augmentation of tumor angiogenesis by a Myc-activated microRNA cluster. Nat Genet 2006; 38(9): 1060-1065.

125. Zhao HY, Ooyama A, Yamamoto M, Ikeda R, Haraguchi M, Tabata S, Furukawa T, Che XF, Iwashita K, Oka T, Fukushima M, Nakagawa M, Ono M, Kuwano M, Akiyama S. Down regulation of c-Myc and induction of an angiogenesis inhibitor, thrombospondin-1, by 5-FU in human colon cancer KM12C cells. Cancer Lett 2008; 270(1): 156-163.

126. Taraboletti G, Benelli R, Borsotti P, Rusnati M, Presta M, Giavazzi R, Ruco L, Albini A. Thrombospondin-1 inhibits Kaposi's sarcoma (KS) cell and HIV-1 Tat- induced angiogenesis and is poorly expressed in KS lesions. J Pathol 1999; 188(1): 76-81.

127. Samols MA, Skalsky RL, Maldonado AM, Riva A, Lopez MC, Baker HV, Renne R. Identification of cellular genes targeted by KSHV-encoded microRNAs. PLoS Pathog 2007; 3(5): e65.

128. Bocci G, Francia G, Man S, Lawler J, Kerbel RS. Thrombospondin 1, a mediator of the antiangiogenic effects of low-dose metronomic chemotherapy. Proc Natl Acad Sci U S A 2003; 100(22): 12917-12922.

129. Hamano Y, Sugimoto H, Soubasakos MA, Kieran M, Olsen BR, Lawler J, Sudhakar A, Kalluri R. Thrombospondin-1 associated with tumor microenvironment contributes to low-dose cyclophosphamide-mediated endothelial cell apoptosis and tumor growth suppression. Cancer Res 2004; 64(5): 1570-1574.

130. Damber JE, Vallbo C, Albertsson P, Lennernas B, Norrby K. The anti-tumour effect of low-dose continuous chemotherapy may partly be mediated by thrombospondin. Cancer Chemother Pharmacol 2006; 58(3): 354-360.

131. Bocci G, Falcone A, Fioravanti A, Orlandi P, Di Paolo A, Fanelli G, Viacava P, Naccarato AG, Kerbel RS, Danesi R, Del Tacca M, Allegrini G. Antiangiogenic and anticolorectal cancer effects of metronomic irinotecan chemotherapy alone and in combination with semaxinib. Br J Cancer 2008; 98(10): 1619-1629.

132. Allegrini G, Falcone A, Fioravanti A, Barletta MT, Orlandi P, Loupakis F, Cerri E, Masi G, Di Paolo A, Kerbel RS, Danesi R, Del Tacca M, Bocci G. A pharmacokinetic and pharmacodynamic study on metronomic irinotecan in metastatic colorectal cancer patients. Br J Cancer 2008; 98(8): 1312-1319.

133. Rico MC, Castaneda JL, Manns JM, Uknis AB, Sainz IM, Safadi FF, Popoff SN, Dela Cadena RA. Amelioration of inflammation, angiogenesis and CTGF expression in an arthritis model by a TSP1-derived peptide treatment. J Cell Physiol 2007; 211(2): 504-512.

134. Punekar S, Zak S, Kalter VG, Dobransky L, Punekar I, Lawler JW, Gutierrez LS. Thrombospondin 1 and its mimetic peptide ABT-510 decrease angiogenesis and inflammation in a murine model of inflammatory bowel disease. Pathobiology 2008; 75(1): 9-21.

135. Thaunat O, Louedec L, Graff-Dubois S, Dai J, Groyer E, Yacoub-Youssef H, Mandet C, Bruneval P, Kaveri S, Caligiuri G, Germain S, Michel JB, Nicoletti A. Antiangiogenic treatment prevents adventitial constrictive remodeling in graft arteriosclerosis. Transplantation 2008; 85(2): 281-289.

136. Castle V, Varani J, Fligiel S, Prochownik EV, Dixit V. Antisense-mediated reduction in thrombospondin reverses the malignant phenotype of a human squamous carcinoma. J Clin Invest 1991; 87(6): 1883-1888.

137. Taraboletti G, Roberts DD, Liotta LA. Thrombospondin-induced tumor cell migration: haptotaxis and chemotaxis are mediated by different molecular domains. J Cell Biol 1987; 105(5): 2409-2415.

138. Shaked Y, Bertolini F, Man S, Rogers MS, Cervi D, Foutz T, Rawn K, Voskas D, Dumont DJ, Ben-David Y, Lawler J, Henkin J, Huber J, Hicklin DJ, D'Amato RJ, Kerbel RS. Genetic heterogeneity of the vasculogenic phenotype parallels angiogenesis;

Implications for cellular surrogate marker analysis of antiangiogenesis. Cancer Cell 2005; 7(1): 101-111.

139. Gordon MS, Mendelson D, Carr R, Knight RA, Humerickhouse RA, Iannone M, Stopeck AT. A phase 1 trial of 2 dose schedules of ABT-510, an antiangiogenic, thrombospondin-1-mimetic peptide, in patients with advanced cancer. Cancer 2008; 113(12): 3420-3429.

140. Allegrini G, Goulette FA, Darnowski JW, Calabresi P. Thrombospondin-1 plus irinotecan: a novel antiangiogenic-chemotherapeutic combination that inhibits the growth of advanced human colon tumor xenografts in mice. Cancer Chemother Pharmacol 2004; 53(3): 261-266.

141. Lih CJ, Wei W, Cohen SN. Txr1: a transcriptional regulator of thrombospondin-1 that modulates cellular sensitivity to taxanes. Genes Dev 2006; 20(15): 2082-2095.

142. Brostjan C, Gebhardt K, Gruenberger B, Steinrueck V, Zommer H, Freudenthaler H, Roka S, Gruenberger T. Neoadjuvant treatment of colorectal cancer with bevacizumab: the perioperative angiogenic balance is sensitive to systemic thrombospondin-1 levels. Clin Cancer Res 2008; 14(7): 2065-2074.

143. Garcia AA, Hirte H, Fleming G, Yang D, Tsao-Wei DD, Roman L, Groshen S, Swenson S, Markland F, Gandara D, Scudder S, Morgan R, Chen H, Lenz HJ, Oza AM. Phase II clinical trial of bevacizumab and low-dose metronomic oral cyclophosphamide in recurrent ovarian cancer: a trial of the California, Chicago, and Princess Margaret Hospital phase II consortia. J Clin Oncol 2008; 26(1): 76-82.

144. Huang H, Campbell SC, Bedford DF, Nelius T, Veliceasa D, Shroff EH, Henkin J, Schneider A, Bouck N, Volpert OV. Peroxisome proliferator-activated receptor gamma ligands improve the antitumor efficacy of thrombospondin peptide ABT510. Mol Cancer Res 2004; 2(10): 541-550.

145. Rofstad EK, Henriksen K, Galappathi K, Mathiesen B. Antiangiogenic treatment with thrombospondin-1 enhances primary tumor radiation response and prevents growth of dormant pulmonary micrometastases after curative radiation therapy in human melanoma xenografts. Cancer Res 2003; 63(14): 4055-4061.

146. Isenberg JS, Maxhimer JB, Hyodo F, Pendrak ML, Ridnour LA, DeGraff WG, Tsokos M, Wink DA, Roberts DD. Thrombospondin-1 and CD47 limit cell and tissue survival of radiation injury. Am J Pathol 2008; 173(4): 1100-1112.

147. Yano K, Oura H, Detmar M. Targeted overexpression of the angiogenesis inhibitor thrombospondin-1 in the epidermis of transgenic mice prevents ultraviolet-B-induced angiogenesis and cutaneous photo-damage. J Invest Dermatol 2002; 118(5): 800-805.

148. Sutton CD, O'Byrne K, Goddard JC, Marshall LJ, Jones L, Garcea G, Dennison AR, Poston G, Lloyd DM, Berry DP. Expression of thrombospondin-1 in resected colorectal liver metastases predicts poor prognosis. Clin Cancer Res 2005; 11(18): 6567-6573.

149. Bergers G, Hanahan D. Modes of resistance to anti-angiogenic therapy. Nat Rev Cancer 2008; 8(8): 592-603.

150. Filleur S, Volpert OV, Degeorges A, Voland C, Reiher F, Clezardin P, Bouck N, Cabon F. In vivo mechanisms by which tumors producing thrombospondin 1 bypass its inhibitory effects. Genes Dev 2001; 15(11): 1373-1382.

151. Fontana A, Filleur S, Guglielmi J, Frappart L, Bruno-Bossio G, Boissier S, Cabon F, Clezardin P. Human breast tumors override the antiangiogenic effect of stromal thrombospondin-1 in vivo. Int J Cancer 2005; 116(5): 686-691.

152. Bajou K, Peng H, Laug WE, Maillard C, Noel A, Foidart JM, Martial JA, DeClerck YA. Plasminogen activator inhibitor-1 protects endothelial cells from FasL-mediated apoptosis. Cancer Cell 2008; 14(4): 324-334.

153. Anderson CR, Hastings NE, Blackman BR, Price RJ. Capillary sprout endothelial cells exhibit a CD36 low phenotype: regulation by shear stress and vascular endothelial growth factor-induced mechanism for attenuating anti-proliferative thrombospondin-1 signaling. Am J Pathol 2008; 173(4): 1220-1228.

154. Simantov R, Febbraio M, Crombie R, Asch AS, Nachman RL, Silverstein RL. Histidine-rich glycoprotein inhibits the antiangiogenic effect of thrombospondin-1. J Clin Invest 2001; 107(1): 45-52.

CHAPTER 14

Novel Antiangiogenic Molecules in Multiple Myeloma

Aldo M. Roccaro and Irene M. Ghobrial

Department of Medical Oncology, Dana-Farber Cancer Institute and Harvard Medical School; 02115, Boston, MA, USA.

Address correspondence to: Dr. Aldo M. Roccaro, Department of Medical Oncology, Dana-Farber Cancer Institute and Harvard Medical School; 02115, Boston, MA, USA; Tel: 001-617-582-8535; Email: aldo_roccaro@dfci.harvard.edu

Abstract: The paradigm for the treatment of multiple myeloma (MM) has significantly changed: therapeutic options have evolved from the introduction of melphalan and prednisone in the 1960s, high-dose chemotherapy and stem cell transplantation in the late 1980s and 1990s, to the rapid introduction of small novel molecules within the last seven years. Based on the understanding of the complex interaction of MM cells with bone marrow microenvironment; and of the role of neoangiogenesis in MM pathogensis, a number of novel therapeutic agents with anti-angiogenic properties are now available, playing a key role in the treatment of MM both in the preclinical settings and as part of clinical trials.

1. INTRODUCTION

The role of angiogenesis in the growth and progression, of both solid tumors and hematologic malignances has already been well established. Indeed, the progression of several cancers of hematopoietic lineage, including non-Hodgkin's lymphomas, lymphoblastic leukemia, B-cell chronic lymphocytic leukemia, acute myeloid leukemia, and multiple myeloma (MM) [1-4], has been correlated with degree of angiogenesis. In particular, it has been shown that bone marrow angiogenesis is a hallmark of MM progression, which correlates with disease activity [5-7]. Subsequently, several preclinical evidences have been supported the idea of using anti-angiogenic molecules as a valid strategy to target plasma cell clone, indirectly, by inhibiting endothelial cell growth.

2. IMMUNOMODULATORY DRUGS (IMIDS): THALIDOMIDE AND LENALIDOMIDE

Thalidomide

Thalidomide was first used as a sedative and hypnotic drug in the 1950's. It was withdrawn from the market because of its teratogenic effects. In 1999 a phase II study showed that thalidomide, used as a single agent in patients with relapsed MM, resulted in an overall response rate (ORR) of 25% [8]. The main activity and efficacy of thalidomide in MM was then elucidated. It has been shown that thalidomide induces *in vitro* growth arrest, blocks the increased secretion of tumor necrosis factor alpha

(TNF-α), and affects the interaction between myeloma cells and BM microenvironment by decreasing the expression of adhesion molecules (E-selectin, L-selectin, ICAM-1, VCAM-1) or inhibiting the paracrine loops of cytokine secretion, such as vascular endothelial growth factor (VEGF) and interleukin (IL)-6; enhances host immune response against MM; and interferes with intracellular growth signaling by inhibiting the constitutive activity of nuclear factor kappa B (NFkB). In addition its anti-angiogenic activity has been demonstrated [9-11] (Fig. **1**). Several studies have then tested the combination of thalidomide with other agents such as dexamethasone and chemotherapeutic drugs in patients with relapsed/refractory MM, and this led to response rates as high as 65% [12-14]. After these encouraging results, thalidomide in combination with dexamethasone entered several phase II clinical trials in newly diagnosed MM patients, and demonstrated a RR of ~ 65% [13-14]. Subsequently, a large phase III clinical trial was performed using thalidomide with dexamethasone versus high-dose dexamethasone alone for newly diagnosed MM patients, resulting in a 63% RR in the thalidomide/dexamethasone arm versus 41% in the dexamethasone arm, although no survival advantage was observed between the two groups [13]. Other phase III trials in elderly patients who were not candidates for autologous stem cells transplant included a randomized study compared melphalan prednisone and thalidomide (MPT) versus melphalan and prednisone (MP), which showed that patients treated with MPT had higher RR (76% versus 48%) and longer event-free survival (EFS) than patients treated with MP alone (54% versus 27%) [15]. Facon and colleagues [16] conducted a large phase III trial of MPT compared to MP or high dose chemotherapy and stem cell transplantation in elderly patients between 65 to 75 years of age and

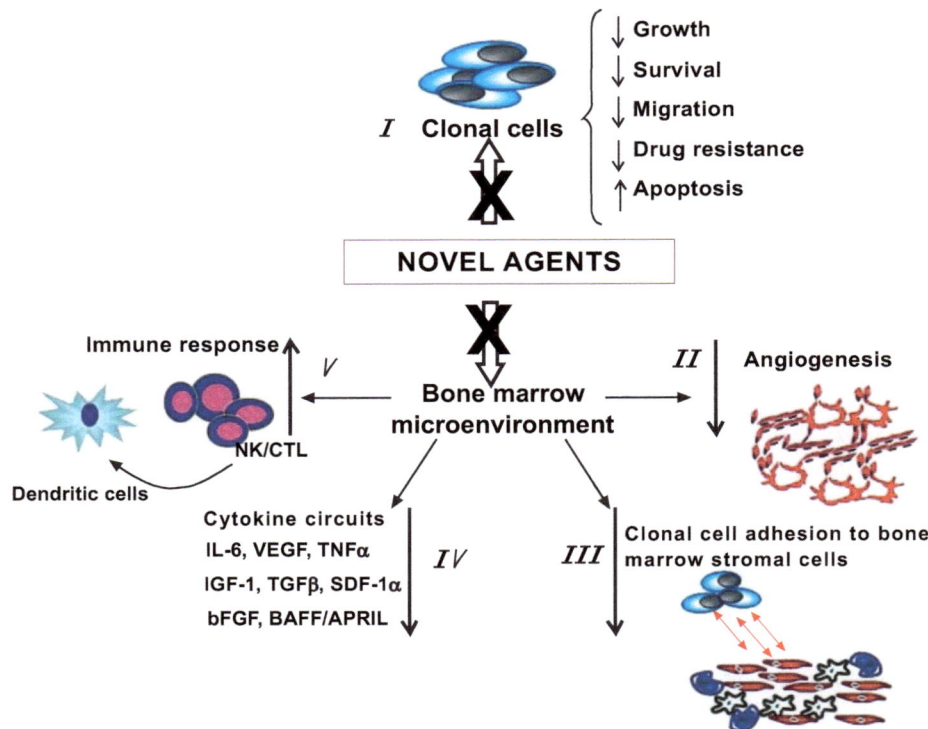

Fig. (1). Mechanisms of action of novel agents:
novel molecules can: I) directly inhibit clonal cells; II) inhibit angiogensis; III) inhibit tumor cell adhesion to bone marrow stromal cells (BMSCs); IV) decrease cytokine production from BMSCs; V) increase host anti-tumor immunity.

showed that patients treated with MPT had a longer overall survival of 54 months compared to 32 months for MP and 39 months for transplant. A randomized study has recently investigated the activity of thalidomide in combination with VAD and doxil, compared to VAD-doxil and it resulted in a higher RR in the arm with thalidomide versus the arm without thalidomide (81% versus 66%) [17]. The toxicities of thalidomide correlate both with dose and length of treatment and include neuropathy and deep vein thrombosis. Other important toxicities include fatigue, somnolence, constipation, rash (including Stevens-Johnson syndrome), and hepatic dysfunction [18].

Lenalidomide

Based on the success of thalidomide, lenalidomide (CC-5013; IMiD-3, Celgene Corp), a more potent immunomodulatory derivative of thalidomide was developed. Lenalidomide overcomes growth and survival advantage conferred by the BM-milieu, downregulates VEGF, and exerts antiangiogenic activities. In addition, lenalidomide co-stimulates T cells, enhances antitumor immunity mediated by interferon (IFN)γ and IL-2, and augments natural killer (NK) cell cytotoxicity [19-21] (Fig. **1**).

Phase I clinical trials using lenalidomide in patients with relapsed and refractory MM, established a dose of 25 mg, and demonstrated a promising RR of 35% [22]. Phase II studies followed and established the optimal schedule of 3 weeks on and 1 week off with once daily dosing [23]. Then, two large randomized phase III studies (MM-009, MM-010) compared lenalidomide and dexamethasone to dexamethasone and placebo for patients with relapsed or relapsed and refractory MM. They both showed comparably favorable results, with RR and time to progression with the lenalidomide/dexamethasone combination signifi cantly greater and more than twice the RR seen with dexamethasone alone [24] Based upon the success of these studies, lenalidomide received FDA-approval for the treatment of relapsed MM in June 2006. A phase II study of the combination of lenalidomide and dexamethasone was performed in 32 newly diagnosed patients with MM and showed an ORR of 91% [25]. A recent study demonstrated the efficacy of lenalidomide in combination with melphalan and prednisone which was associated with a RR of 86% [15]. A Phase III clinical trial using lenalidomide in combination with dexamethasone in newly diagnosed MM patients has been recently completed and showed that lenalidomide plus low-dose dexamethasone is associated with superior OS compared to lenalidomide plus high-dose dexamethasone [26]. The main side effects of lenalidomide include myelosuppression, particularly neutropenia and thrombocytopenia, and deep venous thrombosis especially when it used in combination with high-dose dexamethasone [27].

3.　PROTEASOME INHIBITORS: BORTEZOMIB, NPI-0052

Bortezomib

Bortezomib (PS-341, Millennium Pharmaceuticals, Inc) represents the first in class proteasome inhibitor to have progressed into widespread clinical use in MM patients, based on preclinical data showing its in vitro and in vivo anti-tumor activity in MM cells, by inhibiting proliferation, inducing apoptosis and by targeting the BM microenvironment through its antiangiogenic activity and by inhibiting the binding of MM cells to the BM stromal cells (Fig. **1**). Bortezomib as single agent has been evaluated in patients with advanced, heavily pretreated MM in the SUMMIT study (Study of Uncrontrolled Multiple Myeloma managed with proteasome Inhibition Therapy) [28] which showed an ORR of 35% in 202 patients with relapsed and refractory MM. The CREST (Clinical Response and Efficacy Study of Bortezomib in the Treatment of myeloma) trial, a phase II study randomizing patients to higher (1.3 mg/m3) or lower (1.0 mg/m3) doses of Bortezomib in combination with dexamethasone, revealed positive response rates (33% with low-dose bortezomib alone, 44% with low-dose bortezomib/dexamethasone, 50% with high-dose bortezomib, and 62% with high-dose bortezomib/dexamethasone) [29]. Subsequently, the APEX study (Assessment of Proteasome Inhibition for Extending Remission) compared Bortezomib with high-dose dexamethasone in patients with relapsed/refractory MM, and showed an ORR of 38% in the Bortezomib arm, versus 18% obtained in the high-dose dexamethasone. Moreover, Bortezomib demonstrated superiority over dexamethasone in terms of time to progression and survival [30]. Based on these encouraging data, Bortezomib was FDA-approved in 2003 with full approval in 2005 and numerous trials using Bortezomib in combination with other agents were built. Other combinations included chemotherapies and novel agents [31]. The combination of Bortezomib, thalidomide and dexamethasone (VTD) in patients with relapsed MM showed an overall response rate of 70% including near complete responses in 16%. High responses were also observed in studies of patients with previously untreated MM. Single agent Bortezomib showed an overall response rate of 40% with 10% complete responses in a phase II study of 66 patients with MM. The combination of Bortezomib and dexamethasone led to an overall response rate of 66% to 88% in another phase II trial of newly diagnosed MM [32,33]. In addition, the combination of Bortezomib (V), melphalan (M) and prednisone (P) (MPV) in nontransplant candidates resulted in an overall response rate of 89% [34]. Interestingly, a phase III trial randomizing newly diagnosed MM patients to either VMP or MP, has been recently completed and showed that VMP signifi cantly prolongs survival and is superior for all effi cacy endpoints: specifically VMP induced rapid and durable responses with unprecedented complete response rate (35%); prolonged time to progression (~52% reduced risk of progression), time to next therapy/treatment free interval; and overall survival (~40% reduced risk of death) [35]. Also the combination of Bortezomib, dexamethasone, and cyclophosphamide was shown to be more effective than Bortezomib either used as single agent or with dexamethasone [36]. These encouraging results were subsequently confirmed by a multicenter randomized phase 3 study comparing the combination of doxil and Bortezomib versus Bortezomib alone [37]. Similarly it has been recently demonstrated that liposomal doxorubicin+Bortezomib significantly improves TTP compared to Bortezomib alone, regardless of the number of prior lines of therapy, or anthracycline exposure [38].

New Proteasome Inhibitor, NPI-0052

Based on the significant anti-MM activity of bortezomib, a new proteasome inhibitor (NPI-0052; Nereus Pharmaceuticals, CA) with a different structure and different mechanism of action has been developed. NPI-0052 is an oral proteasome inhibitor that has shown significant anti-neoplastic activity in MM. It also inhibits angiogenesis [39]. Importantly, the combination of NPI-0052 and bortezomib induced significant inhibition of proliferation compared to each agent alone [40,41]. A phase I clinical trial of NPI-0052 in relapsed MM has recently been initiated.

4.　SIGNALING PATHWAYS INHIBI-TORS: ENZASTAURIN, CCI-779, RAD001

Preclinical data have been demonstrated that monoclonal gammopaties are characterized by deregulation of several signaling pathways, as compared to normal plasma cells [42-44]. Moreover there is strong evidence that BM-milieu supports the growth of the clonal cell population. Therefore, this important knowledge has led to the development of several agents that specifically target the neoplastic clone by acting through those upregulated signaling pathways, the BM microenvironment, are able to affect both the clonal cells and the BM-milieu [45].

Protein Kinase C Inhibitor: Enzastaurin

Enzastaurin[H-Pyrrole-2,5-dione,3-(1-methyl-1H indol-3-yl)-4-[1-[-1(2pyridinylmethyl)-4 piperidinyl]-1H-indol- 3-yl], LY 317615; Eli Lilly and company, (Indianapolis, IN) is an oral PKCβ inhibitor, with downstream inhibition of Akt. In MM, enzastaurin has demonstrated specific inhibition of PKC isoforms and Akt activation along with inducing cytotoxicity, apoptosis in MM cells, anti-angiogenesis *in vitro* and *in vivo* [46]. Synergism has been demonstrated when enzastaurin was used in combination with bortezomib. In addition, enzastaurin inhibted MM cell growth in an in vivo xenograft model of these diseases. Based on these exciting preclinical data, enzastaurin alone and in combination with bortezomib entered clinical trials in MM.

Mammalian Target of Rapamycin Inhibitors: CCI-779, RAD001

mTOR inhibitors such as rapamycin and rapamycin analogues, including CCI-779 and RAD001, have demonstrated *in vitro* and *in vivo* activity in MM cell lines and animal model [47]. The combination of rapamycin with active agents in MM such as lenalidomide, bortezomib and 17-AAG have demonstrated synergistic activity in vitro [48,49]. In addition, rapamycin appears to target the BM microenvironment by inhibiting angiogenesis and osteoclast formation in MM *in vitro* [49].

5. NEW SMALL MOLECULES WHICH TARGET PROANGIOGENIG CYTOKINES

Anti-VEGF: Bevacizumab, Pazopanib, Vatalanib

VEGF represents one of the main pro-angiogenic cytokine and its role in the pathogenesis and progression of solid tumor and hematological malignancies, including MM has been widely studied and demonstrated. VEGF is secreted by MM cells and bone marrow stromal cells (BMSCs), and it contributes to BM neoangiogenesis in MM patients [50,51]. Several preclinical evidences provide the rational for using drugs or small molecule which target VEGF. Indeed, it has been shown that Bevacizumab (small monoclonal antibody directed against VEGF) induces survival benefits in patients with metastatic colon cancer, when used in combination with conventional chemotherapeuticals [52]. To date more than 300 clinical trials are evaluating the efficacy of Bevacizumab in both solid tumors and hematologic

malignancies, including multiple myeloma (www.clinicatrials.gov). New small molecules with anti-angiogenic properties are now available, such as Pazopanib (GW786034B). It has been recently demonstrated that Pazopanib exertrs anti-MM; and anti-angiogenic activities, as shown on primary MM endothelial cells [53]. A clinical trial using Pazopanib has been recently completed. The purpose of this study was to evaluate the safety, tolerability, time to progression, time to response and duration of response of Pazopanib in patients with relapsed or refractory MM. Results are not still available to date. Similarly, other clinical trials are evaluating the efficacy of Vatalanib (PTK787/ZK222584), another anti-angiogenic small molecule that inhibits all known vascular endothelial growth factor receptors [54]. There are actually two clinical trials evaluating Vatalanib in either relapsed/refractory MM patients or as post-transplant maintenance therapy in MM patients (www.clinicatrials.gov).

Anti-FGF: SU5402, SU10991, PD173074, PKS412

Basic-fibroblast growth factor (bFGF) represents another cytokine which supports BM neoangiogenesis in MM [55]. Importantly, FGF-receptor 3 (FGFR3) protein is aberrantly expressed in approximately 15% of cases of plasma cell myeloma as a result of t(4;14) [56]. To date, monoclonal antibodies against FGFR3, as well as selective tyrosine kinase inhibitors (SU10991, SU5402, PD173074, PKC412) are available and *in vitro* and *in vivo* evidences have been demonstrated that FGFR3 may represent a therapeutic target in t(4;14) MM patients [57].

6. CONCLUSIONS

The last decade has marked a new era in the treatment of multiple myeloma. Indeed, a new paradigm shift has evolved utilizing novel therapeutic agents targeting the malignant clone and its bone marrow microenvironment. The combination of novel agents with chemotherapeutic drugs and/or glucocorticoids has demonstrated high response rates with complete remission rates comparable to those achieved in the stem cell transplant setting. This has been supported by *in vitro* and *in vivo* evidences showing the anti-tumor activity of these novel agents in MM, as well as in other B-cell malignancies. Many of these novel agents include small molecules that target clonal plasmacells either directly or indirectly by inhibiting BM neonagiogenesis (Figure 1), which is known to support MM cell growth. Together, these therapies should lead to higher response rates, more durable duration of response, less toxicity and prolonged survival for patients, making plasmacell discrasias an increasingly chronic and treatable disease.

7. REFERENCES

1. Lee CY, Tien HF, Hu CY, Chou WC, Lin LI. Marrow ngiogenesis-associated factors as prognostic biomarkers in patients with acute myelogenous leukaemia. Br J Cancer 2007; 97(7): 877-882.

2. Molica S, Vacca A, Ribatti D, Cuneo A, Cavazzini F, Levato D, Vitelli G, Tucci L, Roccaro AM, Dammacco F. Prognostic value of enhanced bone marrow angiogenesis in early B-cell chronic lymphocytic leukemia. Blood 2002; 100(9): 3344-3351.

3. Hazar B, Paydas S, Zorludemir S, Sahin B, Tuncer I. Prognostic significance of microvessel density and vascular endothelial growth factor (VEGF) expression in non-Hodgkin's lymphoma. Leuk Lymphoma 2003; 44(12): 2089-2093.

4. Shih TT, Hou HA, Liu CY, Chen BB, Tang JL, Chen HY, Wei SY, Yao M, Huang SY, Chou WC, Hsu SC, Tsay W, Yu CW, Hsu CY, Tien HF, Yang PC. Bone marrow angiogenesis MR imaging in patients with acute myeloid leukemia: Peak enhancement ratio is an independent predictor for overall survival. Blood 2008; *In press.*

5. Vacca A, Ribatti D, Roncali L, Ranieri G, Serio G, Silvestris F, Dammacco F. Bone marrow angiogenesis and progression in multiple myeloma. Br J Haematol 1994; 87(3): 503-508.

6. Vacca A, Ribatti D, Presta M, Minischetti M, Iurlaro M, Ria R, Albini A, Bussolino F, Dammacco F. Bone marrow neovascularization, plasma cell angiogenic potential, and matrix metalloproteinase-2 secretion parallel progression of human multiple myeloma. Blood 1999; 93(9): 3064-3073.

7. Vacca A, Ria R, Semeraro F, Merchionne F, Coluccia M, Boccarelli A, Scavelli C, Nico B, Gernone A, Battelli F, Tabilio A, Guidolin D, Petrucci MT, Ribatti D, Dammacco F Endothelial cells in the bone marrow of patients with multiple myeloma. Blood 2003; 102(9): 3340-3348.

8. Singhal S, Mehta J, Desikan R, Ayers D, Roberson P, Eddlemon P, Munshi N, Anaissie E, Wilson C, Dhodapkar M, Zeddis J, Barlogie B. Antitumor activity of thalidomide in refractory multiple myeloma. N Engl J Med 1999; 341(21): 1565-1571.

9. Hideshima T, Chauhan D, Shima Y, Raje N, Davies FE, Tai YT, Treon SP, Lin B, Schlossman RL, Richardson P, Muller G, Stirling DI, Anderson KC. Thalidomide and its analogs overcome drug resistance of human multiple myeloma cells to conventional therapy. Blood 2000; 96(9): 2943-2950.

10. Davies FE, Raje N, Hideshima T, Lentzsch S, Young G, Tai YT, Lin B, Podar K, Gupta D, Chauhan D, Treon SP, Richardson PG, Schlossman RL, Morgan GJ, Muller GW, Stirling DI, Anderson KC. Thalidomide and immunomodulatory derivatives augment natural killer cell cytotoxicity in multiple myeloma. Blood 2001; 98(1): 210-216.

11. Mitsiades N, Mitsiades CS, Poulaki V, Chauhan D, Richardson PG, Hideshima T, Munshi NC, Treon SP, Anderson KC. Apoptotic signaling induced by immunomodulatory thalidomide analogs in human multiple myeloma cells: therapeutic implications. Blood. 2002; 99(12): 4525-4530.

12. Rajkumar SV, Fonseca R, Dispenzieri A, Lacy MQ, Lust JA, Witzig TE, Kyle RA, Gertz MA, Greipp PR. Thalidomide in the treatment of relapsed multiple myeloma. Mayo Clin Proc 2000; 75(9): 897-901.

13. Rajkumar SV, Blood E, Vesole D, Fonseca R, Greipp PR; Eastern Cooperative Oncology Group. Phase III clinical trial of thalidomide plus dexamethasone compared with dexamethasone alone in newly diagnosed multiple myeloma: a clinical trial coordinated by the Eastern Cooperative Oncology Group. J Clin Oncol 2006; 24(3): 431-436.

14. Weber D, Rankin K, Gavino M, Delasalle K, Alexanian R. Thalidomide alone or with dexamethasone for previously untreated multiple myeloma. J Clin Oncol 2003; 21(1): 16-19.

15. Palumbo A, Bringhen S, Caravita T, Merla E, Capparella V, Callea V, Cangialosi C, Grasso M, Rossini F, Galli M, Catalano L, Zamagni E, Petrucci MT, De Stefano V, Ceccarelli M, Ambrosini MT, Avonto I, Falco P, Ciccone G, Liberati AM, Musto P, Boccadoro M; Italian Multiple Myeloma Network, GIMEMA. Oral melphalan and prednisone chemotherapy plus thalidomide compared with melphalan and prednisone alone in elderly patients with multiple myeloma: randomised controlled trial. Lancet 2006; 367(9513): 825-831.

16. Facon T, Mary J, Harousseau J, et al. Superiority of melphalan-prednisone (MP) + thalidomide (THAL) over MP and autologous stem cell transplantation in the treatment of newly diagnosed elderly patients with multiple myeloma. J Clin Oncol 2006; 18S: abstract 1.

17. Zervas K, Mihou D, Katodritou I.VAD-doxil vs VAD-doxil plus thalidomide as initial treatment in patients with multiple myeloma: a multicenter randomized trial of The Greek Myeloma Study Group. Blood 2006; 108: abstract 794.

18. Ghobrial IM and Rajkumar SV. Management of thalidomide toxicity. J Support Oncol 2005; 1: 194-205.

19. Hideshima T, Chauhan D, Podar K, Schlossman RL, Richardson P, Anderson KC. Novel therapies targeting the myeloma cell and its bone marrow microenvironment. Semin Oncol. 2001; 28(6): 607-612.

20. Mitsiades CS, Mitsiades N, Poulaki V, Schlossman R, Akiyama M, Chauhan D, Hideshima T, Treon SP, Munshi NC, Richardson PG, Anderson KC. Activation of NF-kappaB and upregulation of intracellular anti-apoptotic proteins via the IGF-1/Akt signaling in human multiple myeloma cells: therapeutic implications. Oncogene. 2002; 21(37): 5673-583.

21. Dredge K, Marriott JB, Macdonald CD, Man HW, Chen R, Muller GW, Stirling D, Dalgleish AG. Novel thalidomide analogues display anti-angiogenic activity independently of immunomodulatory effects . Br J Cancer. 2002; 87(10): 1166-1172.

22. Richardson PG, Mitsiades C, Hideshima T, Anderson KC. Lenalidomide in multiple myeloma. Expert Rev Anticancer Ther 2006; 6(8): 1165-1173.

23. Richardson PG, Blood E, Mitsiades CS, Jagannath S, Zeldenrust SR, Alsina M, Schlossman RL, Rajkumar SV, Desikan KR, Hideshima T, Munshi NC, Kelly-Colson K, Doss D, McKenney ML, Gorelik S, Warren D, Freeman A, Rich R, Wu A, Olesnyckyj M, Wride K, Dalton WS, Zeldis J, Knight R, Weller E, Anderson KC. A randomized phase 2 study of lenalidomide therapy for patients with relapsed or relapsed and refractory multiple myeloma. Blood. 2006; 108(10): 3458-3464.

24. Dimopoulos MA, Anagnostopoulos A, Kyrtsonis MC, Castritis E, Bitsaktsis A, Pangalis GA. Treatment of relapsed or refractory Waldenstrom's macroglobulinemia with bortezomib. Haematologica, 2005; 90(12): 1655-1658.

25. Rajkumar SV, Hayman SR, Lacy MQ, Dispenzieri A, Geyer SM, Kabat B, Zeldenrust SR, Kumar S, Greipp PR, Fonseca R, Lust JA, Russell SJ, Kyle RA, Witzig TE, Gertz MA. Combination therapy with lenalidomide plus dexamethasone (Rev/Dex) for newly diagnosed myeloma. Blood 2005; 106(13): 4050-4053.

26. Rajkumar V, Jacobus S, Callander N, et al. A randomized Trial of Lenalidomide Plus High-Dose Dexamethasone (RD) Versus Lenalidomide Plus Low-Dose Dexamethasone (Rd) in Newly Diagnosed Multiple Myeloma (E4A03): A Trial Coordinated by the Eastern Cooperative Oncology Group. Blood 2007; 110: abstract 74.

27. Rajkumar SV, Blood E. Lenalidomide and venous thrombosis in multiple myeloma. N Engl J Med 2006; 354(19): 2079-2080.

28. A phase 2 study of bortezomib in relapsed, refractory myeloma Richardson PG, Barlogie B, Berenson J, Singhal S, Jagannath S, Irwin D, Rajkumar SV, Srkalovic G, Alsina M, Alexanian R, Siegel D, Orlowski RZ, Kuter D, Limentani SA, Lee S, Hideshima T, Esseltine DL, Kauffman M, Adams J, Schenkein DP, Anderson KC. N Engl J Med 2003; 348(26): 2609-2617.

29. Jagannath S, Barlogie B, Berenson J, Siegel D, Irwin D, Richardson PG, Niesvizky R, Alexanian R, Limentani SA, Alsina M, Adams J, Kauffman M, Esseltine DL, Schenkein DP, Anderson KC.A phase 2 study of two doses of bortezomib in relapsed or refractory myeloma. Br J Haematol. 2004; 127(2): 165-172.

30. Richardson PG, Sonneveld P, Schuster MW, Irwin D, Stadtmauer EA, Facon T, Harousseau JL, Ben-Yehuda D, Lonial S, Goldschmidt H, Reece D, San-Miguel JF, Bladé J, Boccadoro M, Cavenagh J, Dalton WS, Boral AL, Esseltine DL, Porter JB, Schenkein D, Anderson KC; Assessment of Proteasome Inhibition for Extending Remissions (APEX) Investigators.Bortezomib or high-dose dexamethasone for relapsed multiple myeloma. N Engl J Med 2005; 352(24): 2487-2498.

31. Richardson PG, Mitsiades C, Ghobrial I, Anderson K.Beyond single-agent bortezomib: combination regimens in relapsed multiple myeloma. Curr Opin Oncol. 2006; 18(6): 598-608.

32. Jagannath S, Richardson PG, Barlogie B, Berenson JR, Singhal S, Irwin D, Srkalovic G, Schenkein DP, Esseltine DL, Anderson KC; SUMMIT/CREST Investigators.Bortezomib in combination with dexamethasone for the treatment of patients with relapsed and/or refractory multiple myeloma with less than optimal response to bortezomib alone. Haematologica. 2006; 91(7): 929-934.

33. Harousseau JL, Attal M, Leleu X, Troncy J, Pegourie B, Stoppa AM, Hulin C, Benboubker L, Fuzibet JG, Renaud M, Moreau P, Avet-Loiseau H.Bortezomib plus dexamethasone as induction treatment prior to autologous stem cell transplantation in patients with newly diagnosed multiple myeloma: results of an IFM phase II study. Haematologica 2006; 91(11): 1498-1505.

34. Mateos MV, Hernández JM, Hernández MT, Gutiérrez NC, Palomera L, Fuertes M, Díaz-Mediavilla J, Lahuerta JJ, de la Rubia J, Terol MJ, Sureda A, Bargay J, Ribas P, de Arriba F, Alegre A, Oriol A, Carrera D, García-Laraña J, García-Sanz R, Bladé J, Prósper F, Mateo G, Esseltine DL, van de Velde H, San Miguel JF.Bortezomib plus melphalan and prednisone in elderly untreated patients with multiple myeloma: results of a multicenter phase 1/2 study. Blood. 2006; 108(7): 2165-2172.

35. San Miguel J, Schlag R, Khuageva O, et al. MMY-3002: A Phase 3 Study Comparing BortezomibMelphalanPrednisone (VMP) with MelphalanPrednisone (MP) in Newly Diagnosed Multiple Myeloma. Blood 2007; 110: abstract 76.

36. Davies FE, Wu P, Srikanth M, et al. The combination of Cyclophosphamide, Velcade and Dexamethasone (CVD) induces high response rates with minimal toxicity compared to Velcade alone (V) and Velcade plus Dexamethasone. Blood 2006; 108: abstract 3537.

37. Orlowski RZ, Zhuang SH, Parekh T, et al. The combination of pegylated liposomal doxorubicin and bortezomib significantly improves time to progression of patients with relapsed/refractory multiple myeloma compared with bortezomib alone: results from aplanned interim analysis of a randomized phase III study. Blood 2006; 108: abstract 404.

38. Blade J, San Miguel J, Nagler A, et al. The Prolonged Time to Progression with Pegylated Liposomal Doxorubicin + Bortezomib Versus Bortezomib Alone in Relapsed or Refractory Multiple Myeloma Is Unaffected by Extent of Prior Therapy or Previous Anthracycline Exposure. Blood 2007; 110: abstract 410.

39. Chauhan D, Catley L, Li G, Podar K, Hideshima T, Velankar M, Mitsiades C, Mitsiades N, Yasui H, Letai A, Ovaa H, Berkers C, Nicholson B, Chao TH, Neuteboom ST, Richardson P, Palladino MA, Anderson KC. A novel orally active proteasome inhibitor induces apoptosis in multiple myeloma cells with mechanisms distinct from Bortezomib. Cancer Cell. 2005; 8(5): 407-419.

40. Chauhan D, Singh A, Brahmandam M, Podar K, Hideshima T, Richardson P, Munshi N, Palladino MA, Anderson KC. Combination of proteasome inhibitors bortezomib and NPI-0052 trigger in vivo synergistic

cytotoxicity in multiple myeloma. Blood 2008; 111(3): 1654-1664.

41. Roccaro AM, Leleu X, Sacco A, Jia X, Melhem M, Moreau AS, Ngo HT, Runnels J, Azab A, Azab F, Burwick N, Farag M, Treon SP, Palladino MA, Hideshima T, Chauhan D, Anderson KC, Ghobrial IM. Dual targeting of the proteasome regulates survival and homing in Waldenstrom macroglobulinemia. Blood 2008; 111(9): 4752-4763.

42. Hideshima T, Bergsagel PL, Kuehl WM, Anderson KC. Advances in biology of multiple myeloma: clinical applications. Blood 2004; 104(3): 607-618.

43. Hatjiharissi E, Ngo H, Leontovich AA, Leleu X, Timm M, Melhem M, George D, Lu G, Ghobrial J, Alsayed Y, Zeismer S, Cabanela M, Nehme A, Jia X, Moreau AS, Treon SP, Fonseca R, Gertz MA, Anderson KC, Witzig TE, Ghobrial IM. Proteomic analysis of waldenstrom macroglobulinemia. Cancer Res. 2007; 67(8): 3777-3784.

44. Leleu X, Jia X, Runnels J, Ngo HT, Moreau AS, Farag M, Spencer JA, Pitsillides CM, Hatjiharissi E, Roccaro A, O'Sullivan G, McMillin DW, Moreno D, Kiziltepe T, Carrasco R, Treon SP, Hideshima T, Anderson KC, Lin CP, Ghobrial IM. The Akt pathway regulates survival and homing in Waldenstrom macroglobulinemia. Blood 2007; 110(13): 4417-4426.

45. Hideshima T, Catley L, Yasui H, Ishitsuka K, Raje N, Mitsiades C, Podar K, Munshi NC, Chauhan D, Richardson PG, Anderson KC. Perifosine, an oral bioactive novel alkylphospholipid, inhibits Akt and induces in vitro and in vivo cytotoxicity in human multiple myeloma cells. Blood. 2006; 107(10): 4053-4062.

46. Podar K, Raab MS, Zhang J, McMillin D, Breitkreutz I, Tai YT, Lin BK, Munshi N, Hideshima T, Chauhan D, Anderson KC.Targeting PKC in multiple myeloma: in vitro and in vivo effects of the novel, orally available small-molecule inhibitor enzastaurin (LY317615.HCl). Blood 2007; 109(4): 1669-1677.

47. Shi Y, Gera J, Hu L, Hsu JH, Bookstein R, Li W, Lichtenstein A.Enhanced sensitivity of multiple myeloma cells containing PTEN mutations to CCI-779. Cancer Res 2002; 62(17): 5027-5034.

48. Raje N, Kumar S, Hideshima T, Ishitsuka K, Chauhan D, Mitsiades C, Podar K, Le Gouill S, Richardson P, Munshi NC, Stirling DI, Antin JH, Anderson KC. Combination of the mTOR inhibitor rapamycin and CC-5013 has synergistic activity in multiple myeloma. Blood 2004; 104(13): 4188-4193.

49. Francis LK, Alsayed Y, Leleu X, Jia X, Singha UK, Anderson J, Timm M, Ngo H, Lu G, Huston A, Ehrlich LA, Dimmock E, Lentzsch S, Hideshima T, Roodman GD, Anderson KC, Ghobrial IM.Combination mammalian target of rapamycin inhibitor rapamycin and HSP90 inhibitor 17-allylamino-17-demethoxygeldanamycin has synergistic activity in multiple myeloma. Clin Cancer Res. 2006; 12(22): 6826-6835.

50. Ria R, Vacca A, Russo F, Cirulli T, Massaia M, Tosi P, Cavo M, Guidolin D, Ribatti D, Dammacco F.A VEGF-dependent autocrine loop mediates proliferation and capillarogenesis in bone marrow endothelial cells of patients with multiple myeloma. Thromb Haemost 2004; 92(6): 1438-1445.

51. Vacca A, Ria R, Ribatti D, Semeraro F, Djonov V, Di Raimondo F, Dammacco F.A paracrine loop in the vascular endothelial growth factor pathway triggers tumor angiogenesis and growth in multiple myeloma. Haematologica 2003; 88(2): 176-85.

52. Calvani M, Trisciuoglio D, Bergamaschi C, Shoemaker RH, Melillo G. Differential involvement of vascular endothelial growth factor in the survival of hypoxic colon cancer cells. Cancer Res 2008; 68(1): 285-291.

53. Podar K, Tonon G, Sattler M, Tai YT, Legouill S, Yasui H, Ishitsuka K, Kumar S, Kumar R, Pandite LN, Hideshima T, Chauhan D, Anderson KC. The small-molecule VEGF receptor inhibitor pazopanib (GW786034B) targets both tumor and endothelial cells in multiple myeloma. Proc Natl Acad Sci U S A 2006; 103(51): 19478-19483.

54. Sini P, Samarzija I, Baffert F, Littlewood-Evans A, Schnell C, Theuer A, Christian S, Boos A, Hess-Stumpp H, Foekens JA, Setyono-Han B, Wood J, Hynes NE.Inhibition of multiple vascular endothelial growth factor receptors (VEGFR) blocks lymph node metastases but inhibition of VEGFR-2 is sufficient to sensitize tumor cells to platinum-based chemotherapeutics. Cancer Res 2008; 68(5): 1581-1592.

55. Vacca A, Ribatti D, Presta M, Minischetti M, Iurlaro M, Ria R, Albini A, Bussolino F, Dammacco F. Bone marrow neovascularization, plasma cell angiogenic potential, and matrix metalloproteinase-2 secretion parallel progression of human multiple myeloma. Blood 1999; 93(9): 3064-3073.

56. Lauring J, Abukhdeir AM, Konishi H, Garay JP, Gustin JP, Wang Q, Arceci RJ, Matsui W, Park BH. The multiple myeloma associated MMSET gene contributes to cellular adhesion, clonogenic growth, and tumorigenicity. Blood 2008; 111(2): 856-864.

57. Paterson JL, Li Z, Wen XY, Masih-Khan E, Chang H, Pollett JB, Trudel S, Stewart AK.Preclinical studies of fibroblast growth factor receptor 3 as a therapeutic target in multiple myeloma. Br J Haematol 2004; 124(5): 595-603.

Index

www.ingramcontent.com/pod-product-compliance
Lightning Source LLC
Chambersburg PA
CBHW041715210326
41598CB00007B/660